Introduction to clinical radiology

A CORRELATIVE APPROACH TO DIAGNOSTIC IMAGING

Introduction to clinical radiology

A CORRELATIVE APPROACH TO DIAGNOSTIC IMAGING

RICHARD H. DAFFNER, M.D.

Associate Professor of Radiology,
Duke University School of Medicine;
Chief, Radiology Service,
Veterans Administration Hospital,
Durham, North Carolina

with **614** illustrations

The C. V. Mosby Company

SAINT LOUIS   1978

The C. V. Mosby Company
11830 Westline Industrial Drive, St. Louis, Missouri 63141

Library of Congress Cataloging in Publication Data

Daffner, Richard H
  Introduction to clinical radiology.

  Bibliography: p.
  Includes index.
  1. Diagnosis, Radioscopic. I. Title.
RC78.D28   616.07'572   78-5680
ISBN 0-8016-1203-9

GW/CB/CB 9 8 7 6 5 4 3 2 1

To
AL MARSCO

Preface

This book is intended for the medical student beginning clinical rotations. The concept for this book originated in the series of lectures I have given over the years to medical students. All the material is from this series of teaching sessions.

In writing this book, I have chosen an orientation based on clinical problem solving. Many of the radiology texts for medical students list the radiographic signs of certain conditions as isolated facts without attempting to correlate them with the pathophysiology that produces them. It is my goal to make that correlation and to show that by recognition of a radiographic pattern, it is possible to define the pathophysiologic process producing that pattern.

The first three chapters are of an introductory nature, outlining the scope of diagnostic radiology (imaging), explaining the physical basis of image formation, and discussing the use of radiographic contrast agents. The remainder of the book is devoted to a discussion of the radiographic aspects of the lungs, heart, gastrointestinal tract, urinary tract, skeleton, and central nervous system.

Each of the clinical chapters is divided into four sections: technical considerations, anatomic considerations, pathologic considerations, and case studies.

The technical considerations portion of each chapter includes the types of examinations performed for that portion of the body, the use of special views, and a description of how that particular examination may be of help in clinical problem solving. Technical considerations begin with the proper identification of the film with regard to the patient. The patient's name or identifying number should be on the film. Identification should be a permanent part of any study and should not be added after the examination. This is the standard accepted practice medicolegally. Other data that should be contained on the film include the date of the examination and the time the study was done. This is especially important in patients who have multiple examinations done the same day.

Other signs helpful in establishing the film's identity, whenever it is in doubt, include matching certain anatomic landmarks on several films: ribs and clavicles on chest examinations, vertebral bodies and pelvis on abdominal examinations, and teeth, sella, and orbits on skull examinations. The presence of metallic foreign bodies such as surgical clips, wire sutures, or bullets also aids in identification.

Technical considerations should also include an analysis of the film density (blackness). Films that are too dark or too light are difficult to interpret and often obscure important pathologic findings. Motion is another technical problem that distorts the anatomy and obscures the borders of structures.

The anatomic considerations portion reviews pertinent anatomy of the region being studied. No attempt is made to be encyclopedic; rather, the approach is very brief, but covering all the essentials. It is important for you to recognize that a radiograph is a two-dimensional representation of three-dimensional structures. You must remember the adage that if you know what the gross appearance of a structure is, you can easily predict its radiographic appearance.

The pathologic considerations include those pathophysiologic alterations of normal anatomic structures that result in radiographic abnormalities. Logic tells us that there are a limited number of ways for disease to affect an organ. Similarly, there are limitations on the way an organ responds to that disease process. For example, in the gastrointestinal tract a mucosal tumor appears the same whether it is located in the esophagus, stomach, small intestine, or colon. The same holds true for other lesions of this system. Furthermore, an extrapolation may be made to other tubular structures in the body—airways, urinary tract, and blood vessels. It is my premise that once readers know the pattern of a lesion, they will recognize it anywhere in the body, even if it is in an unusual location.

The final section of each clinical chapter is a series of case studies designed to illustrate the points made earlier in the text. With the exception of the chest and skeletal case studies, the approach is to present groups of patients with similar "chief complaints." The task of the reader is to then decide which imaging studies should be performed based on an analysis of the history, physical findings, economics, and good judgment. Please remember that these studies are expensive. All the cases presented are of the "bread and butter" type and could easily be seen every day in a busy clinic or office practice.

Finally, it is my hope that the book will be easily read and understood. Learning should be fun. It has been my intent to keep it that way in this book.

In the production of this book many individuals provided help in various capacities. I would like to acknowledge the following people who provided that aid: Hazel Underwood, who devoted many hours of her own time to typing the manuscript; Ronald Mitchell, Chief of the Medical Media Production Service, Veterans Administration Hospital, Durham, North Carolina, and his staff, Evelyn Sauerbier, James Henderson, David Hong, Ronald Kovacs, Linda Kohl-Orton, and Donald Powell, for the excellent photography and original artwork; Charles Putman, Chairman, Department of Radiology, Duke University Medical Center, for encouragement, advice, and support of the project; colleagues in the Department of Radiology, Duke University Medical Center, who reviewed and critiqued portions of the book—Collins Baber, James Chen, Herman Grossman, David Merten, Carlisle Morgan, Fearghus O'Foghludha, Robert Older, James Reed, and William Thompson; and Alva Daffner, my understanding wife, who reviewed the manuscript and provided encouragement, advice, and consolation during the many months of production.

Richard H. Daffner

Contents

PART ONE

Introduction to diagnostic radiology: an overview

1 Introduction to diagnostic imaging

The realm of diagnostic radiology encompasses a variety of modalities of imaging that may be used individually or, more commonly, in combination to provide the clinician with enough information to aid in making a diagnosis. Diagnostic imaging includes plain film radiography, contrast-enhanced radiography, computed tomography, nuclear imaging, and diagnostic ultrasound. The first three of these imaging forms utilize x-rays. Nuclear radiology involves the detection of emissions from radioactive isotopes in various parts of the body; ultrasound does not have any associated ionizing radiation. A brief introduction to each type of examination is necessary at this point for the reader to understand how these modalities are used in clinical problem solving.

PLAIN FILM RADIOGRAPHY

Plain film radiography is the bread and butter of the diagnostic radiologist. The term "plain film" means that no contrast material is used to enhance various body structures. In performing plain film examinations the natural contrast between the basic four radiographic densities—air, soft tissue (water), fat, and bone—is relied on to define abnormalities. Examples of plain film studies with which you are familiar include chest radiographs, plain films of the abdomen, and skeletal films.

Plain film radiography has its special components: fluoroscopy, tomography, and stereoscopy. Fluoroscopy is a useful modality for visualizing the diaphragm, heart motion, valve calcification within the heart, and localization of chest masses (Fig. 1-1).

Conventional tomography is a mode of imaging in which the x-ray tube and the film move in concert to produce a blurred image. The focal point, or fulcrum, however, remains in sharp focus (Fig. 1-2). Tomography blurs out unwanted structures while keeping the object of interest in clearer focus. It is most useful in evaluating the lungs (Fig. 1-3), kidneys, gallbladder, and bony structures. Tomography will improve contrast. However, it will not create contrast where there is none to begin with.

Stereography is a unique method of plain film diagnosis wherein the x-ray tube is shifted several degrees after an initial examination, and a second exposure is made.

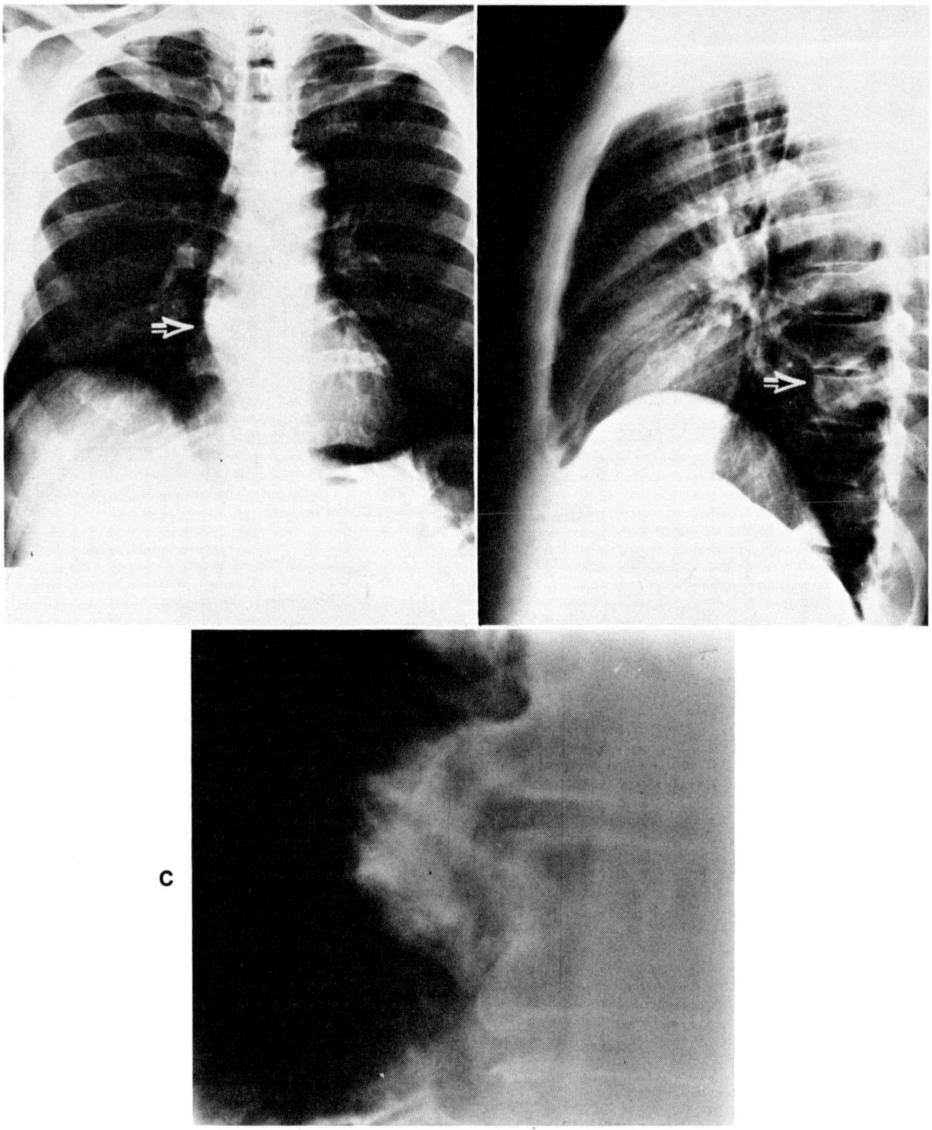

Fig. 1-1. Value of chest fluoroscopy. **A,** Routine PA chest film shows "mass" through cardiac shadow to right of midline (arrow). **B,** Lateral film shows "mass" to be posterior (arrow). **C,** Fluoroscopic spot film shows density in question to be bony spurs bridging thoracic vertebral bodies. There was no tumor.

When viewed either through a stereoscopic viewer or by the observer crossing the eyes, a "three-dimensional" image is obtained. This is most useful for localizing calcifications within the skull.

Mammography is the radiographic study of the breast. At the present time, it is the most effective method of examining the intact breast for suspected pathologic conditions. The technique involves using x-ray film or xerographic plates to record x-ray images of the breast tissues. Mammography is essentially a form of plain film diagnosis.

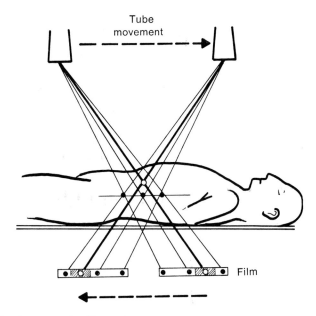

Fig. 1-2. Principle of tomography. X-ray tube and film move in opposite directions. Focal point (clear dot) remains in sharp focus, whereas remaining shadows are blurred.

CONTRAST EXAMINATIONS

Plain film radiography is adequate for situations where natural radiographic contrast exists between body structures such as heart and lungs or bones and adjacent soft tissues. To examine structures that do not have inherent contrast differences from the surrounding tissues, it is necessary to use one of a variety of contrast agents. The vast majority of contrast studies are of the gastrointestinal tract, urinary tract, and blood vessels.

The most common contrast material used for gastrointestinal examinations is a preparation of barium sulfate mixed with other agents to produce a uniform suspension. These products are available as premixed powders or liquids in unit packages or in bulk form to be mixed and measured in the radiology department. They may be administered alone or in combination with air, water, or an effervescent mixture that produces carbon dioxide. These gas-enhanced studies are referred to as "air contrast" studies (Fig. 1-4). Administration of these preparations is either by mouth (antegrade) or by rectum (retrograde).

In addition to barium preparations, water-soluble agents are available for studying the gastrointestinal tract whenever there is a possibility of extravasation of the contrast material beyond the bowel wall. Barium, which is an inert substance, produces a severe desmoplastic reaction in tissues into which it is introduced. Water-soluble agents, on the other hand, do not produce this type of reaction and are absorbed from the rupture site to be excreted through the kidneys. The water-soluble agents, however, are not without hazard, since they can cause a severe chemical pneumonia if aspirated or extravasated into the respiratory tract. Water-soluble agents also cost more and hence are not used on a routine basis.

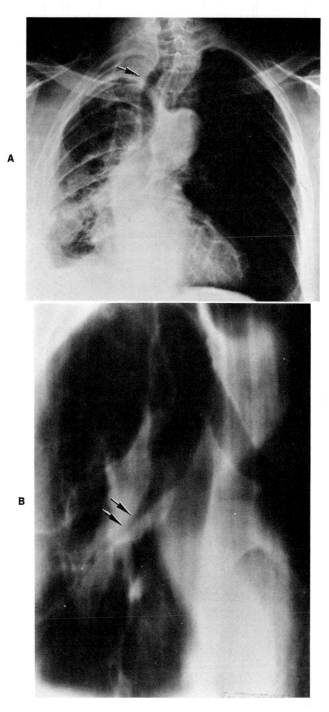

Fig. 1-3. Use of tomography. **A,** PA chest film shows mass in right hilar region. There is peripheral pneumonia. Note deviation of trachea (arrow) to right. **B,** Tomogram through hilum demonstrates mass encroaching on bronchus intermedius (arrows). This carcinoma resulted in obstructive atelectasis of right lung.

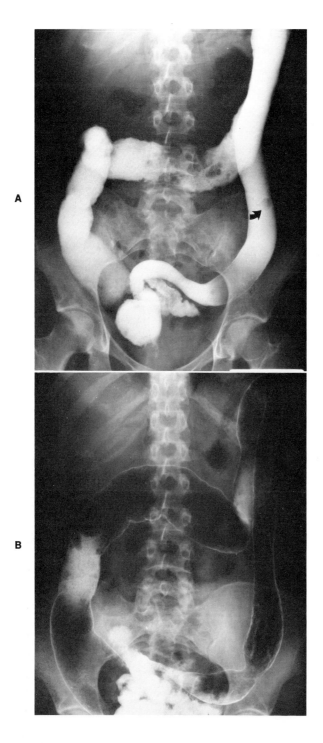

Fig. 1-4. Contrast examinations of gastrointestinal tract. **A,** Barium enema in patient with ulcerative colitis. Polyp is present (arrow). **B,** Air contrast barium enema in same patient. Note outlining of bowel wall.

Continued.

Gallbladder studies are performed either by oral administration or intravenous infusion of drugs that are removed from the bloodstream, conjugated by the liver, excreted in the bile, and transported to the gallbladder, where concentration takes place. This results in visualization of this structure.

Urography is the radiographic study of the urinary tract. The contrast agents used for this study are primarily the water-soluble sodium and methyl glucamine salts of

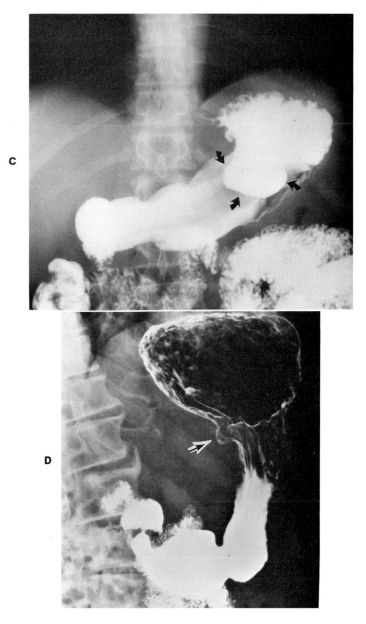

Fig. 1-4, cont'd. C, Upper gastrointestinal (upper GI) examination of stomach. Large gastric ulcer is present (arrows). **D,** Air contrast upper GI examination in patient with healing gastric ulcer (arrow).

diatrizoic or iothalamic acids. The common term for this study is the IVP. Contrast agents may also be introduced into the urinary tract in a retrograde manner. I will discuss the physiology of these agents in a later chapter.

Angiography is the study of the vascular system. Water-soluble agents similar to those used for urography are injected either arterially or intravenously, and a rapid sequence exposure is made to follow the course of the contrast material through the blood vessels (Fig. 1-5).

The lymphatic system may be studied by injecting an iodinated compound of poppy-seed oil into the lymph vessels on the dorsum of the foot or the hand. The resultant study shows the flow of lymph from the limb to the regional lymph nodes and thence to the deep lymphatic system (Fig. 1-6). These studies are used to stage patients with malignancies.

Contrast studies of the larynx and tracheobronchial tree are performed to evaluate patients for mass lesions, obstructions, and changes of bronchiectasis (Fig. 1-7).

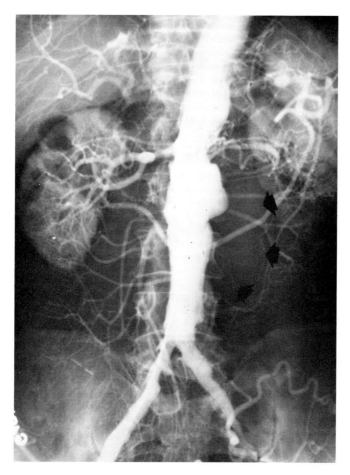

Fig. 1-5. Aortogram in patient with abdominal aortic aneurysm. Extent of aneurysm is outlined by arrows. This represents clot within aneurysm. (From Daffner, R. H.: New Physician **22:**173, 1973. Reproduced with permission of the publisher.)

The contrast agent used for these studies is an iodinated oil, Dionosil, that is introduced into the anesthetized respiratory tract via catheter.

A sinogram (fistulogram) involves the injection of contrast material through an abnormal sinus tract into the body. Water-soluble agents are commonly used for these studies. In evaluating an empyema cavity in the chest where there is a danger that a bronchopleural fistula may be present, an oil-soluble material such as Dionosil is used because water-soluble contrast material entering the bronchial tree could produce a severe and often fatal chemical pneumonia.

Sialography is the study of the salivary glands to evaluate patients with suspected salivary tumors or ductal obstructions. An oily contrast material (iodinated poppyseed oil) is injected into the duct, which has been cannulated.

Diseases encroaching on the spinal canal may be studied by myleography. The main indication is evidence of cord or nerve root compression. The most common lesion is a herniated nucleus pulposus from a lumbar disc. Myelography is performed by inserting a needle between the spinous processes of a lumbar vertebra and enter-

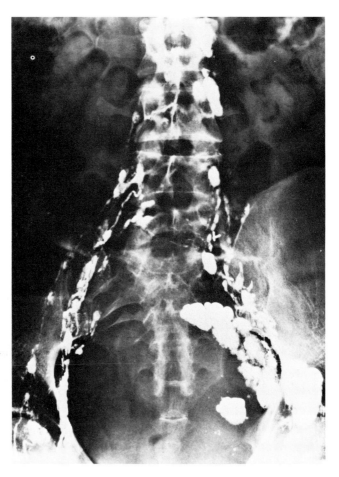

Fig. 1-6. Lymphangiogram in patient with lymphocele following renal transplant. Contrast medium is pooling in lymphocele on left. Contrast medium may be seen within lymphatics bilaterally and in para-aortic chain.

ing the subarachnoid space. It may also be performed by puncture of the cisterna magna when there is a complete block within the vertebral canal and it is necessary to inject contrast medium above the lesion. Cerebrospinal fluid may be removed for study at this time. Pantopaque, an iodinated, water-insoluble compound, is then injected under fluoroscopic monitoring in varying amounts, and the patient is positioned for the study. Recently a water-soluble compound has been introduced for myelography. Fig. 1-8 shows a myelogram taken in a patient with a herniated lumbar disc. Note the compression of the thecal sac by the herniated material.

The cerebral ventricles, cisterns, and subarachnoid space may be studied by the injection of air either directly into a ventricle or through a needle into the subarachnoid space at the lumbar level. The conventional manner of pneumoencephalography utilizes the lumbar puncture technique similar to that performed for

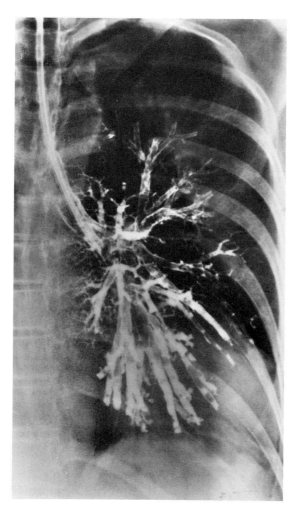

Fig. 1-7. Bronchogram in patient with tubular bronchiectasis. Contrast medium fills bronchial tree on left.

myelography. Small amounts of air are then injected and allowed to rise and fill the basal cisterns and ventricular system. Films are taken in various positions to outline these internal cavities of the brain. The procedure is quite painful, however, and carries a greater risk than many other diagnostic procedures. One of the risks is possible herniation of the cerebellar tonsils through the foramen magnum. In patients in whom elevated cerebrospinal fluid pressure is suspected, the study is performed by injecting the air through trephine holes directly into a lateral ventricle (ventriculography).

Cisternography is a specialized form of this procedure using positive contrast material to study the basal cisterns and, in particular, the cerebellopontine angle cisterns in patients suspected of having an acoustic neuroma. Contrast medium is introduced into the subarachnoid space as in myelography, and the patient is positioned with the head down to allow the heavier contrast material to flow into the cranial vault through the foramen magnum.

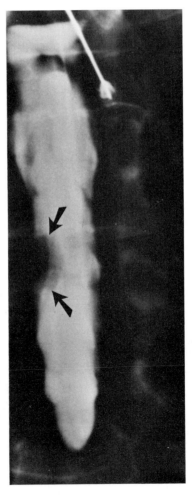

Fig. 1-8. Myelogram in patient with herniated intervertebral disc. Rounded filling defect (arrows) is present.

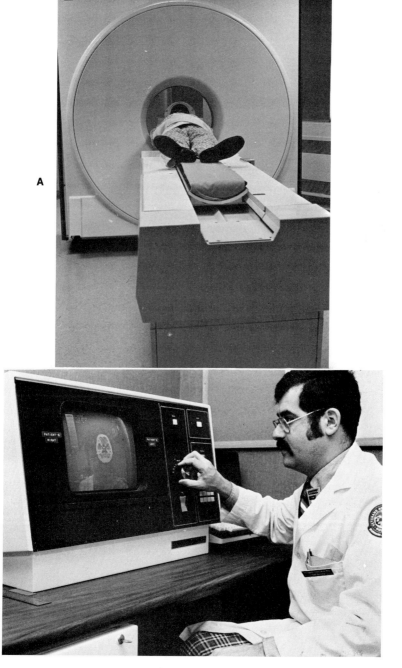

Fig. 1-9. Components of CT scanner. **A,** Gantry and table. **B,** Viewing console. All scans in this book were made on this machine. (Courtesy General Electric.)

Computed tomography has reduced the number of air studies of the brain considerably. Neuroradiologists are now able to accurately define the location and extent of intracranial tumors without having to resort to pneumoencephalography as frequently as in the past.

COMPUTED TOMOGRAPHY

Computed tomography (CT) is the newest modality of diagnostic imaging available to radiologists. The principle, which will be discussed in greater detail in the next chapter, is the measurement of x-ray absorption of various tissues by a paired moving x-ray tube and detector system (hence the term "tomography"). A computer is used to reconstruct the image based on these density measurements according to a prescribed mathematical "recipe," the algorithm. The resulting image, which is displayed on a television monitor (cathode ray tube [CRT]), is a representation of what would be seen with the patient cut open on a transverse plane. After the tube and detector make a complete revolution the table top moves the patient automatically to image a second level or "slice." An average examination of the head is 8 to 10 slices and of the body, 12 to 15 slices. Fig. 1-9 shows the major components of a total body scanner.

To enhance the appearance of certain viscera or vascular neoplasms, contrast material is injected intravenously. The contrast agent used is identical to that used in urography or arteriography.

Head scanning is performed for the evaluation of patients with a variety of neurologic findings. This study is particularly useful in defining and localizing brain tumors

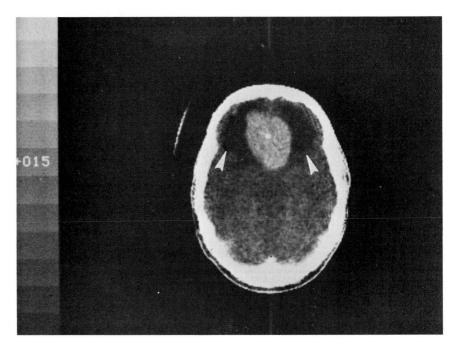

Fig. 1-10. CT scan in patient with meningioma of sphenoid ridge. Tumor is represented by large dense area in center anteriorly. It is surrounded by zone of edema (arrowheads).

(primary or metastatic) and in evaluating patients with neurologic emergencies such as intracerebral hemorrhage or subdural hematoma. Fig. 1-10 shows the head scan in a patient with a meningioma. Notice how well the tumor is defined against the normal brain tissue. Fig. 1-11 shows a patient with cerebral atrophy. Note the deep convolutional changes and enlargement of the ventricular system.

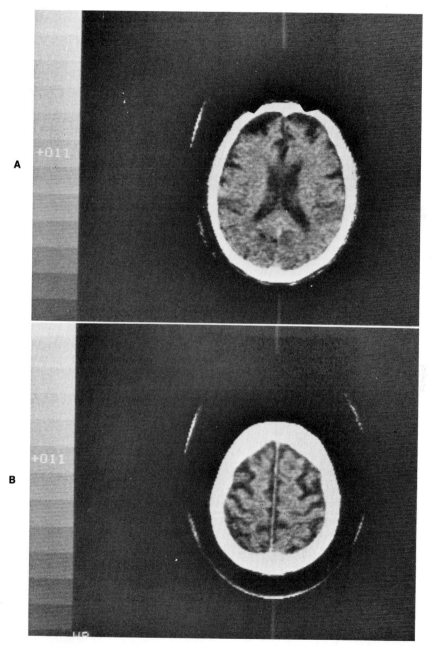

Fig. 1-11. Cerebral atrophy. CT scans demonstrate widening of cerebral sulci. This is most notable in frontal region, **A.**

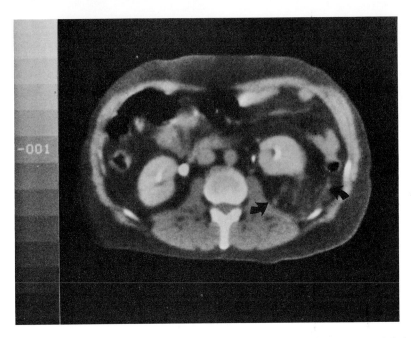

Fig. 1-12. Renal carcinoma. CT scan shows mass extending into perirenal tissues on left (arrows). On this and all other scans in this book, patient is viewed from his feet, that is, his right is to your left, etc.

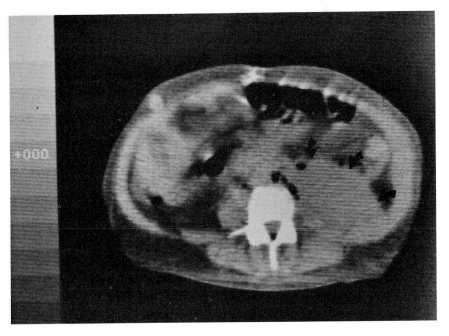

Fig. 1-13. Periaortic abscess. This patient developed abscess following aortic bypass surgery. Abscess is seen as mass in left flank (arrows). Multiple lucencies within mass represent gas within abscess.

Scanning of the remainder of the body is particularly useful in evaluating visceral neoplasms. Other uses include studies of patients with obstructive jaundice, investigation of patients with suspected pancreatic disease, mediastinal studies for defining the extent of tumors, and evaluation of patients with Hodgkin disease/lymphoma for staging purposes. Fig. 1-12 shows the total body scan of a patient with renal carcinoma. Notice that the tumor has extended beyond the confines of the kidney. This information is quite useful to the referring surgeon. Fig. 1-13 shows a patient who had persistent fever and back pain following surgery for an aortic aneurysm. A large gas-containing abscess dissecting into the left psoas muscle and left flank is present.

NUCLEAR IMAGING

Nuclear medicine traditionally has two divisions: diagnostic imaging and laboratory analysis. The diagnostic radiologist is concerned with the imaging aspect. The use of isotopes for laboratory purposes and for evaluation of physiologic functions will not be discussed. However, the reader should be aware that the laboratory aspect of nuclear medicine is an area equally as important as the imaging aspect.

The principles of nuclear imaging depend on the selective uptake of certain compounds by different organs of the body. These compounds may be labeled with a radioactive substance of sufficient energy level to allow detection outside the body. The ideal isotope is one that may be administered in low doses, is nontoxic, has a short half-life, is readily incorporated into "physiologic" compounds, and is relatively inexpensive. At the present time, technetium-99m fulfills most of these requirements.

The half-life of an element is the time necessary for its degradation to one half of its original activity. There are actually three types of half-lives: physical half-life, biologic half-life, and effective half-life. The *physical half-life* is that time period in which the element would "decay" on its own. This occurs naturally whether the element is sitting in a bottle on the laboratory shelf or has been administered to a patient. *Biologic half-life* concerns the normal physiologic removal of the substance to which the isotope has been attached. For example, the sodium pertechnetate commonly injected for brain scanning is excreted in the urine and into the GI tract. Although the physical half-life of technetium-99m is approximately 6 hours, the biologic half-life is less. The *effective half-life* is a mathematical derivation based on a formula combining biologic and physical half-lives. It measures the actual time the isotope remains effective within the body.

Table 1. Isotope scans and common indications

Type of scan	Common indications
Brain (Fig. 1-14)	Tumors, subdural hematoma
Lung (Fig. 1-15)	Pulmonary embolism
Liver (Fig. 1-16)	Metastases, masses
Bone (Fig. 1-17)	Metastases
Thyroid (Fig. 1-18)	"Goiter," nodules
Liver/lung	Subdiaphragmatic abscess
Heart/lung (Fig. 1-19)	Pericardial effusion

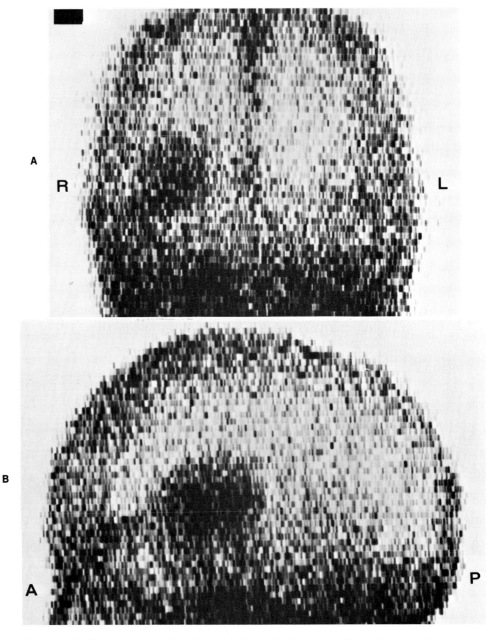

Fig. 1-14. Rectilinear brain scan in patient with right frontal lobe tumor. Tumor is represented by dense area of increased tracer uptake. **A,** Lateral view. **B,** AP view.

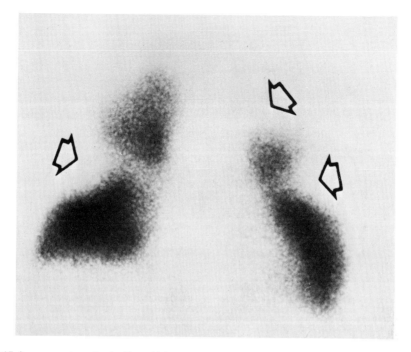

Fig. 1-15. Lung scan in patient with multiple pulmonary emboli. Perfusion defects in AP projection are outlined by arrows.

Fig. 1-16. Liver scan in patient with multiple metastases. AP view shows multiple "filling defects" represented as light areas.

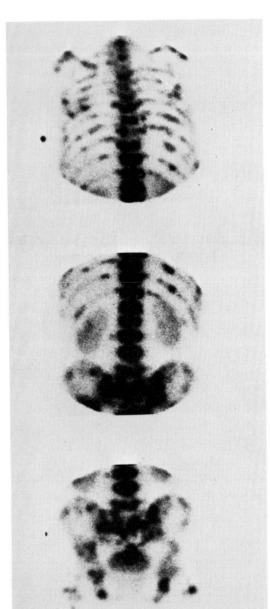

Fig. 1-17. Bone scan in patient with carcinoma of breast. Abnormal areas of increased tracer activity are seen on all three views.

Nuclear imaging is performed either on a static or on a dynamic basis. Static studies include the brain scan, thyroid scan, liver scan, and renal scan. Dynamic studies include rapid sequence flow to the brain and perfusion-diffusion studies of the lung. Table 1 illustrates (Figs. 1-14 to 1-19) common types of scans. Equipment for detecting the uptake of isotopes and for recording their images includes the

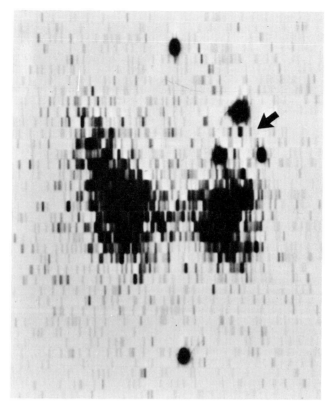

Fig. 1-18. Thyroid scan. Nonfunctioning nodule is present in upper pole on left (arrow). Three dots near arrow represent palpable extent of nodule.

rectilinear scanner (Fig. 1-20), the gamma camera (Fig. 1-21), and the tomographic scanner.

There are basically five mechanisms of isotope concentration within the body:

1. Blood pool or compartmental localization, for example, cardiac scan
2. Physiologic incorporation, for example, thyroid scan, bone scan
3. Capillary blockage, for example, lung scan
4. Phagocytosis, for example, liver scan
5. Cell sequestration, for example, spleen scan

DIAGNOSTIC ULTRASOUND

Diagnostic ultrasound is a noninvasive imaging technique utilizing sonic energy in the frequency range of 1 to 10 MHz (1,000,000 to 10,000,000 cps). It is a nonionizing form of energy. Echoes or reflections of the ultrasound beam from interfaces between tissues with different acoustic properties yield information on the size, shape, and internal structure of organs and masses. However, ultrasound is reflected by air–soft tissue interfaces, limiting its use in the chest.

Both pulsed and continuous wave (CW) ultrasound are used. Pulsed ultrasound is used principally for static cross-sectional images in the abdomen or pelvis. The

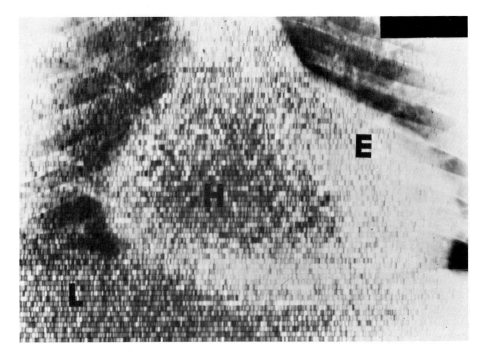

Fig. 1-19. Heart/lung scan in patient with pericardial effusion. Enlarged cardiac shadow with effusion *(E)* is seen as light area. Dark area in center represents cardiac blood pool *(H)*. Liver *(L)* is dark area to lower right. Scan superimposed on chext x-ray film for correlation.

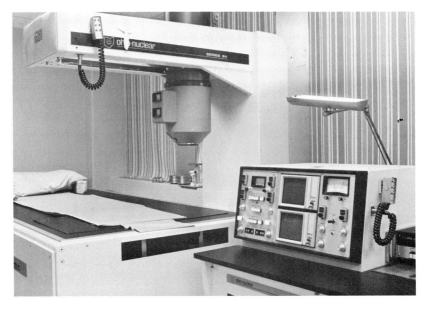

Fig. 1-20. Rectilinear nuclear scanner. (Courtesy Ohio Nuclear.)

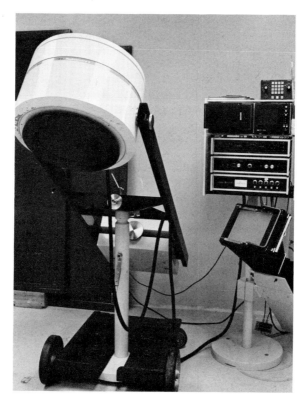

Fig. 1-21. Gamma camera isotope scanner. (Courtesy General Electric.)

transducer transmits ultrasound waves for approximately 1 microsecond and then acts as a receiver for the returning echoes for approximately 1 millisecond. More recently, *real-time ultrasound* techniques have been used to perform dynamic imaging of moving objects such as the fetus in utero or the pulsating aorta. This technique also permits rapid and efficient screening of a body region. The CW or Doppler method is used primarily as a nonimaging modality to record the dynamics in periodically changing regions such as the fetal heart or blood vessels. Fig. 1-22 shows the components of an ultrasound machine.

Three display modes are commonly used (Fig. 1-23). In amplitude mode (A-mode), information is displayed on a CRT as vertical spikes. The height or amplitude of a spike is related to the size of the echo; the distance from the initial or transducer spike is related to the depth of the reflecting interface from the transducer. A-mode is used principally for echoencephalography to detect any shift of midline brain structures.

In brightness mode (B-mode), information is displayed as dots, the brightness of which corresponds to the strength of the corresponding echo. The location of the dot is proportional to the distance of the reflecting interfaces from the transducer. Since this constitutes only a single line on the CRT (corresponding to the line of sight of the transducer), one can build up a cross-sectional image or B-scan by a composite of many such lines obtained during a scan. The images can be displayed over a wide range of gray scale or shading (Figs. 1-24 and 1-25). In particular the difference in

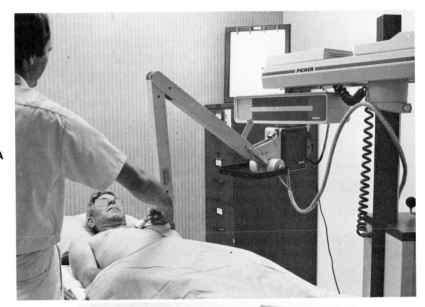

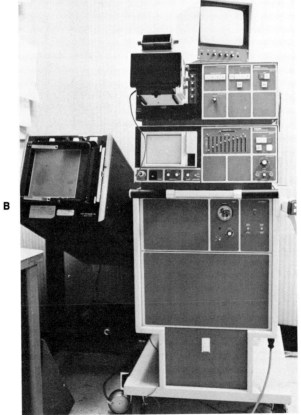

Fig. 1-22. A and **B,** Ultrasound equipment. In **A** technologist is using transducer. (Courtesy Picker Corporation.)

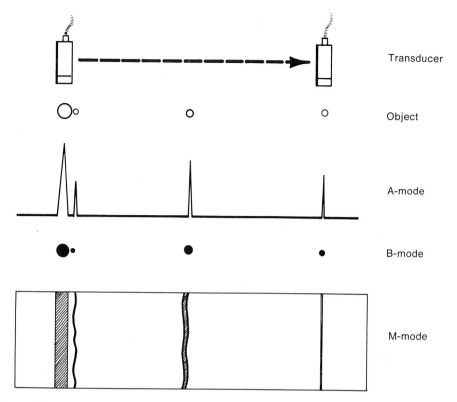

Transducer

Object

A-mode

B-mode

M-mode

Fig. 1-23. Ultrasound display modes. Three modes of ultrasound display are demonstrated when transducer passes over objects of varying size.

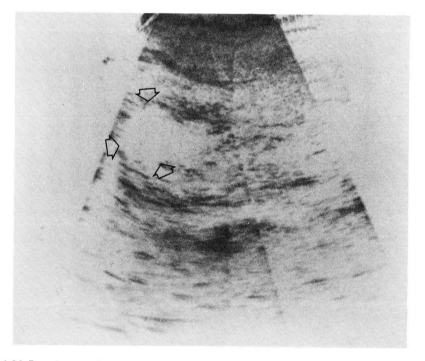

Fig. 1-24. B-mode scan of renal cyst in longitudinal plane. Arrows outline echo-free zone representing cyst in upper pole of this patient's kidney.

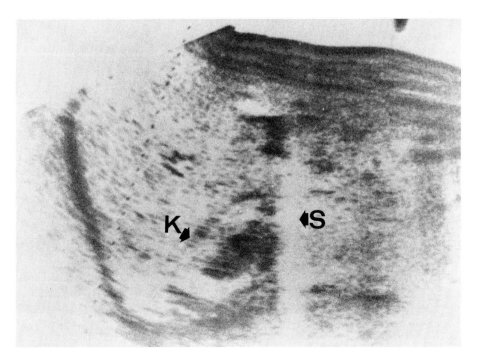

Fig. 1-25. Gallstones. Gallstones within gallbladder cast linear acoustic shadow *(S)*. Right kidney is also demonstrated *(K)*.

acoustic properties of various tissues is seen as a difference in the gray scale display of these tissues.

Motion mode (M-mode), is used in echocardiography to study the dynamic changes of the cardiac structures. Essentially the baseline of B-mode is moved at a constant rate on the CRT screen. The cardiac structures form patterns in the M-mode relating to their motion.

Recently, comparisons have been made between ultrasound and computed tomography. An important advantage of ultrasound is the absence of ionizing radiation and the relatively lower cost of the equipment. However, a great deal of technical skill is required to perform a study. Ultrasound does not, however, image air-containing organs well and penetrates bone very poorly. These limitations do not extend to computed tomography, and thus CT has potential benefit throughout the chest. Comparisons of the relative efficacies of these two imaging modalities have shown their complementary nature.

SUMMARY

The spectrum of imaging forms that makes up the world of the diagnostic radiologist has been covered. In your medical career, you will utilize all these modalities to help you diagnose your patient's problems. You should be cautioned, however, that imaging examinations and laboratory tests are not a substitute for a thorough history and physical examination. When you order a diagnostic study, you should have a specific reason for doing so. They are costly and in some instances carry a degree of risk for the patient.

References

Ambrose, J.: Computerized transverse axial scanning (tomography): part 2. Clinical application, Br. J. Radiol. **46:**1023, 1973.

Dalrymple, G. V., and Slayden, J. E.: Radiology in primary care, St. Louis, 1975, The C. V. Mosby Co.

Evens, R. G.: New frontier for radiology: computed tomography, Am. J. Roentgenol. **126:**1117, 1976.

Frankel, G., and Rosenfeld, D. D.: Xeroradiographic detection of occult breast cancer, Cancer **35:**542, 1975.

Hall, F. M.: Overutilization of radiologic examinations, Radiology **120:**443, 1976.

Hounsfield, G. N.: Computerized transverse axial scanning (tomography): part 1. Description of system, Br. J. Radiol. **46:**1016, 1973.

Littleton, J. T.: Tomography: physical principles and clinical applications, Baltimore, 1976, The Williams & Wilkins Co.

O'Mara, R. E.: Bone scanning in osseous metastatic disease, J.A.M.A. **229:**1915, 1974.

Peck, D. R., and Lowman, R. M.: Mammography: current application, J.A.M.A. **236:**1886, 1976.

Rigler, L. G.: Is this radiograph really necessary? Radiology **120:**449, 1976.

Squire, L. F.: Fundamentals of radiology, Cambridge, Mass., 1975, Harvard University Press.

Thompson, T. T.: Primer of clinical radiology, Boston, 1973, Little, Brown & Co.

Wolfe, J. N.: Xeroradiography: image content and comparison with film roentgenographs, Am. J. Roentgenol. **117:**690, 1973.

Wolfe, J. N.: Mammography, Radiol. Clin. North Am. **12:**189, 1974.

2 Physical foundations of diagnostic imaging

The first chapter considered the various forms of diagnostic imaging. A logical continuation is to describe the principles involved in obtaining diagnostic images.

X-RAYS
Definition

X-rays, or roentgen rays, are a form of electromagnetic radiation or energy of extremely short wavelength. The spectrum of electromagnetic radiation is illustrated in Fig. 2-1. X-rays in the diagnostic range are in the spectrum of short wavelengths. The shorter the wavelength of an electromagnetic radiation form, the greater its energy and, as a rule, the greater its ability to penetrate various materials.

X-rays are described in terms of particles or packets of energy called quanta or photons. Photons travel at the speed of light. The amount of energy carried by each photon depends on the wavelength of the radiation. The energy of an x-ray photon may be determined if its wavelength is known according to the formula

$$E = \frac{12.4}{\lambda}$$

where E equals the energy in electron volts and λ is the wavelength in angstroms. Thus it is apparent that the shorter the wavelength, the greater the energy.

The energy carried by x-rays is measured in electron volts. An electron volt is the amount of energy an electron gains as it is accelerated through a potential of 1 volt. In diagnostic work, x-rays with energies up to 125,000 electron volts (125 keV) are used.

An atom is ionized when it has lost an electron. Any photon that has about 15 or more electron volts of energy is capable of producing ionization in atoms and molecules (ionizing radiation). X-rays, gamma rays, and certain types of ultraviolet radiation are all typical ionizing radiation forms.

Production

X-rays used in diagnostic radiology require a vacuum and the presence of a high potential difference between a cathode and an anode. In the basic x-ray tube, electrons are boiled off the cathode (filament) by heating it to a very high temperature. To

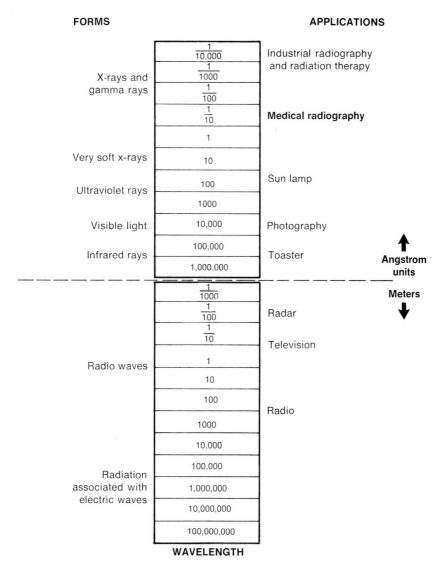

Fig. 2-1. Spectrum of electromagnetic radiation. Numbers represent wavelength of the particular radiation. The shorter the wavelength, the greater the energy associated with that radiation.

move these electrons toward the anode at an energy sufficient to produce x-rays a high potential, up to 125,000 volts (125 kV), is used. When the accelerated electrons strike the tungsten anode, x-rays are produced in two ways: bremsstrahlung and characteristic radiation.

Bremsstrahlung is produced when the electron passes near the nucleus of a tungsten atom and is deflected sharply from its original course (Fig. 2-2). The electron loses energy in the encounter, and this energy is given off in the form of an x-ray photon.

The second form of x-ray production occurs when an electron approaching a tungsten atom strikes an electron in the K shell of that atom and displaces it from its

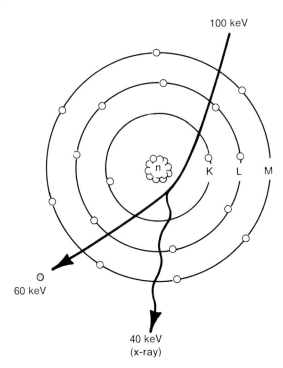

100 keV

n

K L M

60 keV

40 keV
(x-ray)

Fig. 2-2. Bremsstrahlung production. High speed electron passing near tungsten nucleus is deviated from its course. This deviation results in loss of energy, which is given off as an x-ray.

normal orbit around the nucleus. This results in an ionized tungsten atom. An electron from an L shell transfers immediately into the vacant orbit in the K shell, resulting in a discharge of the difference in energy between the K shell and the L shell (Fig. 2-3). This energy is given off as an x-ray that is termed a *characteristic x-ray* because its energy will be the same every time a K-shell vacancy is filled by an L-shell electron for that particular type of atom. For tungsten the energy given off as characteristic radiation is 57.9 keV.

Both Bremsstrahlung and characteristic radiation collisions are relatively rare, however. In about 99% of all encounters the electrons simply heat the anode without producing x-radiations. The anode therefore is made of tungsten because of its high melting point. Tungsten is also more efficient than other substances in producing useful x-rays of energies in the diagnostic range.

Production of images

Image production by x-rays results from attenuation of those x-rays by the material through which they pass. Attenuation is the process by which x-rays are removed from a beam through absorption and scatter. In general, the greater the density of a material, that is, the number of grams per cubic centimeter, the greater its ability to absorb or scatter x-rays (Fig. 2-4). Absorption is also influenced by the atomic number of the structure. The denser the structure, the greater the attenuation, which results in less blackening of the film (fewer x-rays strike the film). Less

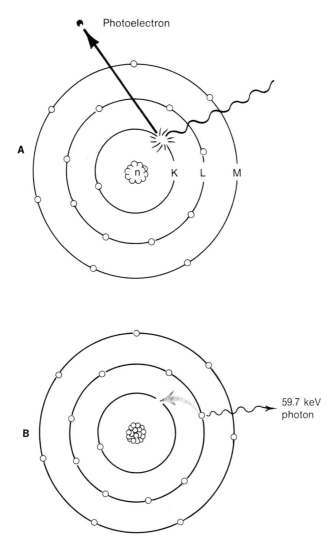

Fig. 2-3. Characteristic radiation production utilizing photoelectric effect. **A,** Incoming photon displaces K-shell electron (photoelectron). **B,** Electron from outer shell fills vacancy in K shell. Difference in energy level between outer shell and vacant shell is given off as x-ray photon. Amount of energy of this x-ray will be same or "characteristic" of that element each time orbital electron of particular shell moves to vacant inner shell.

dense structures attenuate the beam to a lesser degree and result in more blackening of the film (more x-rays strike the film) (Fig. 2-5).

It is important to differentiate between two types of "density" that you will hear mentioned when discussing radiographs with radiologists or other colleagues: physical density and radiographic density. *Physical density* is the type of density just described. *Radiographic density* is a term that refers to the degree of blackness of a film. *Radiographic contrast* is the difference in radiographic densities on a film. The radiographic density of a substance is related to its physical density. The effect on film or other recording media occurs "paradoxically"; structures of high physical density produce less radiodensity and vice versa. Structures that produce more

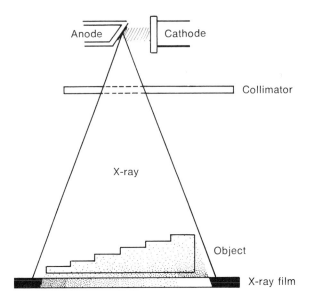

Fig. 2-4. Relationship between density and absorption of x-ray. The denser a particular material is, the greater its ability to absorb x-rays. Net result of greater absorption is less darkening of film.

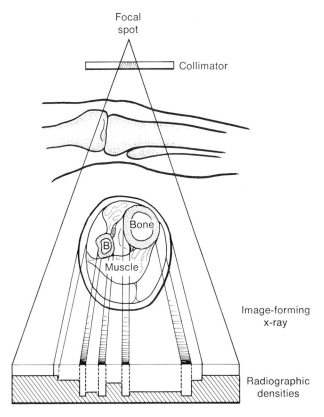

Fig. 2-5. Differential absorption of x-rays depends on composition of various tissues. Denser tissues absorb more x-rays; less dense tissues transmit more x-rays. Resultant radiographic image is essentially a "shadowgram."

blackening on film are referred to as being *radiolucent;* those that produce less blackening are called *radiopaque or radiodense.* There are four types of radiographic densities; these are, in increasing order of physical density, gas (air), fat, water, and bone (metal). Radiographically these appear as black, gray-black, gray, and "white," respectively.

Recording media

The type of recording medium with which you are most familiar is x-ray film. X-ray film consists of a plastic sheet coated with a thin emulsion containing silver bromide and a small amount of silver iodide. This emulsion is sensitive to light and radiation. A protective coating covers the emulsion. When the film is exposed to light or to ionizing radiation and then developed, chemical changes take place within the emulsion, resulting in the deposition of metallic silver, which is black. The amount of blackening on the film depends entirely on the amount of radiation reaching the film and therefore on the amount attenuated or removed from the beam by the subject.

Other recording media include the Xerox plate, the fluoroscopic screen/image intensification system, photoelectric detector crystals, and xenon detector systems.

Xerography is a recording method that uses an electrostatically charged plate to record the image. X-ray photons that strike this plate change the charge on the plate in proportion to the amount of radiation reaching it; this amount, in turn, depends on the degree of absorption in the tissue through which the x-ray beam passed. The pattern of charges left on the plate is translated into a visible image by blowing an electrostatically charged powder across the plate. An image is formed wherever the powder sticks to the plate, and this image is transferred onto paper or plastic by heat.

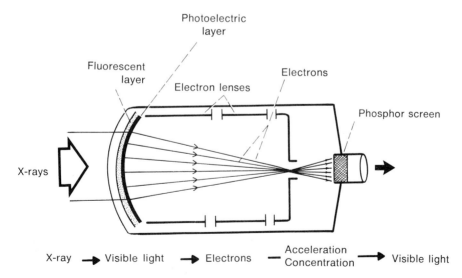

Fig. 2-6. Image intensifier. X-rays striking fluorescent layer give off visible light, which in turn is converted into electron stream. This is accelerated, focused, and concentrated onto output phosphor screen that converts electronic image back into visible light. Original brightness is magnified approximately 50,000 times.

A fluoroscopic screen is a screen coated with a substance (phosphor) that gives off visible light (or "fluoresces") when it is irradiated. The brightness of the light is proportional to the intensity of the x-ray beam striking the plate and depends on the amount of radiation removed from the beam by the object irradiated. In its most common use today the fluorescent screen is combined with an electronic device that converts the visible light into an electron stream that amplifies the image (makes it brighter) by converting the electron pattern back into visible light (Fig. 2-6). This system allows the radiologist to see the image clearly without necessitating dark adaptation of the eyes, as is necessary in "conventional" (non-image-enhanced) fluoroscopy. The development of image amplification has been one of the major breakthroughs in diagnostic radiology over the past 25 years.

The detection of photons emitted by radioisotopes is accomplished with sodium

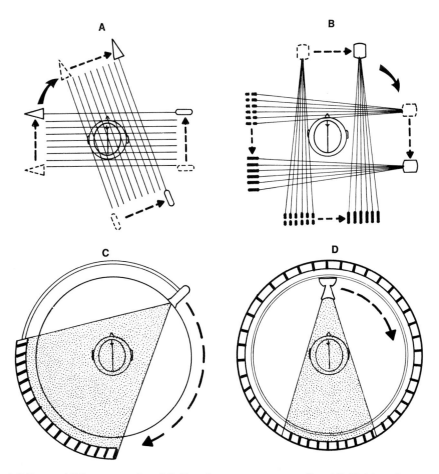

Fig. 2-7. Types of CT scanners. **A** and **B**, Translate-rotate scanners. **C** and **D**, Rotate-only scanners. **A**, Single x-ray tube and single detector. This was prototype of all CT scanners. **B**, Single x-ray tube with multiple detectors. Scanning times in this system range from 4½ minutes to 18 seconds. **C**, Rotate-only scanner with tube and detector arc rotating. Scanning time is 2 to 5 seconds. All CT scans in this book were made on this type of scanner. **D**, Rotate-only scanner. X-ray tube is only moving part; 360-degree detector array remains stationary. Scanning time is 1 to 6 seconds.

iodide crystals. These crystals respond, when irradiated, by emitting light whose brightness is related to the energy of the photons striking them. Photodetectors convert the light into an electronic signal, which is then amplified and converted into a variety of display images.

Under ordinary circumstances the fleshy organs of the body such as the heart, kidneys, liver, spleen, and pancreas are considered to be of uniform radiographic density, like water, which produces a gray appearance on conventional radiographs. However, these tissues vary in their chemical properties, and it is possible, using computer techniques, to measure these differences, magnify them, and display them in varying shades of gray or in color; this is the basis of computed tomography (CT).

In CT an x-ray beam and a detector system move in synchrony. The beam-detector system moves through an arc of 360 degrees, irradiating the subject with a highly collimated beam, and allows the detector to measure the intensity of radiation passing through the subject. The data from these measurements are analyzed by a computer system where various shades of gray (CT numbers) are assigned to different structures based on their absorption or attenuation coefficients. The computer reconstructs a picture based on geometric plots of where these measurements were taken. Although this system of diagnosis was developed in the early 1970's, the reader may be interested to know that the mathematical formula for the reconstruction of images based on measurements of their points in space was actually worked out in 1917 by the mathematician Radon. Four types of scan systems are shown in Fig. 2-7.

The information obtained with CT systems is displayed on a television screen (CRT) and recorded on magnetic tape. Once the information has been recorded, it is possible to alter the visual intensities of the various densities on the reading console (Fig. 2-8). The data from the television screen may be recorded further on Polaroid film, conventional photographic film, or x-ray film using a device known as a multiformat camera.

Nature of the radiographic image

As mentioned previously, the degree of darkening on the developed x-ray film will depend on the number of x-rays actually striking that film. To ensure that only the part of interest is irradiated, beam-restricting devices are used to control the actual shape of the radiation stream as it strikes the body. These restricting devices are referred to as collimators. In CT the beam is very highly collimated to a narrow width, approximately 1 cm or less.

There are physical and geometric factors that affect the radiographic image. These include thickness of the part being irradiated, motion, scatter, magnification, and distortion.

The *thickness* of the part will determine how much of the beam is removed or attenuated. This was explained earlier. Thus an obese patient requires more x-rays for adequate penetration than does a thin patient; bone requires more x-rays for penetration than does the surrounding muscle.

Motion of a part being radiographed results in a blurred nondiagnostic image. Motion may be overcome by shortening the exposure time. One way of decreasing the time of exposure is to enhance the effectiveness of the recording medium. This may be done by using intensifying screens. An intensifying screen is a device coated

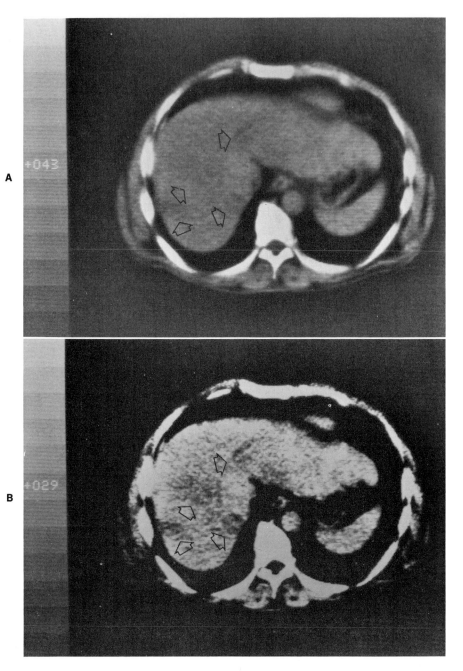

Fig. 2-8. CT scan image manipulations. Ability to enhance certain areas of scan slice is one of functions of CT scanner. This is illustrated in patient with multiple hepatic metastases. All four pictures are of same slice. Number in middle represents CT number or absorption value of that particular shade of gray. **A,** Window width 150. Metastatic lesions are barely visible as areas of low density (arrows). **B,** Window width 30. By lowering width of window, low density areas are "enhanced" (arrows). Compare to **A. C,** Use of interrogation mode. Machine is asked to identify all areas of CT No. 29. Note that metastases identify at 29 (arrow). **D,** Identifying CT value of normal liver shows metastatic lesions as negative defects (arrows).

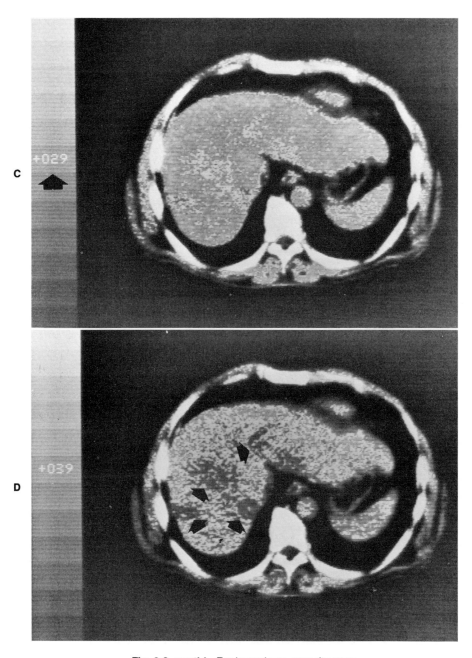

Fig. 2-8, cont'd. For legend see opposite page.

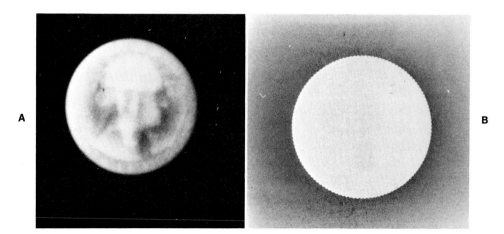

Fig. 2-9. Screen technique vs cardboard technique. Radiographs of a coin were made using identical exposure factors. **A** was made by using intensifying screens; **B,** by direct exposure without screens. Note that for given exposure there is greater degree of penetration using intensifying screens. Image on coin is clearly visible in **A,** whereas there has not been enough penetration in **B.** However, note detail of ribbed edge of coin seen on film made with cardboard technique. This detail is absent on exposure made using screens.

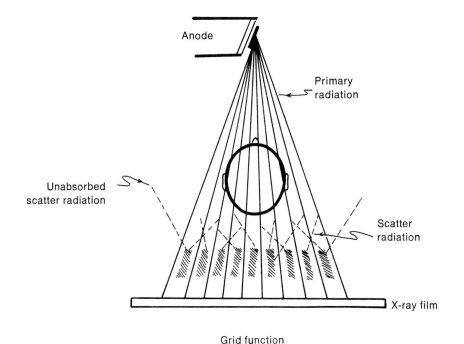

Fig. 2-10. Grid function. Grid absorbs scattered radiation. Angling of lead strips in grid permits only primary beam to pass through.

with a fluorescent material that gives off visible light when struck by x-rays. This light exposes the film. Cassettes (film holders) containing screens are used for about 90% of diagnostic x-ray work. This has the advantage of reducing the exposure time during which motion could occur. However, a disadvantage of intensifying screens is that detail is often lost. Fortunately, most radiographic examinations do not require a great amount of very fine detail, and screen technique is usually adequate.

Nonscreen technique, also referred to as "cardboard" technique, utilizes x-ray film in a light-tight (cardboard) container. No intensifying screen is used, and only the x-ray beam itself darkens the film. This has the advantage of producing a highly detailed film of the structure radiographed but has the disadvantage of requiring longer exposure times. Cardboard technique is used mainly for examinations of the hand or foot, where fine bony detail must be seen. It also has been used in mammography, where exquisite detail of breast structure is necessary. Fig. 2-9 compares the images using screen and cardboard technique.

Scatter is produced by deflection of some of the primary radiation beam; this can produce fog on the film and is undesirable. To eliminate as much scatter as possible, a grid that has alternating angled slats of very thin radiolucent material combined with thin lead strips is used (Fig. 2-10). This results in the removal of much of the scatter. To prevent the lead strips from casting their own shadows as they absorb radiation, the whole grid is moved very quickly during the exposure, eliminating these lines. This system is known as the Bucky-Potter system, after the two men who invented it.

The radiographic image is a two-dimensional representation of a three-dimensional structure. Consequently, some structures will be farther from the film

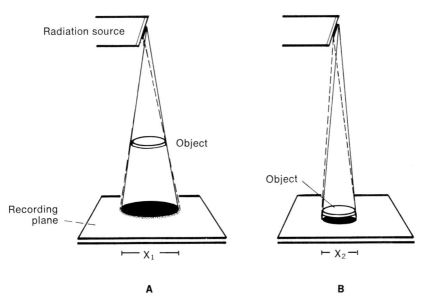

Fig. 2-11. Effect of magnification. **A,** Object is farther from film, resulting in larger image. However, its margin is not as distinct as in **B. B,** Object is closer to film, resulting in smaller and sharper image than in **A.**

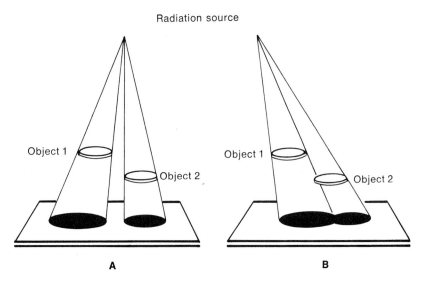

Fig. 2-12. Distortion. Radiographic shape of object depends on angle at which radiographic beam strikes it. **A,** Two objects of similar size cast distinct shadows when x-ray beam is nearly perpendicular. Difference in size is result of magnification. **B,** Angling x-ray beam while objects remain in same relationship to one another results in overlapping shadow that is not true representation of actual object. **C** and **D,** Distortion may be illustrated in this patient with right middle lobe pneumonia. **C** is PA radiograph of chest. **D** was made with patient bending backward toward film (lordotic view). Note change in appearance of heart, ribs, and infiltrate, which now appears as mass adjacent to heart on right (arrow).

than others. Geometrically, x-rays behave similar to light. Hence *magnification* of objects will occur when they are some distance from the film. The farther an object is from the film, the greater the magnification; the closer the object is to the film, the less the magnification (Fig. 2-11). This has considerable importance in evaluating structures such as the heart on chest radiographs. On the standard chest radiograph the x-ray beam enters through the back of the patient and exits from the front (posterior to anterior [PA]). Since the heart is located anteriorly, there will be relatively little magnification. However, on an anterior to posterior (AP) radiograph of the chest the beam enters from the patient's front and exits through the back. Hence there is somewhat greater magnification of the heart because of its distance from the film. The best rule to follow to reduce the undesirable effect of magnification is to have the part of greatest interest closest to the film. This will give the least magnification, that is, the truest image, of the region of interest.

Distortion occurs when the object being radiographed is not perfectly perpendicular to the beam. The radiographic shadow of an object depends on the sum of the shadow produced by that object when x-rayed. Changes in the relationship of that object to the x-ray beam may distort its radiographic image (Fig. 2-12). For diagnostic clarity, therefore, it is best to have the part of major interest closest and as perpendicular to the film as possible.

ULTRASOUND PHYSICS

Diagnostic ultrasound employs high frequency (1 to 10 MHz or cps) sonic energy. This is well above the normal ear response of 20 to 20,000 Hz. The radiation is

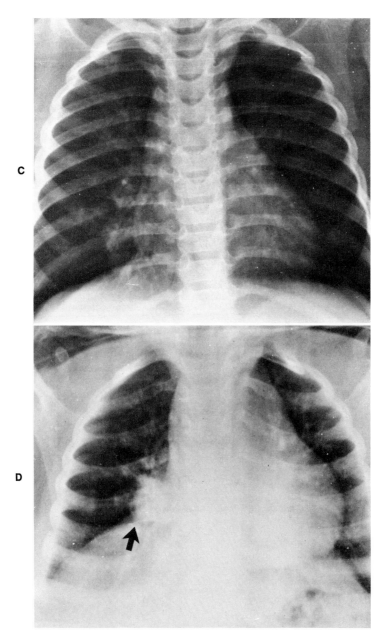

Fig. 2-12, cont'd. For legend see opposite page.

nonionizing. Mechanically the energy is transmitted through a medium by temporal variations in the local pressure. Sound cannot exist in a vacuum. The sound is generated by the periodic mechanical vibration of a crystal that is set in motion by a frequency-tuned electrical circuit. The crystal oscillates 1 microsecond and then functions as a tuned receiver for approximately 1 millisecond. In its receiver mode the crystal is set into mechanical oscillation by an echo created by the reflection of the ultrasound from an interface between media with different acoustic properties. The mechanical oscillations can then be converted into an electrical signal, the size of which is related to the strength of the echo.

The amount of sonic energy that is reflected at acoustic interfaces is related to the differences in the acoustic impedances of the media. The acoustic impedance (z) is defined as the density (ρ) of the medium times the velocity (v) of sound in that medium $(z = \rho v)$. As the density of the medium increases, v also increases. The velocity of sound in air is 331 m/sec; in water, 1497 m/sec; and in average soft tissue, 1540 m/sec. Quantitatively the fraction of the incident energy that is reflected (R) at an interface is determined by the equation

$$R = \frac{(z_1 - z_2)^2}{(z_1 + z_2)^2}$$

where z_1 and z_2 are the acoustic impedances of the two media. It can be seen that where z_1 and z_2 are nearly the same (as in similar soft tissues) there is little reflection, whereas when z_1 and z_2 are markedly different (as between air and soft tissues) the reflection is large and may comprise nearly all the incident sonic energy. Since the angle of reflection of the sonic wave (defined as the angle between the reflected wave front and a wave perpendicular to the interface) is equal to the angle of incidence, the transducer should at some point in its motion be perpendicular to the interface, so that the reflected wave travels directly back to the transducer.

Frequency and wavelength are related by the equation

$$v = \lambda f$$

where λ is the wavelength and f is the frequency. V is the velocity of the wave. Since v is constant in a particular medium, λ increases as f decreases and vice versa. Thus high frequency waves have short wavelengths of the order of 1 mm in diagnostic ultrasound. This allows adequate spatial resolution along the line of site of the transducer. However, the frequency cannot be made too high, since the penetrating ability of sound falls drastically with increasing frequency.

SUMMARY

This chapter has briefly discussed the production and nature of x-rays, the production of the diagnostic image, and the various ways of recording that image. Factors affecting the diagnostic image such as thickness, motion, scatter, magnification, and distortion were discussed as well as means of preventing or correcting these occurrences.

References

Carlsen, E. N.: Ultrasound physics for the physician. A brief review, J. Clin. Ultrasound 3:69, 1975.
Christensen, E. E., Curry, T. S. III, and Nunnally, J.: An introduction to the physics of diagnostic radiology, Philadelphia, 1972, Lea & Febiger.
The fundamentals of radiography, Rochester, N.Y., 1968, Eastman Kodak Co.
Gottschalk, A., and Potchen, E. J.: Diagnostic nuclear medicine, Baltimore, 1976, The Williams & Wilkins Co.
Maynard, C. D.: Clinical nuclear medicine, ed. 2, Philadelphia, 1978, Lea & Febiger.

3 Radiographic contrast agents

We are able to recognize various structures within the body either because of their inherent radiographic density (such as bone distinguished from muscle) or because they contain one of the basic natural contrast materials (air). However, since most of the internal viscera are of the radiographic density of water or close to it, it is necessary to introduce into these structures a material that will outline walls, define anatomy, and demonstrate any pathologic conditions. The first chapter briefly mentioned these agents and some of the studies for which they are used. This chapter will deal with their physiology and pharmacology, define indications and contraindications for their use, and discuss the treatment of reactions to contrast agents.

Barium preparations

Barium sulfate (USP) in one of its many forms, provides the mainstay for radiographic examination of the gastrointestinal (GI) tract. Barium is of high atomic weight, which results in considerable absorption of the x-ray beam, thus providing excellent radiographic contrast. In the usual preparation, finely pulverized barium mixed with dispersing agents is suspended in water. When administered orally or rectally, it provides adequate coating of the gastrointestinal tract.

Although barium itself is chemically inert, when extravasated outside the GI tract, it produces a severe desmoplastic reaction. This is most likely to occur when there is a perforation of the GI tract. In the past, barium mixed with fecal material was deemed to be a rapidly lethal mixture when introduced into the peritoneal cavity. However, studies have shown that the combination of barium and feces is no more lethal than the introduction of feces alone into the peritoneum. However, because of the tendency to produce severe granulomas and adhesions, barium should not be used whenever a suspected perforation exists. In these situations a water-soluble contrast material should be used.

Barium preparations are safe to use as long as the entire GI tract is patent. Oral barium may be used if an obstruction is present proximal to the ileocecal valve, since the contents of the small intestine remain fluid up to that point. If the obstruction is distal to the ileocecal valve, the patient is best examined with a retrograde study (barium enema) because once the bowel contents enter the cecum, water is rapidly absorbed. If barium is allowed to remain within the colon for a long period of time behind an obstruction, it may inspissate.

Water-soluble contrast materials

Water-soluble contrast agents are used predominantly for urography, angiography, and contrast enhancement of CT studies. The most common agents used are the sodium or meglumine salts of diatrizoic or iothalamic acid in concentrations of 60% to 90%.

These agents are hypertonic, resulting in a fluid shift from the extracellular to the intravascular space. Although normal individuals may not suffer any severe long-lasting effects from this shift, patients who are dehydrated or in a precarious state of cardiac and fluid balance are at special risk. Secondary effects from the changes in viscosity and tonicity of the blood include platelet aggregation, changes in blood pressure, changes in cardiac output, and changes in pulse rate. As the serum osmolality rises, there may be changes in blood coagulation, with a resultant bleeding tendency.

The extent and severity of these changes will depend on the volume injected, the speed of injection, and the tonicity and viscosity of the agent. Rapid injection, high volume injection, and high tonicity and viscosity of the agent are associated with more severe reactions. Fortunately the majority of these agents are used for urography, where a slower injection rate prevents many of these effects. Occasionally a vagal reaction occurs in which there is vasodilatation and systemic hypotension. Bradycardia is encountered rather than tachycardia.

Cardiac changes include bradycardia, a fall in systemic blood pressure, flattening of the T waves, and decreased cardiac output. This occurs especially if the contrast agent is injected directly into the heart. In the kidneys, especially in a dehydrated patient, glomerular and tubular damage that results in temporary impairment of renal function and oliguria occasionally occurs.

Excretion of these agents is by pure glomerular filtration within the kidney. The material is removed intact by the glomeruli. In patients with chronic renal failure, however, the material may be secreted into the small bowel by a process known as "vicarious excretion."

In addition to their use in angiography and urography, these same agents may be injected into sinus tracts or used in diluted form to examine the GI tract when there is a suspected perforation. They do not cause any of the undesirable side effects that barium is known to produce when outside the GI tract. However, there is one important contraindication for water-soluble contrast media: suspected communication between the GI tract and the tracheobronchial tree (tracheoesophageal fistula). As mentioned in Chapter 1, water-soluble materials are extremely irritating to the tracheobronchial mucosa and produce a severe chemical pneumonia that may result in death. A barium or oil-soluble preparation should be used when airway communication is suspected.

Agents used to visualize the biliary tree

The agent most commonly used for cholecystography is iopanoic acid (Telepaque). Other agents used are iocetamic acid (Cholebrine), sodium tyropanoate

(Bilopaque), and calcium or sodium ipodate (Oragrafin). These agents are ingested orally, absorbed in the duodenum, conjugated as a glucuronide salt in the liver, and excreted in the bile. The material is then stored and concentrated within the gallbladder. In their native form, these agents are not water soluble, allowing their absorption from the GI tract. In the conjugated form, they are water soluble and are not absorbed on passage through the bowel.

Meglumine iodipamide (Cholografin) is a water-soluble contrast medium for intravenous cholangiography and cholecystography. On slow intravenous injection, it is carried to the liver where it is excreted within the bile, permitting visualization of the biliary tree and gallbaldder. A small amount is excreted by the kidneys.

• • •

Oil-soluble agents such as propyliodone (Dionosil) are used for bronchography. The material is inert within the tracheobronchial tree and provides adequate coating and definition of the structures. Excess oil is decanted from the bottle to reduce the possibility of lipid pneumonia.

Ethiodized oil (Ethiodol) is an oily agent used for lymphangiography. It also may be used for sialography.

• • •

An excellent discussion of indications, types, and usages of contrast material is contained in the *Physician's Desk Reference for Radiology and Nuclear Medicine*. The reader is referred to that source for a more in-depth discussion.

ADVERSE REACTIONS TO CONTRAST MATERIAL AND THEIR MANAGEMENT

The incidence of reaction to iodinated contrast material is variable and unpredictable. The Subcommittee on Treatment of Adverse Reactions of the Committee on Contrast Media from the International Society of Radiology reviewed the data from 150,000 case reports. They found that the overall incidence of reactions was 5%. Interestingly, there was a lower incidence of reactions in those patients who had a methylglucamine salt administered as compared with those who had been given sodium salts. Serious reactions were reported to vary between 1:1000 and 1:2000, with fatalities occurring from 1:13,000 to 1:40,000. Although many reactions occur in patients with no previous allergic history, the study found that in a patient with a history of allergy the risk of reaction was twice that of the general population. If the patient had a history of a previous reaction to contrast media, the chances of another reaction were three times greater than that of the general population. Pretesting with a small injection of the contrast medium was found to have little or no value in identifying patients who would later react. Similarly, pretreatment with antihistamines and steroids in patients with known allergies to contrast material were shown to be ineffective.

Types of reaction

There are three basic types of reaction: mild, intermediate, and severe. *Mild* or *minor reactions* (nausea, vomiting, sneezing, flushing, diaphoresis, and occasional

Table 2. Signs and symptoms of reactions to contrast material

Type	Cardiovascular	Respiratory	Cutaneous	Gastro-intestinal	Nervous	Urinary
Mild	Pallor Diaphoresis Tachycardia	Sneezing Coughing Rhinorrhea	Erythema Feeling of warmth	Nausea Vomiting Metallic taste	Anxiety Headache Dizziness	
Interme-diate	Bradycardia Palpitations Hypotension	Wheezing Acute asthma attack	Urticaria Pruritis	Abdominal cramps Diarrhea	Agitation Vertigo Slurred speech	Oliguria
Severe	Acute pulmonary edema Shock Congestive heart failure Cardiac arrest	Laryngospasm Cyanosis Laryngeal edema Apnea	Angioneurotic edema	Paralytic ileus	Disorien-tation Stupor Coma Convul-sions	Acute renal failure

headache) resolve without therapy. *Intermediate reactions* are those that require therapy for the patient's symptoms but are not life-threatening. These include urticaria, angioneurotic edema, and wheezing. *Severe reactions* include cardiovascular collapse, which may be associated with pulmonary edema, laryngeal edema, and apnea. There may be central nervous system depression. Death may result if proper treatment is not instituted immediately.

Table 2 lists signs and symptoms of contrast reactions in order of increasing severity.

Treatment of reactions to contrast material

Before instituting treatment the severity of the reaction and the body systems involved should be carefully evaluated. The patient's vital signs should be monitored. Once a determination has been made regarding the organ system involved and the nature and severity of the reaction, proper treatment may be instituted. After successful treatment of a reaction of any kind, the type of reaction, severity, and mode of treatment should be noted in the patient's permanent record. In addition, a notation should be made on the patient's x-ray folder that he has had an allergic reaction, and the type of reaction should be stated. Furthermore, the patient's referring physician should be notified immediately whenever a reaction occurs.

Mild reactions require careful observation of the patient and reassurance. Most of these symptoms will pass within a few minutes. Anxiety is believed to play a key role in the development of minor reactions.

The intermediate reactions are treated by intravenous administration of 25 to 50 mg of diphenhydramine (Benadryl). This may be augmented by 0.3 to 0.5 ml of a 1:1000 solution of epinephrine subcutaneously. In the majority of cases the patient will respond favorably within several minutes; hives begin to fade, wheezing subsides, and the patient appears less apprehensive. The use of steroids for intermediate types of reaction is controversial. Some authorities believe that a 100 mg bolus of

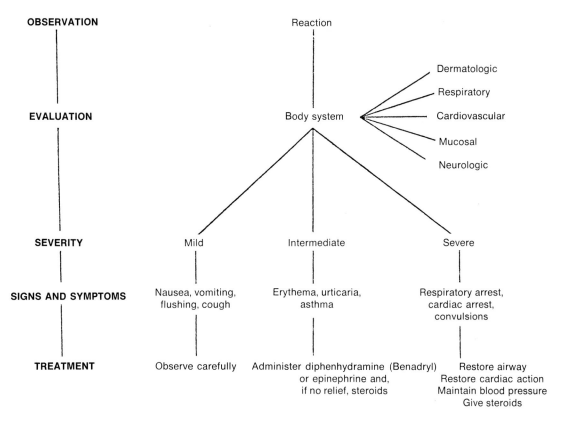

Fig. 3-1. Flow chart for management of reactions to radiographic contrast material.

prednisolone is useful in the more severe type of intermediate reaction. Use your own judgment in this situation.

Severe reactions require immediate recognition and evaluation of the patient's cardiopulmonary status. Cardiopulmonary resuscitation (CPR) equipment should be readily at hand in any area where contrast materials are used. Furthermore, the radiologist and the technical staff should be well trained in the technique of CPR. In general the radiologist is the first physician called to the scene when a reaction occurs. Proper treatment of a severe reaction follows the "ABCD system":

A Airway open
B Breathing restored
C Circulation maintained
D Drug and definitive therapy

Once the initial CPR has begun, a code/crash team should be summoned. The principles and practice of CPR are a subject with which the reader should be familiar and will not be covered further in this book. The reader should never inject contrast agents unless familiar with CPR and the management of reactions.

Recently a vagal type of reaction has been recognized as a distinct complication of the use of contrast material. This reaction may be recognized by noting hypotension and bradycardia rather than tachycardia, as found in the anaphylactoid reactions.

Treatment of patients with vagal reactions is by the use of 0.5 to 1.0 mg of atropine intravenously.

Adjunctive procedures to be performed before the patient has a reaction and that may aid in the later treatment of a reaction include recording the patient's pulse and blood pressure and noting the cardiac rhythm. In addition, the use of a scalp vein–type needle-tubing combination that is taped in place to the forearm will ensure a ready channel of access to the patient's bloodstream in the event of an emergency.

Fig. 3-1 is a flow chart of steps to follow in managing a patient who has had a reaction to contrast material.

SUMMARY

The basic types of radiographic contrast materials have been discussed with their indications and uses. Of prime importance is the recognition that these agents, when injected intra-arterially or intravenously, may cause severe life-threatening reactions. The types of reactions, their recognition, and their treatment were briefly discussed. The reader is advised to be thoroughly familiar with the technique of CPR.

References

Andrews, E. J.: The vagus reaction as a possible cause of severe complications of radiological procedures, Radiology 121:1, 1976.

Ansell, G.: Adverse reactions to contrast agents. Scope of problem, Invest. Radiol. 5:374, 1970.

Berg, G. R., Hutter, A. M., Jr., and Pfister, R. C.: Electrocardiographic abnormalities associated with intravenous urography, N. Engl. J. Med. 289:87, 1973.

Committee on Drugs: Prevention and management of adverse reactions to intravascular contrast media, Chicago, 1977, American College of Radiology.

Daffner, R. H.: Experimental barium and fecal peritonitis: a reevaluation, J. Ky. Med. Assoc. 74:229, 1976.

Davidson, A. J.: Radiologic diagnosis of renal parenchymal disease, Philadelphia, 1977, W. B. Saunders Co.

Fischer, H. W., and Doust, V. B.: An evaluation of pre-testing in the problem of serious and fatal reactions to excretory urography, Radiology 103:497, 1972.

Higgins, C. B.: Effects of contrast media on the conducting system of the heart, Radiology 124:599, 1977.

Lasser, E. C., Lang, J., Sovak, M., Kolb, W., Lyon, S., and Hamlin, A. E.: Steroids: theoretical and experimental basis for utilization in prevention of contrast media reactions, Radiology 125:1, 1977.

Lindgren, P.: Hemodynamic responses to contrast media, Invest. Radiol. 5:424, 1970.

Miller, R. E., and Skukas, J.: Radiographic contrast agents, Baltimore, 1977, University Park Press.

Physicians desk reference for radiology and nuclear medicine, Oradell, N.J., 1978, Medical Economics Co.

Shehadi, W. H.: Adverse reactions to intravascularly administered contrast media. A comprehensive study based on a prospective survey, Am. J. Roentgenol. 124:145, 1975.

Stadalnik, R. C., Vera, Z., DaSilva, O., Davies, R., Kraus, J. F., and Mason, D. T.: Electrocardiographic response to intravenous urography: prospective evaluation of 275 patients, Am. J. Roentgenol. 129:825, 1977.

Standards for cardiopulmonary resuscitation (CPR) and emergency cardiac care (ECC), J.A.M.A. 227:833, 1974.

Stanley, R. J., and Pfister, R. C.: Bradycardia and hypotension following use of intravenous contrast media, Radiology 121:5, 1976.

Witten, D. M.: Reactions to urographic contrast media, J.A.M.A. 231:974, 1975.

Witten, D. M., Hirsch, F. D., and Hartman, G. W.: Acute reactions to urographic contrast medium. Incidence, clinical characteristics and relationship to history of hypersensitivity states, Am. J. Roentgenol. 119:832, 1973.

PART TWO Introduction to diagnostic radiology: clinical application

4 Pulmonary radiology

The chest radiograph is the examination you will be requesting and observing with the greatest frequency. In addition, it is the examination that you will most likely be reviewing alone. Chest radiographs account for more than half of all the examinations performed in any radiology practice. One of the reasons for this is that the chest is the "mirror of health or disease." Besides giving information about the patient's heart and lungs, the chest film provides valuable information about adjacent structures such as the GI tract, the thyroid gland, or the bony structures around the thorax. Furthermore, metastatic disease from the abdominal viscera frequently manifests itself in the lungs.

TECHNICAL CONSIDERATIONS

Once you have assured yourself that the radiograph presented is that of the correct patient, the film should be analyzed for density, motion, and rotation. A determination should be made whether the entire thorax is displayed. Be sure that the technologist has not cut the costophrenic angles off the film. On a properly exposed radiograph the thoracic spine should be barely discernible through the shadow of the heart. The clavicular shadows should be equidistant from the patient's midline, indicating no rotation.

The next step is to decide what type of examination has been performed. The ordinary chest radiograph is made with the patient in the erect position with the anterior portion of the chest against the film cassette. The x-ray tube is positioned 6 feet behind the patient, and the horizontal beam enters from the back (posterior) and exits through the front (anterior): the PA radiograph. If the patient turns completely around and the beam enters from the front, the film is termed an AP film. Fig. 4-1, *A*, is a PA erect film of a young patient; Fig. 4-1, *B*, is an AP erect film of the same patient. Note the differences.

In general the following are features commonly seen on PA chest radiographs: identification markings, if present, are oriented so that the observer may read them without reversing the film; the clavicles are superimposed over the upper lungs and are slanted with the medial aspect lower than the lateral; and the posterior portions of the cervical and thoracic vertebrae (neural arch, articular processes, apophyseal joints, and laminae) are more clearly visible. The following findings suggest an AP

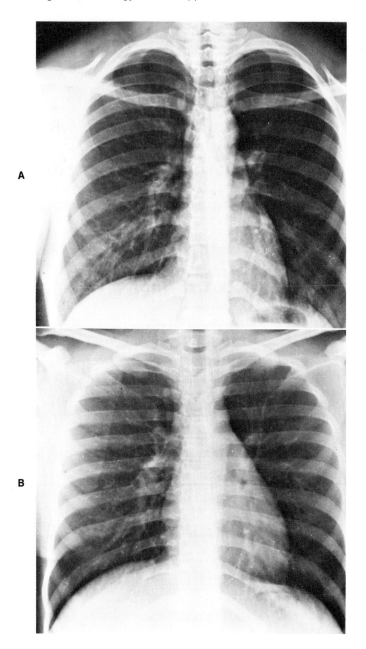

Fig. 4-1. Normal chest. **A,** PA view. **B,** AP view. Note differences described in text.

film: identification marks and writing are reversed; the heart appears slightly large; the clavicles are usually higher; and there is demonstration of the bodies and Luschka joints of the lower cervical vertebrae.

One of the most important technical considerations in evaluating the chest radiograph is the determination of whether or not the film is in optimal inspiration. Fig. 4-2 is a film of a healthy man that was deliberately made in forced expiration. Failure

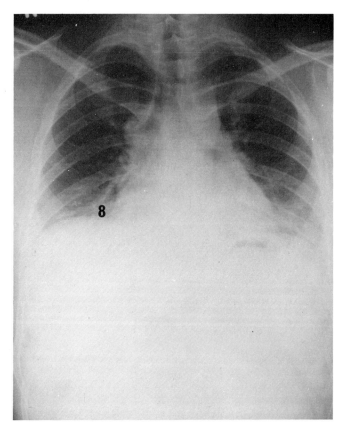

Fig. 4-2. Expiratory chest film. Film was made deliberately in poor inspiration to demonstrate effects of poor inspiratory result. Cardiac silhouette appears enlarged, and this patient could easily be diagnosed as being in congestive heart failure. Diaphragm is at level of eighth rib posteriorly. Compare with Fig. 4-3. (From Daffner, R. H., Gehweiler, J. A., and Carden, T. S., Jr.: Case studies in radiology, New York, 1975, Appleton-Century-Crofts. Reproduced with permission of the publisher.)

to note the fact that the film was a poor inspiratory *result* could easily lead to a mistaken diagnosis of congestive heart failure. After all, the heart appears large and rather poorly defined, the pulmonary vessels appear slightly prominent, and there is apparent blunting of both lung bases, suggesting fluid. Fig. 4-3 is a maximal inspiratory film of the same individual; it is perfectly normal.

There are many reasons why a film may not be obtained in full inspiratory expansion. Massive obesity is a mechanical cause; pain in a patient postoperatively results in voluntary restriction; the cardiac patient with congestive heart failure is unable to displace the edema fluid in the "waterlogged" lungs; and the patient with chronic restrictive lung disease cannot expand to expected maximum because of scarring and loss of compliance in the lung tissues. For all these reasons the term *"poor inspiratory result"* is used rather than *"poor inspiratory effort."* In most instances, these patients will have made a good inspiratory *effort,* but the *result* is poor.

A film is considered to be in optimal inspiratory result when we are able to see the diaphragm crossing the tenth rib or interspace posteriorly or the eighth rib an-

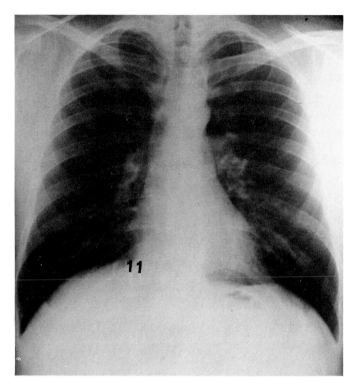

Fig. 4-3. Full inspiratory PA chest radiograph. This is same individual as in Fig. 4-2. Note difference between two radiographs. Diaphragm is at level of eleventh rib posteriorly. (From Daffner, R. H., Gehweiler, J. A., and Carden, T. S., Jr.: Case studies in radiology, New York, 1975, Appleton-Century-Crofts. Reproduced with permission of the publisher.)

teriorly. The reader is cautioned not to fall into the pitfall of diagnosing nondisease in a patient with a poor inspiratory film.

Interestingly enough there are certain circumstances in which it is desirable to have a film deliberately made in expiration. These include evaluation of the patient with a suspected foreign body of a bronchus, a "ball valve" type of bronchial obstruction, or a suspected pneumothorax. In the first instance (Fig. 4-4) the PA inspiratory film is normal; the expiratory film demonstrates no change in the volume of the lung on the obstructed side. The normal lung decreases in volume, and the mediastinum swings *toward* the normal side. In the second instance the pneumothorax is enhanced by the decrease in lung volume (Fig. 4-5).

Rotation of the patient or angulation may result in distortion of normal anatomic shadows. As mentioned previously, you should be able to detect rotation by observing the position of the medial ends of the clavicles.

Occasionally a debilitated patient who is examined by portable technique will sag down against the pillow, with the result that a lordotic view of the chest is obtained. This is easy enough to detect because the heart assumes an egg-shaped configuration, the ribs appear tapered, and the clavicles are seen above the ribs.

Lordotic views have been advocated as a means of examining lesions in the lung apices. The examination is made by having the patient lean backward toward the

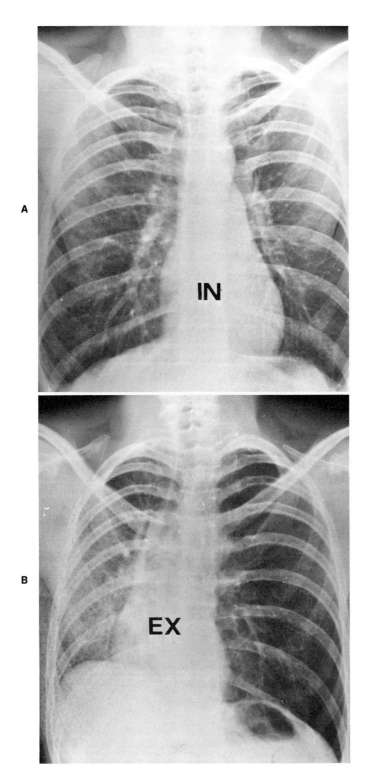

Fig. 4-4. Value of inspiratory and expiratory films in patient with endobronchial obstructing lesion on left. **A,** The inspiratory *(IN)* film appears normal. **B,** On expiration *(EX)* there is appropriate volume loss and mediastinal shift to normal right side. There is no change in volume on obstructed left side. (From Daffner, R. H., Gehweiler, J. A., and Carden, T. S., Jr.: Case studies in radiology, New York, 1975, Appleton-Century-Crofts. Reproduced with permission of the publisher.)

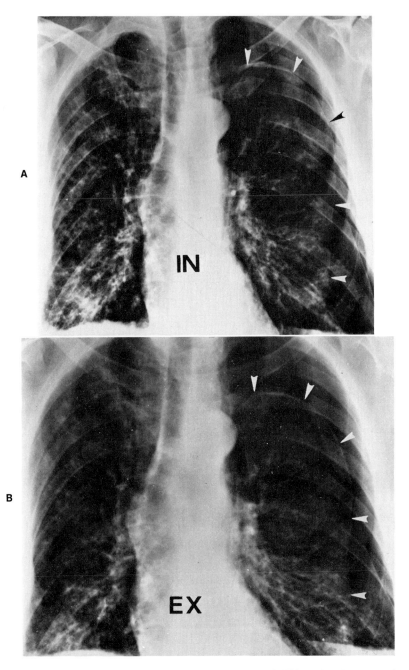

Fig. 4-5. Value of expiratory film in patient with pneumothorax. **A,** This patient has extensive chronic lung disease. Pneumothorax is present on left (arrowheads). *IN,* Inspiratory film. **B,** Expiratory *(EX)* film enhances effect of the pneumothorax (arrowheads).

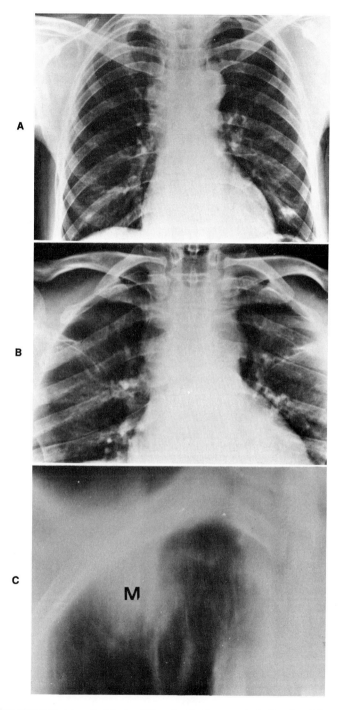

Fig. 4-6. Value of tomography. **A,** PA chest film of patient suspected of having right upper lobe tumor. There is faint increase in density in right upper lobe, particularly under first rib. **B,** Lordotic film, which clears clavicle and first rib off of lung apices, is normal. **C,** Tomogram of right upper lobe shows large mass *(M)*. Diagnosis: bronchogenic carcinoma.

film while a horizontal beam is used to make the exposure. We do not use this view frequently because anterior lesions are often not demonstrated by this technique. In these cases a kyphotic (reversed lordotic) view is used. Fig. 4-6, *A*, shows the PA chest film of a patient suspected to have a right upper lobe lesion. A lordotic film (Fig. 4-6, *B*) was normal. Tomograms demonstrated a 3 cm carcinoma far anterior in the right upper lobe (Fig. 4-6, *C*). An alternative to a lordotic view, a coned-down view of the apex of the lung, was unremarkable in this particular patient.

A final technical consideration regards the analysis of films made by portable technique. Studies of this kind are performed on severely debilitated or gravely ill patients who are unable to come to the x-ray department. In reviewing these films, it is important to recognize the circumstances under which they were made. There may be slight motion on the film (the patient cannot hold the breath), the patient may be rotated, or the patient may be in a slight lordotic position. Some portable films are made with the patient supine. This can result in a redistribution of blood to the upper lobes of the lung. Since this is an early sign of congestive heart failure, the reader again is cautioned to make note of whether this film was performed with the patient in the upright position or in the supine position. The presence or absence of an air-fluid level in the gastric air bubble may aid in determining upright versus supine positioning.

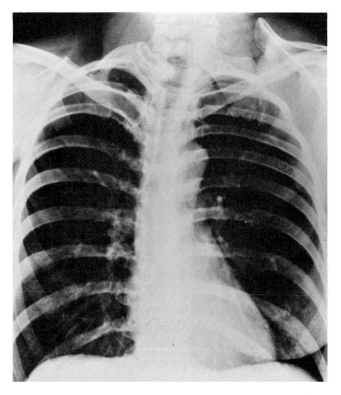

Fig. 4-7. Routine chest film in patient who has had right radical mastectomy and who also has anomaly of left shoulder. Analysis should be in logical order, as denoted in text. Note absence of right breast shadow. Note also bony anomaly in left shoulder and lower left neck region.

ANATOMIC CONSIDERATIONS

A logical approach to the interpretation of chest radiographs is predicated on the observer developing an orderly system for scanning films. It matters not whether this review begins from the outside and proceeds inward or vice versa. What is important is that the method be reproduced each and every time that particular type of study is reviewed. Working from the inside outward, observe the following:

1. Trachea and mediastinum
2. Heart and great vessels
3. Lungs
4. Costophrenic angles
5. Diaphragm
6. Bones and soft tissues

The order of visual scan is illustrated in Fig. 4-7, showing a patient who has had a right radical mastectomy and has a congenital anomaly of the left shoulder. Analysis of this film is as follows: "The heart and mediastinal structures are normal. The pulmonary vessels and aorta are normal. The lungs are clear. The costophrenic angles are clear. The diaphragm is regular. The patient has had a right radical mastectomy as indicated by the absence of the right breast shadow and increased lucency (radiability) from the missing pectoralis muscle. A bony anomaly is present in the left shoulder: elevation of the scapula, the presence of an omovertebral bone, and a cleft vertebra at C6. This particular type of anomaly is called Sprengel deformity."

The lateral chest film should receive the same attention as the PA film and is analyzed in a similar fashion. Consider the lateral chest film in a patient with known esophageal carcinoma (Fig. 4-8): ". . . on the lateral chest film the trachea is deviated anteriorly by a soft tissue mass that contains an air-fluid level (arrow). This is most consistent with the diagnosis of an obstructing esophageal carcinoma. The cardiac silhouette is normal. The lungs are clear. The costophrenic angles and posterior recesses are clear. The diaphragm is normal. There are no significant abnormalities in the spine."

An anatomic review of the structures seen in the chest under normal circumstances now will be covered in the same order as the film analysis.

The trachea is a midline structure whose air shadow stands out in bold contrast to the surrounding soft tissues of the neck and mediastinum. On a well-penetrated film the carina (bifurcation of the trachea) may be seen at the level of the T4-5 interspace on the frontal film. On the lateral film the tracheal air column may be seen slowly angling down from the upper portion of the chest. The soft tissue line seen on its posterior wall should not be bowed and should not exceed 3 mm in thickness (arrow, Fig. 4-9).

The mediastinum, the extrapleural space between the lungs, is the midregion of the thorax. Contained within it are the heart, pericardium, great vessels, trachea, thoracic duct, and numerous smaller blood vessels, nerves, and lymphatic vessels. Traditionally the mediastinum has been divided into four components—two superior and two inferior—of which there are three subdivisions—anterior, middle, and posterior. We may make this division by drawing a horizontal line from the sternal angle (of Louis) back to the T4-5 intervertebral disc (Fig. 4-10). In the living patient, this line cuts through the midportion of the aortic arch. Any structures above this line lie

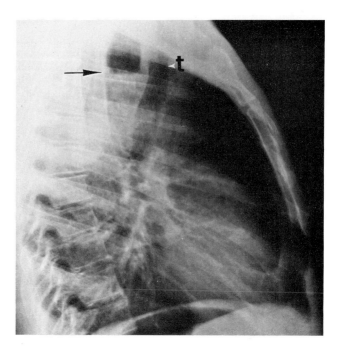

Fig. 4-8. Lateral chest film in patient with obstructive carcinoma of middle third of esophagus. There is anterior bowing of tracheal air shadow *(t)* by retrotracheal mass that contains air-fluid level (arrow). Remainder of analysis should be as stated in text.

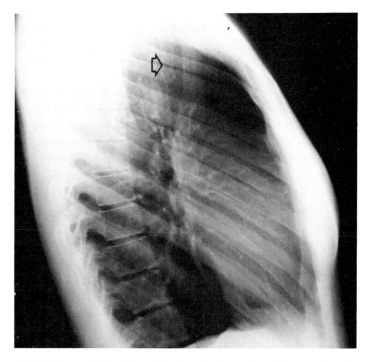

Fig. 4-9. Normal lateral chest. Retrotracheal area (arrow) is not widened.

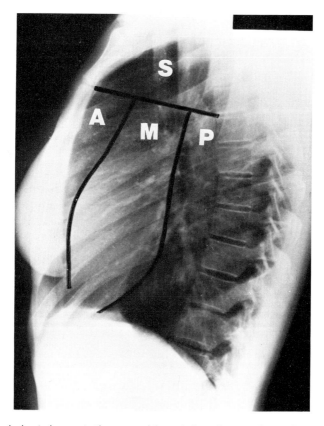

Fig. 4-10. Lateral chest demonstrating normal boundaries of anatomic mediastinum. *S,* Superior mediastinum; *A,* anterior mediastinum; *M,* middle mediastinum; *P,* posterior mediastinum. Text describes delineation of these boundaries.

in the superior mediastinum, and any below are in the inferior mediastinum. The anatomic anterior mediastinum is bounded by the sternum anteriorly and by the pericardium posteriorly. The middle mediastinum is located between the anterior and posterior pericardium. The posterior mediastinum is bounded anteriorly by the posterior pericardium and posteriorly by the spine. All three subdivisions of the anatomic inferior mediastinum are bounded inferiorly by the diaphragm.

Although this division may prove satisfactory for the anatomist, radiologists and surgeons prefer to use the *"roentgen mediastinum,"* a concept proposed by Felson that is far more useful in clinical practice than the anatomic mediastinum, especially when dealing with neoplasms. Tumors of the mediastinum tend to spread in a craniocaudal manner rather than anteroposteriorly.

To delineate the three parts of the roentgen mediastinum, the following lines may be imagined on a lateral radiograph (Fig. 4-11). Line A-A' begins at the diaphragm just behind the shadow of the inferior vena cava and extends upward along the back of the heart and in front of the trachea to the neck. The second line, B-B', runs across the body of each thoracic vertebra 1 cm from its anterior margin and extends upward. The area anterior to line A-A' is the anterior mediastinum; the area between lines A-A' and B-B' is the middle mediastinum, and the area posterior to line B-B' is

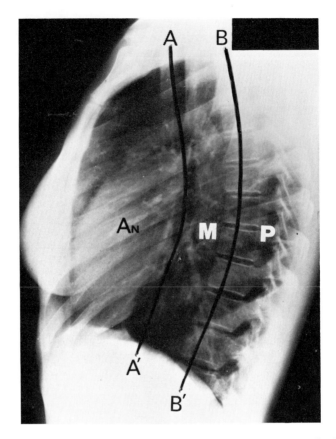

Fig. 4-11. Normal lateral chest delineating roentgen mediastinum. *An,* Anterior mediastinum; *M,* middle mediastinum; *P,* posterior mediastinum. Construction of lines *A-A'* and *B-B'* is described in text.

the posterior mediastinum. Pathologic aspects of these compartments will be discussed in the following section.

The anatomy of the heart and great vessels will be described in the next chapter. It is sufficient to say at this point, however, that all lung markings seen on the normal chest radiograph are made by pulmonary arteries and veins and not by bronchi. After all, the blood-filled vessels are of water density; air-filled bronchi, which normally have thin walls, provide no significant contrast to the aerated lungs.

There are three lobes in the right lung and two in the left. Each lobe is divided into anatomic segments supplied by its own bronchus and blood vessels. In the right upper lobe are the apical, anterior, and posterior segments; the middle lobe has medial and lateral segments. The right lower lobe contains a superior segment and, in clockwise fashion, posterior, medial, anterior, and lateral basal segments.

The left upper lobe consists of a fused apical-posterior segment, an anterior segment, and superior and inferior lingular segments. The left lower lobe is similar to the right lower lobe except that the anterior and medial basal segments are fused. A knowledge of the location of these segments is important in localizing disease. The reader is advised of the fact that there is a significant portion of lung contained in the costophrenic recess posteriorly. This recess extends as far down as the level of L2.

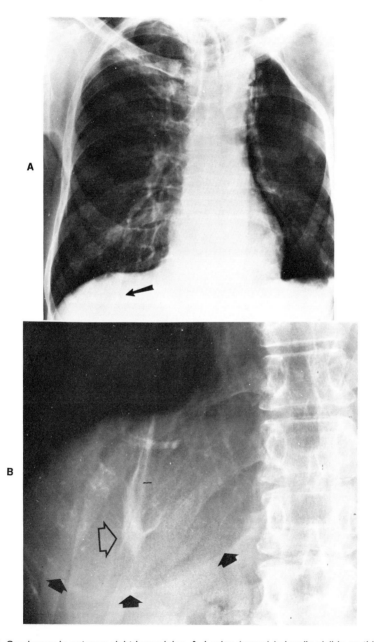

Fig. 4-12. Carcinoma in extreme right lower lobe. **A,** Lesion (arrow) is hardly visible on this PA chest radiograph. Patient has also had previous left-sided thoracotomy. **B,** Detailed view of abdominal film shows stellate lesion in extreme right lower lobe (open arrow). Extent of emphysematous right lower lobe is outlined by solid arrows.

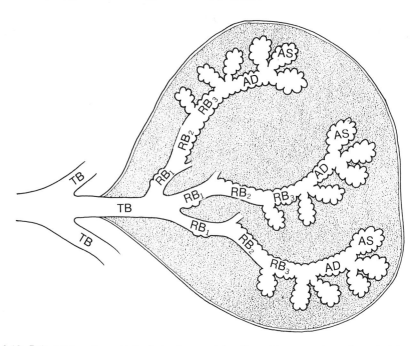

Fig. 4-13. Pulmonary acinus. Unit of structure and function of lung consists of terminal bronchiole *(TB)* and series of progressively smaller respiratory bronchioles *(RB)*, leading finally to alveolar duct *(AD)* and ending in alveolar sacs *(AS)*. Grouping of three to five acini together forms pulmonary lobule.

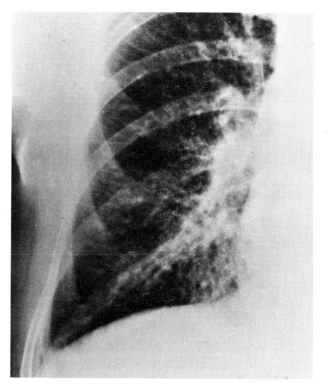

Fig. 4-14. Kerley lines. Fine linear striations extending obliquely and horizontally are septal lines. Ordinarily, these lines are not seen until they become thickened or edematous.

Occasionally, tumors occur within the lung in this location. These lesions often will not be seen on chest radiographs but may be detected on an abdominal radiograph (Fig. 4-12).

The basic anatomic and functional pulmonary unit is the *acinus*, the portion of lung distal to the terminal bronchiole where gas exchange takes place. It contains respiratory bronchioles, alveolar ducts, alveolar sacs, and alveoli. Anatomically and radiographically a consistently recognizable structure results from the grouping of three to five acini together to form the pulmonary lobule. The usual lobule is approximately 1 cm in diameter in the adult. Each of these lobules is surrounded by its own interlobular septa and interstitial structures (Fig. 4-13). Diseases that affect the air spaces are referred to as having an "acinar or alveolar type pattern"; diseases that affect the interstitial tissues are referred to as having an "interstitial pattern."

The interlobular septa are not seen under normal circumstances. However, when they become edematous or thickened by other pathologic processes, they become visible as faint linear lines known as septal (Kerley) lines (Fig. 4-14).

There are microscopic communications between the distal portions of the bronchiolar tree and surrounding alveoli known as the canals of Lambert. They provide an accessory route for air passage from the bronchioles to the alveoli. Another connection, the pores of Kohn, are small openings in the alveolar wall 10 to 15 μ in diameter. These permit the lung distal to an obstructed bronchus or bronchiole to be ventilated by a process known as collateral air drift.

The pleura consists of two layers: the visceral pleura and the parietal pleura. The visceral pleura encases the lungs. Under normal circumstances the pleura is not visualized with the exception of the normal interlobar fissures. On the right there are two fissures, the oblique (major) and the horizontal (minor). The left lung contains an oblique fissure only. The oblique fissure begins at the level of the fourth thoracic vertebra, extending obliquely downward and forward and ending approximately at the level of the sixth rib anteriorly. The horizontal fissure begins roughly at the level of the sixth rib laterally and extends anteriorly and slightly downward to end near the medial portion of the fourth rib. Occasionally an accessory fissure may be seen bordering a segment of lung that has become partially or completely separated from its adjacent segments. The best known of these is the azygos fissure, which is created by the downward migration of the azygos vein through the apical pleura of the right upper lobe. In doing so the vein invaginates a portion of pleura and results in a comma-shaped structure seen in the vicinity of the right upper lobe (Fig. 4-15). It is a normal variant.

The pleura is frequently involved in inflammatory and traumatic insults to the chest. These may result in areas of thickening along the pleural surface or in the costophrenic or cardiophrenic angles. They may distort these anatomic boundaries.

The diaphragm, which separates the thoracic from the abdominal cavities, is most often seen as a smooth dome-shaped structure on either side. There may be scalloping or irregularities along the diaphragmatic surface, a frequent finding considered to be of little significance. The right hemidiaphragm is slightly higher than the left. Occasionally, gaseous distention of the stomach or colon produces elevation of the left hemidiaphragm above the right. The reason for the lower left hemidiaphragm is the contiguity of the left ventricle with it and not the mass of the liver elevating the right hemidiaphragm.

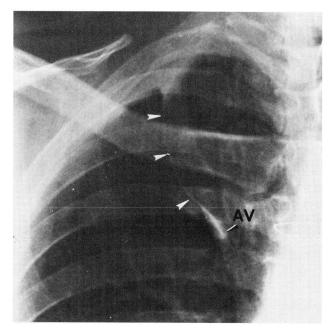

Fig. 4-15. Azygos fissure (arrowheads). Azygos vein *(AV)* is small density at base of linear fissure.

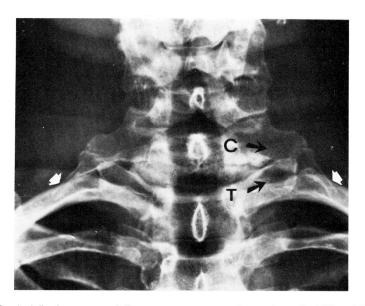

Fig. 4-16. Cervical ribs (open arrows). Transverse processes of seventh cervical *(C)* and first thoracic *(T)* vertebrae are identified (arrows). Occasionally, these anomalous ribs may impinge on neurovascular structures in subclavian region.

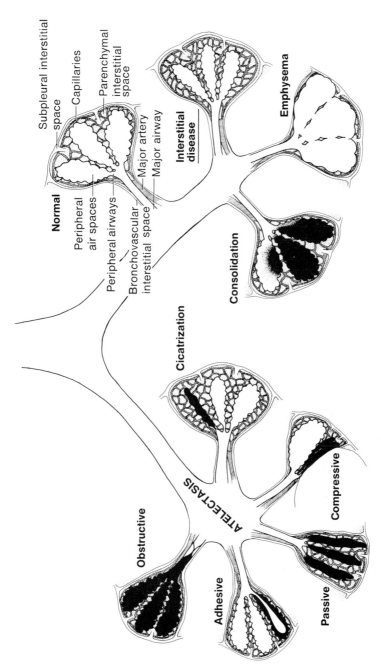

Fig. 4-17. Graphic representation of pathologic alterations that may be seen in the lung.

Soft tissue shadows commonly seen on the routine chest radiograph are the anterior axillary fold produced by the bulk of the pectoral muscles, companion shadows along the upper surfaces of the clavicles, shadows of the sternomastoid muscles in the neck, and breast shadows. In addition, nipple shadows are frequently seen over the lower chest radiographs in men.

Bony structures seen on the chest radiograph include the ribs, thoracic spine, lower cervical vertebrae, clavicles, scapulae, and occasionally the heads of the humeri. In addition, the sternum is clearly visible on the lateral chest film. Occasionally the manubrium projects as a prominence just to the right of the midline. It should not be mistaken for a pulmonary mass. Occasionally, cervical ribs are encountered. An abnormal-appearing rib in the cervicothoracic region can be considered a cervical rib if the transverse process to which it is articulating points inferiorly. Cervical transverse processes point down; thoracic transverse processes point up (Fig. 4-16).

PATHOLOGIC CONSIDERATIONS

This section will discuss six pathologic patterns that may alter the normal appearance of the lung. The reader should be aware that any or all of these may be seen at one time in the same patient. Furthermore, any of these entities may be combined with abnormalities of the heart and pulmonary vessels. The six abnormalities are as follows:

1. Air space disease—consolidation
2. Atelectasis
3. Pleural fluid
4. Masses
5. Emphysema
6. Interstitial changes

Fig. 4-17 illustrates several of these changes.

Air space disease—consolidation

When the air spaces become filled with fluid (inflammatory exudate, blood, or edema), they lose their normal lucency and become opaque. In pneumonia the inflammatory infiltrate usually follows normal anatomic planes and has a segmental distribution. By knowing the location of the lung segments and their relationship to the mediastinum and diaphragm, it is possible to accurately localize an area of consolidation by noting the loss of these normal anatomic landmarks.

The basis for visualization of the border of a structure depends on its contiguity with another structure of different radiographic density. Hence we see the silhouette of the mediastinal structures and the diaphragm because they are of water density and are outlined by the adjacent air density in the lung. Consolidations adjacent to these borders result in the loss of the normal-appearing shadows or silhouettes. This concept was first described by Fleischner and popularized by Felson as the *"silhouette sign."*

Fleischner's famous experiment demonstrating the silhouette sign is illustrated as follows (Fig. 4-18): An empty film box was tilted on end; liquid paraffin was poured into it and allowed to congeal into a triangular density. A second empty film box was taped behind the first box, and both were radiographed (Fig. 4-18, A). The gray shadow of the solid paraffin represents a "cardiac border," and the blackness of the air within both boxes represents "aerated lung," creating a model for demonstration

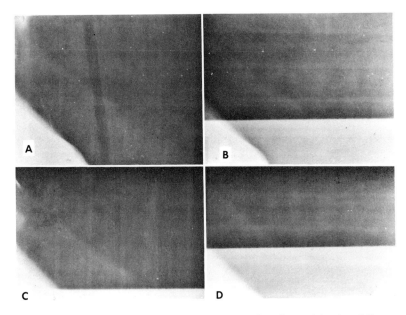

Fig. 4-18. Experiment to demonstrate silhouette sign. See text for description.

of the effects of consolidation on the silhouette. The boxes were again radiographed in the upright position after mineral oil (of approximately the same radiographic density as solid paraffin) was poured into the empty box behind the one containing the paraffin (Fig. 4-18, *B*). Note the air-fluid level at the border between the mineral oil and the air in the second box. More importantly, the shadow of the "heart" is still clearly visible because of the air adjacent to its border. Thus an area of consolidation behind the cardiac silhouette does not cause obliteration of its border.

The mineral oil was then poured out of the back box and into the box containing the paraffin. A radiograph of this (Fig. 4-18, *C*) shows obliteration of a portion of the border of the "heart" shadow because of the contiguity of the two structures of similar radiographic density. This is analogous to pneumonia in a middle lobe or in the lingula obliterating the cardiac border (Fig. 4-19).

Finally, mineral oil was poured into the second box, with the resultant radiograph shown in Fig. 4-18, *D*. Note the obliteration of the lower "cardiac" border by the "consolidated" area adjacent to it. However, the upper "cardiac" border is clearly visible along with an air-fluid level behind it because this upper border is still surrounded by air.

In summary, an intrathoracic lesion that is contiguous with the border of the heart, aorta, or diaphragm will result in the loss of that border on the radiograph. This border will not be obliterated unless the lesion is anatomically contiguous with it. These principles apply not only to the PA chest radiograph but also to the lateral view and, in addition, to certain abdominal diseases such as loss of the psoas margin in a retroperitoneal inflammatory process or hemorrhage.

The following lesions are illustrated: right middle lobe consolidation (Fig. 4-19), right upper lobe consolidation (Fig. 4-20), lingular consolidation (Fig. 4-21), and left lower lobe consolidation (Fig. 4-22).

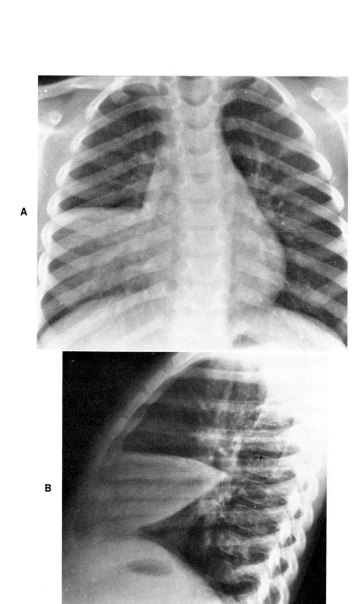

Fig. 4-19. Right middle lobe consolidation. **A,** PA film shows loss of right cardiac border (silhouette sign). **B,** Lateral view confirms anterior location of infiltrate adjacent to heart.

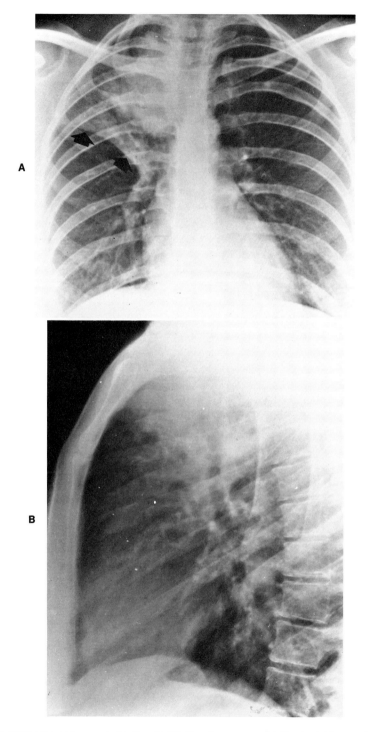

Fig. 4-20. Right upper lobe consolidation. **A,** PA film shows consolidation in right upper lobe obliterating mediastinal structures on right. Extent of lesion is delineated by minor fissure inferiorly that is slightly elevated because of atelectasis (arrows). **B,** Lateral film shows anterior location of infiltration.

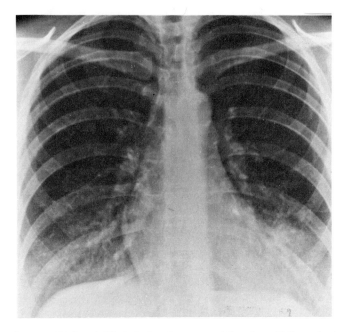

Fig. 4-21. Lingular consolidation. Infiltrate in lingula causes obliteration of left cardiac border. Location is anterior, similar to that seen in right middle lobe. Note preservation of left diaphragmatic shadow (posteriorly located).

On the lateral film, we can identify each hemidiaphragm because of a normal-appearing silhouette sign. The anterior portion of the cardiac border lies in contiguity with the left hemidiaphragm. Therefore the anterior one third of the left diaphragmatic shadow will be obliterated by the cardiac border. This is the most reliable way to identify the hemidiaphragms (Fig. 4-23). A summary of localization using the silhouette sign is in Table 3. Although the localizing signs are extremely useful, the reader is cautioned that they are not always infallible. For example, an area of consolidation in the lateral segment of the right middle lobe will not always obliterate the right cardiac border. It is therefore important to use two views at all times when evaluating patients with lung disease.

The *cervicothoracic sign*, a variant of the silhouette sign, is useful in determining whether a mass lesion that is seen above the level of the clavicles is wholly intrathoracic or mediastinal. If this lesion is seen in its entirety, it must lie *posteriorly* because it is surrounded by air and therefore must be entirely within the thorax. If it is located anteriorly, its border will be obliterated by the shadows of the neck. Therefore it is cervicothoracic, lying partially in the anterior part of the mediastinum and partially in the neck. Fig. 4-24 illustrates this in a patient with a prominent brachiocephalic artery.

Another useful sign to indicate consolidation within the lung is the *air bronchogram*. As previously mentioned, normal bronchi are not visible on the chest radiograph. This is because of their thin walls, the fact that they contain air, and the fact that they are surrounded by air within the lung parenchyma. However, parenchymal consolidation that results in a water density in the alveolar spaces in the lung may

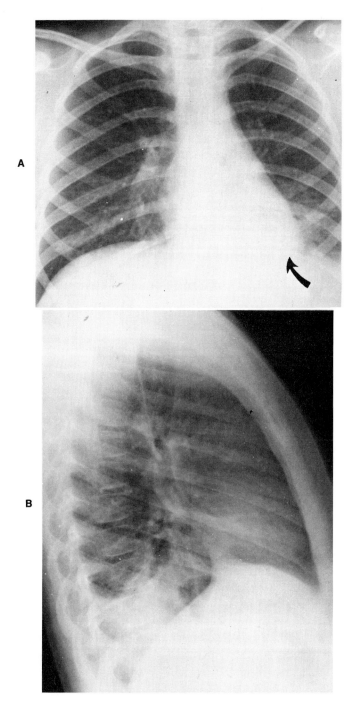

Fig. 4-22. Left lower lobe consolidation. **A,** PA view of chest shows obliteration of diaphragmatic shadow on left (arrow). **B,** Lateral view shows consolidation posteriorly.

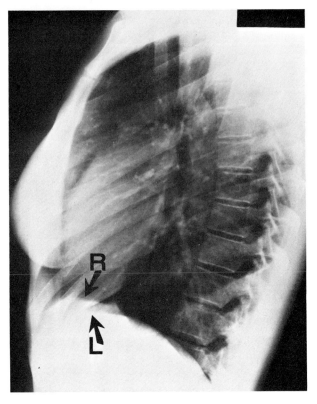

Fig. 4-23. Normal lateral chest. Right hemidiaphragmatic shadow *(R)* is clearly visible. Left hemi-diaphragmatic shadow *(L)* disappears anteriorly because of contiguity of adjacent heart shadow (silhouette sign).

cause the demonstration of adjacent bronchi, since the air within their lumens will stand out in stark contrast to the dense lung (Fig. 4-25). The formation of the air bronchogram sign is illustrated in Fig. 4-26. Plastic tubing sealed at each end was placed in an empty plastic container and radiographed (Fig. 4-26, *A*). The walls are barely discernible, since the tubing contains air and there is air surrounding it. Water was then added to the container to cover the tubing (Fig. 4-26, *B*). The wall is barely visible. However, the air within the tubing defines its lumen (air bronchogram). Water was then poured into the tubing with the resultant radiographic appearance shown in Fig. 4-26, *C*. In this illustration there is no difference between the contrast medium inside the tube and the outside (no air bronchogram).

The air bronchogram is a valuable sign that, when present, is virtually diagnostic of acinar disease. A pleural or mediastinal lesion may be excluded because there are no bronchi traversing these lesions. Similarly, a mass lesion of the lung would engulf, occlude, or displace bronchi, and therefore the air bronchogram would not be seen within these lesions. If an air bronchogram is seen within a round pulmonary density, the lesion is most likely an inflammatory process, an infarct, a contusion, or, more rarely, an alveolar cell carcinoma or lymphoma. All these are acinar lesions. Rare exceptions to this rule are bronchiectasis and chronic bronchitis, in which thickening of the bronchial walls may result in tubular air profiles (Fig. 4-27).

Table 3. Localization using the silhouette sign

Structure	Obliteration/ overlap by shadow	General	Anatomic location
Heart	Obliteration	Anterior	Middle lobe Lingula Anterior mediastinum Anterior segment of an upper lobe Lower end of oblique fissure Anterior portion of pleural cavity
	Overlap	Posterior	Lower lobe Posterior mediastinum Posterior portion of pleural cavity
Ascending aorta (right border)	Obliteration	Anterior	Anterior segment right upper lobe Right middle lobe Right anterior mediastinum Anterior portion, right pleural cavity
	Overlap	Posterior	Superior segment right lower lobe Posterior segment right upper lobe Posterior mediastinum Posterior pleural cavity
Aortic knob (left border)	Obliteration	Posterior	Apical-posterior segment left upper lobe Posterior mediastinum Posterior pleural cavity
	Overlap	Anterior	Anterior segment left upper lobe Far posterior portion mediastinum or pleural cavity
Descending aorta	Obliteration	Posterior	Superior and posterior basal segments of left lower lobe

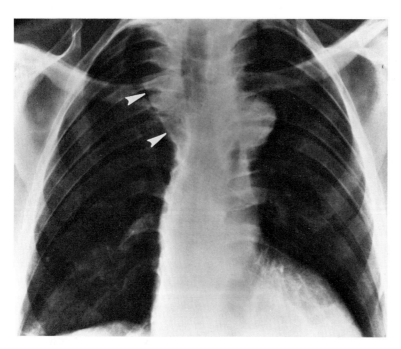

Fig. 4-24. Cervicothoracic sign. Shadow of tortuous brachiocephalic artery (arrowheads) disappears as vessel enters neck at level of clavicle.

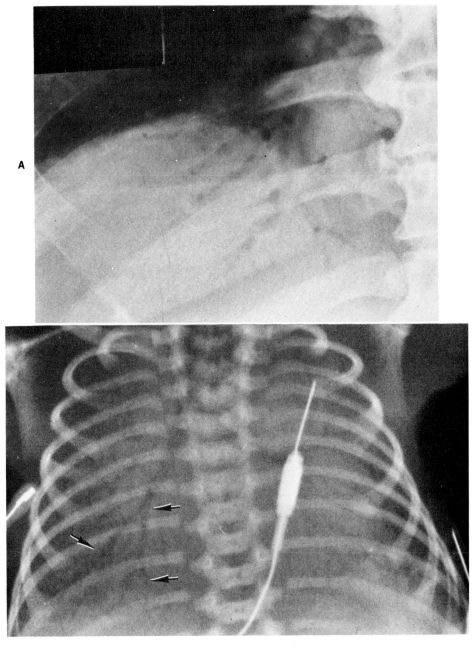

Fig. 4-25. Air bronchograms. **A,** Detail film of patient with right lower lobe pneumonia. Air bronchogram is represented by dark tubular shadows. Note branching pattern. **B,** Patient with hyaline membrane disease. Note air bronchogram in right lower lobe. Once again, the branching black shadows of air-filled bronchi are plainly visible (arrows).

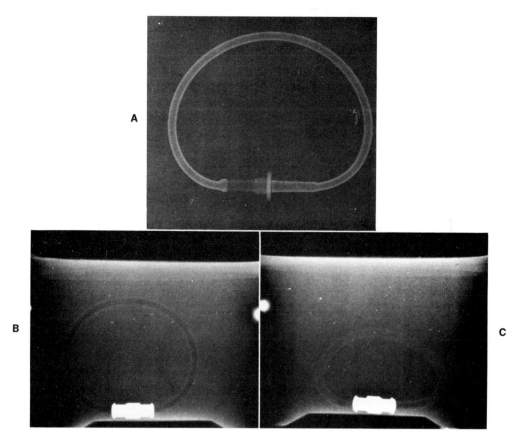

Fig. 4-26. Air bronchogram demonstration. **A,** Radiograph of plastic tube in air. Wall and lumen are clearly visible. **B,** Following immersion of tube in water, outer wall is not as well seen. However, lumen persists as dark ring. **C,** Tube was filled with water and reimmersed in container of water. There is no differentiation between lumen and surrounding water. Wall of tube is faintly visible.

Atelectasis

Atelectasis is a condition of volume loss of some portion of the lung. It may be massive with complete collapse of an entire lung or, more commonly, less extensive and involving a lobe, segment, or subsegment. Atelectasis results from a number of causes, which are illustrated in Fig. 4-17.

Obstructive atelectasis, the most common type, results when a bronchus is obstructed by a carcinoma, foreign body, mucous plug, or inflammatory debris (Fig. 4-28). Quite often there is associated pneumonia distal to the site of obstruction.

Compressive atelectasis is a purely physical phenomenon in which lung is compressed by a tumor, emphysematous bulla, pleural effusion, or enlarged heart (Fig. 4-29).

Cicatrization atelectasis is produced by organizing scar tissue (Fig. 4-30). This occurs most often in healing tuberculosis and other granulomatous diseases as well as in entities such as pulmonary infarct and pulmonary trauma.

Adhesive atelectasis is a unique type of volume loss that occurs in the presence of

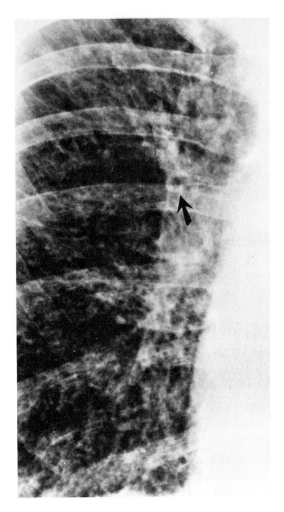

Fig. 4-27. Bronchial thickening in patient with bronchiectasis. Thickened bronchial walls are visible as ringlike shadows. Thickening of large bronchus is also apparent (arrow).

patent airways. The mechanism involved is believed to be the inactivation of surfactant. A common example of this is hyaline membrane disease.

Passive atelectasis results from the normal compliance of the lung in the presence of either pneumothorax or hydrothorax. The airways remain patent (Fig. 4-31).

The radiographic signs of lobar and segmental collapse are of two types: *direct* and *indirect*. Of the direct signs, displacement or deviation of a fissure is the most reliable, indicating compensatory hyperinflation in an adjacent lobe to take the place of some of the collapsed lung. Other direct signs of collapse are increased opacity, crowding of vessels, and presence of a silhouette sign. In any case, one or all of these signs may be seen (Fig. 4-32).

Of the indirect signs the most reliable is displacement of the hilar vessels, which shift in the direction of the collapse. Other indirect signs include a shift of the mediastinum, elevation of the hemidiaphragm, compensatory emphysema, hernia-

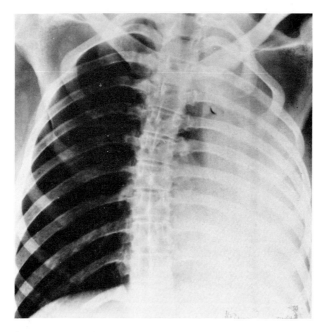

Fig. 4-28. Obstructive atelectasis. There is total atelectasis of left lung secondary to mucous plug in left main stem bronchus in patient postoperatively. Note shift of mediastinum to left, increased density of left hemithorax, and approximation of ribs, all indicating volume loss. This appearance may be seen in obstruction secondary to carcinoma.

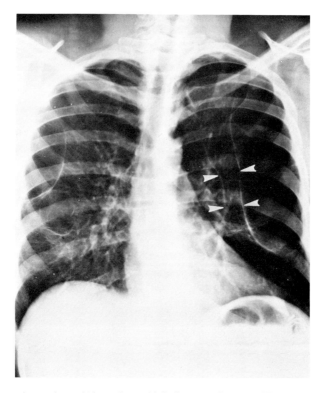

Fig. 4-29. Compressive atelectasis in patient with bullous emphysema. There is compression of uninvolved lung bilaterally by large emphysematous bullae. This is more marked on left, where arrowheads delineate compressed lung.

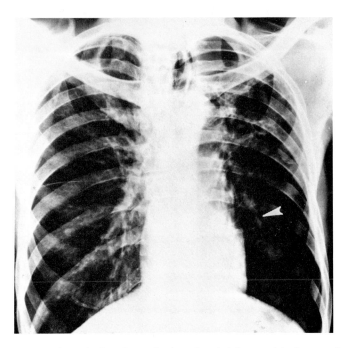

Fig. 4-30. Cicatrization atelectasis. Scarring and volume loss in left upper lobe has resulted in crowding of lung markings and upward shift of pulmonary vessels. Compensatory hyperinflation on left is illustrated by difference in lucency between two lower lobes. Upward-shifted left lower lobe pulmonary artery is outlined (arrowhead).

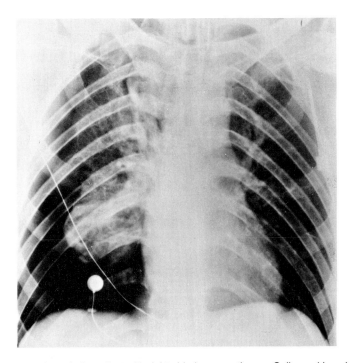

Fig. 4-31. Passive atelectasis in patient with right-sided pneumothorax. Collapsed lung is responsible for density seen to right of cardiac border.

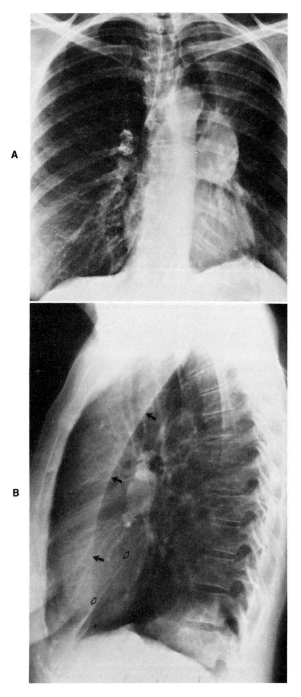

Fig. 4-32. Fissure shift in patient with left upper lobe atelectasis. **A,** Large central carcinoma has resulted in left upper lobe collapse. Note hilar mass and upward displacement of vessels on left. **B,** Lateral view demonstrates anterior shift of oblique fissure on left (solid arrows). Normal position of oblique fissure on right is shown by open arrows.

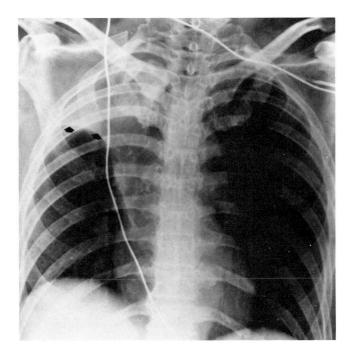

Fig. 4-33. Right upper lobe collapse secondary to mucous plug. There is upward shift of minor fissure (arrows). Note increased density in right upper lobe.

tion of lung across the midline, and approximation of the ribs. This last sign generally indicates that the collapse has been long-standing. As with the direct signs, any or all of these may be seen in a particular case.

In general the upper lobes collapse medially, upward, and anteriorly. On the right side the most reliable signs are increase in density with obliteration of the upper mediastinal shadows on the right and shift of the minor fissure obliquely upward. On the left the most reliable sign is the presence of increased density near the midline, with preservation of the aortic knob. In both instances the diaphragm is usually elevated. On the lateral view the major fissure is displaced anteriorly and superiorly (Fig. 4-32 and 4-33).

The right middle lobe and lingula collapse downward and medially, producing haziness adjacent to the cardiac border on the frontal film. A lordotic view orients the atelectatic segment of lung more perpendicularly to the direction of the x-ray beam and allows better visualization. On the lateral film a triangular-shaped density is seen overlying the cardiac silhouette (Fig. 4-34).

The lower lobes collapse posteriorly, medially, and downward. On a frontal radiograph the classic lower lobe collapse is a triangular-shaped density behind the cardiac shadow. On the lateral film a fissure shift may be appreciated. In total collapse a wedge-shaped density occurs posteriorly and inferiorly, extending down to the diaphragm (Fig. 4-35). In some instances, lower lobe collapse is difficult to detect on the frontal radiograph. Oblique films are quite useful in making this diagnosis.

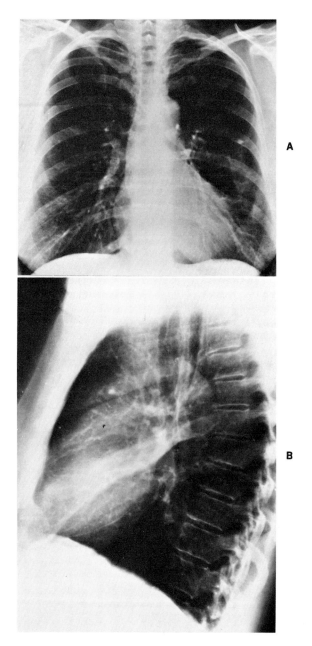

Fig. 4-34. Atelectasis of lingula. **A,** PA view shows haziness along left cardiac border. **B,** Lateral view shows increased density overlying cardiac shadow.

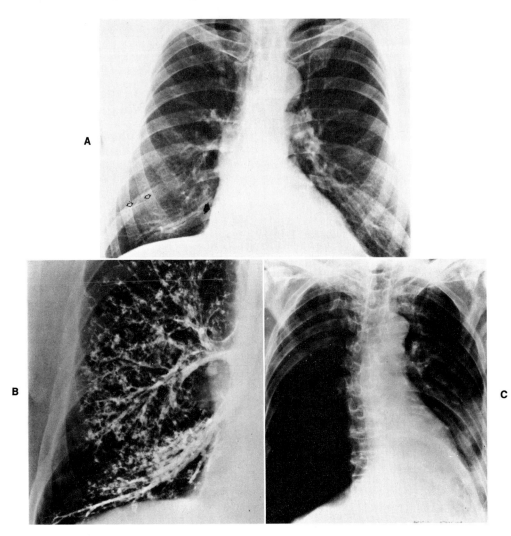

Fig. 4-35. Lower lobe collapse. **A,** Right lower lobe collapse. Atelectatic right lower lobe appears as straight density adjacent to cardiac border (solid arrow). Displaced minor fissure is outlined by open arrows. **B,** Bronchogram of same patient. Note compression and crowding of right lower lobe bronchi. **C,** Left lower lobe collapse. The following signs are apparent: increased density, silhouette sign, and shift of cardiac shadow to left.

Pleural fluid accumulation

Pleural effusion is a sign rather than a disease and occurs in a variety of pathologic conditions, including infection, embolism, neoplasm, congestive heart failure, and trauma. Pleural fluid may be either free or loculated within the pleural space. Free pleural fluid occupies the most dependent portion of the pleural cavity and may be demonstrated on a decubitus film (Fig. 4-36, *A*). It also can be seen as a meniscus and elevation of the "diaphragm" on an upright film (Fig. 4-36, *B*) or as an increase in the overall opacity of one hemithorax on a recumbent film.

Loculation of pleural fluid occurs when fibrous adhesions form. Occasionally the

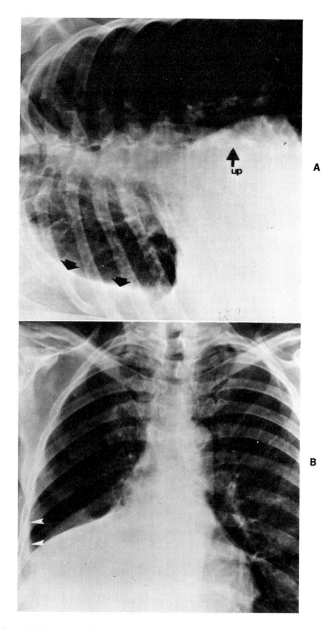

Fig. 4-36. Right pleural effusion. **A,** Right lateral decubitus film shows fluid to layer out along right costal gutter (arrows). **B,** PA film shows subpulmonic collection of fluid on right, obliterating right cardiac border. Note meniscus (arrowheads).

fluid will collect in a fissure to form a "pseudotumor" or "phantom tumor" (Fig. 4-37). This usually occurs in patients with congestive heart failure and clears with resolution of that condition. A pseudotumor may be recognized by its tapered margins at a fissure.

Other signs of pleural effusion include widening of the pleural space, blunting of

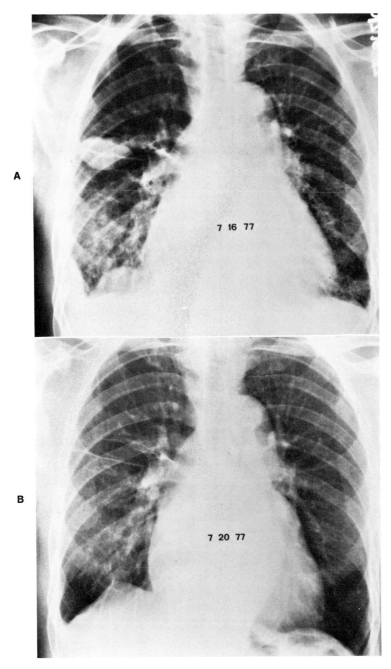

Fig. 4-37. Pseudotumor. **A,** Patient is in congestive heart failure. "Mass" density is present in right mid-lung field. There are bilateral pleural effusions. **B,** Four days later, congestive heart failure has improved considerably. "Mass" is no longer present. Effusions have cleared as well.

the costophrenic angle, and mediastinal shift in massive effusion. It is estimated that up to 300 ml of pleural fluid may accumulate in the costophrenic sinus posteriorly before an effusion is apparent on the frontal radiograph.

Patients with unexplained pleural effusions should be carefully studied for neoplasm. In addition to cytologic studies of the fluid itself, it is desirous to clear those portions of the lung that would be obscured by the fluid. To do this a decubitus or Trendelenberg position (head down) is used to make the fluid flow away from the lung bases. A more useful technique, however, is to employ CT, in which the patient may be turned to various positions to allow redistribution of the fluid (Fig. 4-38).

Mass lesions

Mass lesions of the lung and mediastinum are a very important group of diseases. In general a variety of clinical, historic, and radiologic findings are used to predict the nature of the lesion. Ultimately the diagnosis rests in the hands of the pathologist. The most common etiologies of the solitary pulmonary nodule are either tumors or granulomas.

In the evaluation of solitary pulmonary nodules the following studies are useful: an old chest film, chest fluoroscopy, chest tomography, and, rarely, bronchography. The most valuable study a patient can have for evaluation of a solitary nodule is an old chest film. The reader should be cautioned, however, that in evaluating patients with serial chest films, it is necessary to examine not only the most recent old chest film but also one dating back a considerable period of time to measure the size of the

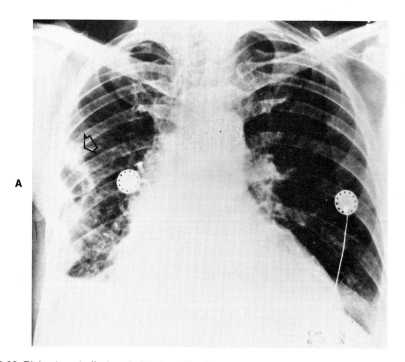

Fig. 4-38. Right pleural effusion. **A,** PA chest film demonstrates right pleural effusion. Pulmonary mass is also present (arrow).

Continued.

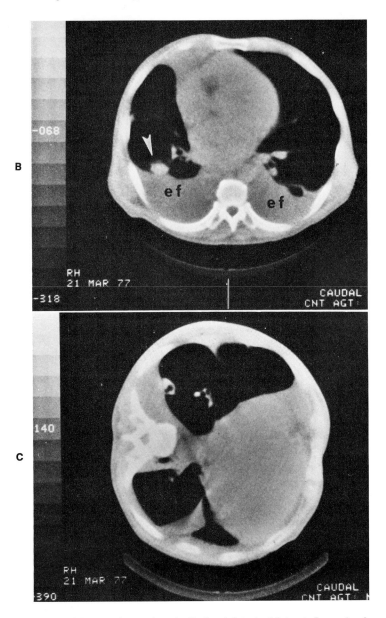

Fig. 4-38, cont'd. B, CT scan shows pleural effusion *(ef)* to be bilateral. Second pulmonary nodule is seen in right lower lobe (arrowhead). **C,** Nodule may be better delineated by placing patient in left lateral decubitus position.

lesion. A very slowly growing lesion may not appear to have grown from one study to the next. However, in comparing films *out of sequence*, the difference may be quite dramatic. Fig. 4-39 is a series of circles, each differing in diameter by 1 mm. It is difficult to tell the difference between consecutive circles. However, by comparing drawings out of sequence a significant difference is apparent. A change in size also represents a change in *volume*, which increases by the cube of the radius. Thus a lesion that doubles in its diameter has actually increased eightfold in volume.

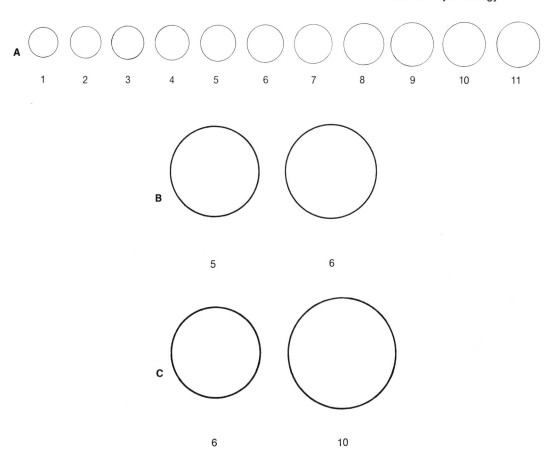

Fig. 4-39. When comparing pulmonary lesions, it is necessary to compare films out of sequence. **A,** Diameters of circles differ by 1 mm. **B,** Comparing circles 5 and 6 there is little apparent difference. Lesion of similar size may possibly be reported as undergoing no change. **C,** Comparing circles 6 and 10, an out-of-sequence comparison, difference in size is grossly apparent.

Chest fluoroscopy is an important examination for a patient with lung nodules. The fluoroscopist should first make sure that the nodule is not an artifact such as hair braids, a button on a nightgown, or a skin lesion. The next step is to determine the location of the lesion, especially whether it is in the lung or is a bony abnormality such as an osteochondroma, a healing rib fracture, or spinal osteophytes (Fig. 4-40).

Tomographic examination provides additional important information. First, it defines the border of the lesion. A smooth, round, and well-defined border favors a benign lesion; a poorly defined, lobulated, spiculated, or hazy border suggests a malignant lesion with invasion. A spiculated margin on a pulmonary lesion (Fig. 4-41) is quite similar to spiculation seen at the border of a mammary carcinoma on a mammogram (Fig. 4-42). Tomography may also demonstrate calcification within or around the lesion. Calcification is considered almost pathognomonic of a benign lesion, especially when it is centrally located or "popcorn shaped" (Fig. 4-43). The reader is cautioned, however, in using calcification as the sole criterion of the nature of the lesion, since a scar carcinoma may engulf a calcified granuloma. In these instances the calcification may be eccentric.

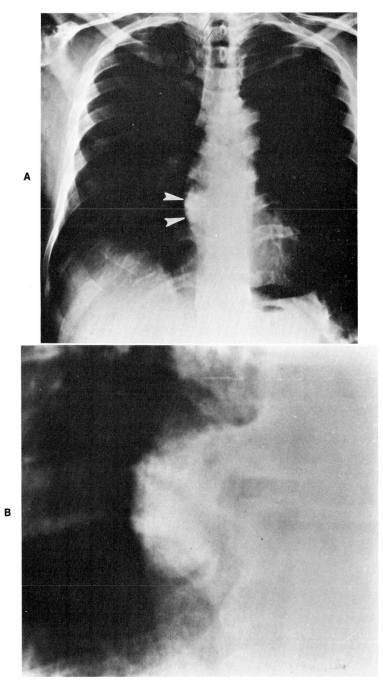

Fig. 4-40. Spinal osteophyte appearing as pulmonary "mass." **A,** PA radiograph of chest shows density posterior to cardiac shadow (arrowheads). **B,** Fluoroscopic spot film shows "mass" to be in fact spinal osteophyte.

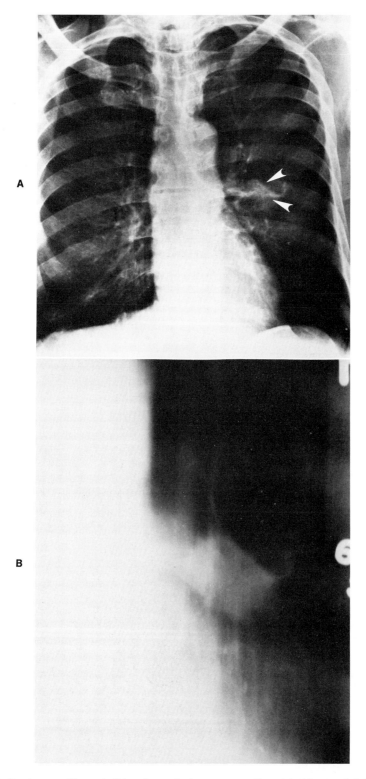

Fig. 4-41. Carcinoma of lung. **A,** PA radiograph shows mass adjacent to hilum on left (arrowheads). **B,** Tomogram of tumor shows irregular border that is somewhat spiculated.

Tomography is also useful in delineating satellite lesions, a common finding in histoplasmosis; in revealing cavitation; and in defining vessels going to or from a lesion. This is particularly useful in evaluating arteriovenous malformations or even pulmonary sequestrations, which often appear as mass lesions. The demonstration of these vessels supports the diagnosis.

Bronchography, especially if combined with *bronchial brush biopsy*, may be of use in large central lesions. However, if a lesion is small or peripheral, bronchography is not too helpful.

CT proved useful in evaluating patients with pulmonary and mediastinal masses. The information gained includes evidence of mediastinal invasion, chest wall invasion, and presence of peripheral nodules. Fig. 4-44 illustrates a patient with a large central carcinoma.

Patients with solitary pulmonary nodules are often submitted to a battery of diagnostic studies, including upper GI, barium enema, intravenous urography, and metastatic bone surveys. These are performed before histologic confirmation of the lesion in the hope that a primary lesion will be found, thus indicating that the pulmonary lesion is metastatic. The yield from this process is extremely low and results in longer hospitalization and expense to the patient. The final diagnosis rests on tissue examination. It is now possible to biopsy these lesions percutaneously or trans-

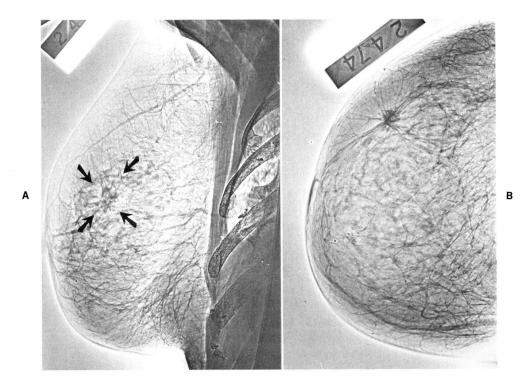

A

B

Fig. 4-42. Carcinoma of breast with spiculation. Stellate appearance is quite apparent on these mammograms (arrows in **A**). This appearance may be seen in any infiltrating carcinoma regardless of location.

bronchially under fluoroscopic or CT control. If either of these studies fails to provide an adequate answer, thoracotomy with excision of the lesion in toto is the next step.

Mediastinal masses are sometimes difficult to separate from pulmonary parenchymal masses. However, most show extraparenchymal signs such as sharp margins, tapered borders, and convexity toward the lung. The majority of all primary mediastinal masses occur in the anterior compartment; one third occur in the middle compartment; and the remainder occur in the posterior compartment. Most patients with mediastinal masses are asymptomatic. Table 4 lists abnormalities found in each compartment of the roentgen mediastinum. The most common lesions of the anterior mediastinum are lymphomas (Fig. 4-45), thymic lesions (Fig. 4-46), and teratomas. Other anterior lesions that may be seen include foramen of Morgagni hernias (Fig. 4-47) and pericardial cysts (Fig. 4-48).

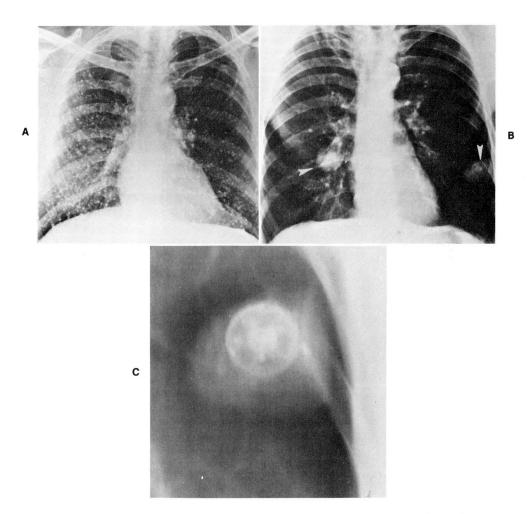

Fig. 4-43. Calcified granulomas in histoplasmosis. **A,** Diffuse pulmonary calcifications. **B,** Localized calcification in two granulomas (arrowheads). **C,** Detail tomogram of left-sided lesion shows calcification within nodule.

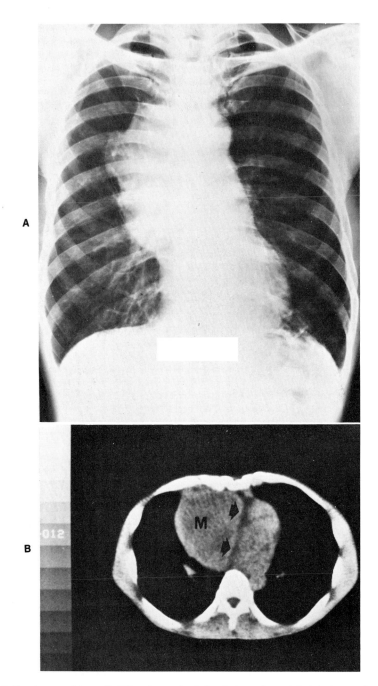

Fig. 4-44. Carcinoma of lung. **A,** PA radiograph of chest shows large lobulated mass in anterior and middle mediastinum on right. **B,** CT scan shows cleavage plane (arrows) between mass *(M)* and adjacent mediastinal structures.

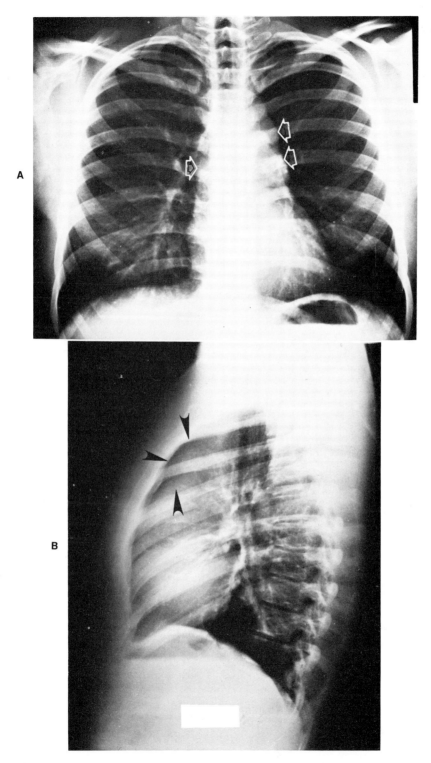

Fig. 4-45. Lymphoma of anterior mediastinum. **A,** PA radiograph shows lobular mediastinal mass (arrows). **B,** Lateral film shows mass to be located in anterior mediastinum (arrowheads).

Table 4. Conditions found in each compartment of the roentgen mediastinum

Condition	Compartment		
	Anterior	Middle	Posterior
Neoplasms	Lymphoma Thymic lesion Thyroid lesion Parathyroid Teratoma Carcinoma (lung)	Lymphoma Carcinoma (lung, esophagus) Metastases	Neurogenic tumor Lymphoma Carcinoma (lung) Pheochromocytoma Myeloma
Cystic lesions	Thymic cyst Pericardial cyst	Bronchogenic cyst Esophageal duplication cyst	Neurenteric cyst Thoracic duct cyst Lateral meningocele

Vascular ab-
normalities
	Buckled brachiocephalic
	  artery
	Anomalous or dilated superior
	  vena cava
	Aortic aneurysm
	Cardiac aneurysm
	  (including sinus of Valsalva)
		Aneurysm of aorta or
		  great vessels
		Right aortic arch
		Aortic ring
		Azygos vein enlargement
			Aortic aneurysm

Other	Foramen of Morgagni hernia
	Hematoma
	Mediastinitis
	Abscess
	Postoperative esophageal
	  bypass
		Hiatal hernia
		Enlarged lymph node
		  (other than lymphoma)
		Mediastinitis
		Abscess
		Hematoma
			Bochdalek hernia
			Extramedullary
			  hematopoiesis
			Hematoma
			Abscess

The majority of masses arising in the middle mediastinum are lymph nodes representing lymphoma, metastatic disease, sarcoidosis (Fig. 4-49), or response to infection.

The most likely cause of a posterior mediastinal mass is a neurogenic tumor (Fig. 4-50). These generally appear as a paraspinous mass and are often associated with changes in the spine or of the posterior ribs. Neurofibromas frequently enlarge the neural foramina. Calcification may occur in neuroblastomas in children.

Bronchogenic carcinoma may appear as a mediastinal mass in any compartment. This should always be considered in any adult with a mediastinal mass.

Multiple pulmonary nodules may be granulomas or metastases. If the lesions contain calcium and are widely disseminated (Fig. 4-51), the diagnosis is most likely a granulomatous disease. Multiple large nodules, particularly of varying sizes (Fig. 4-52) usually are metastases. Metastases may also occur in a "lymphangitic" form, resulting in a prominent interstitial pattern (Fig. 4-53).

Emphysema

One does not need a chest radiograph to make a diagnosis of emphysema. There are adequate physical findings for that. However, there are certain radiographic findings that corroborate those of the physical examination. A better use of the chest film in the emphysematous patient is to detect localized bullae, peribronchial infiltrates, and pneumothorax or pneumomediastinum.

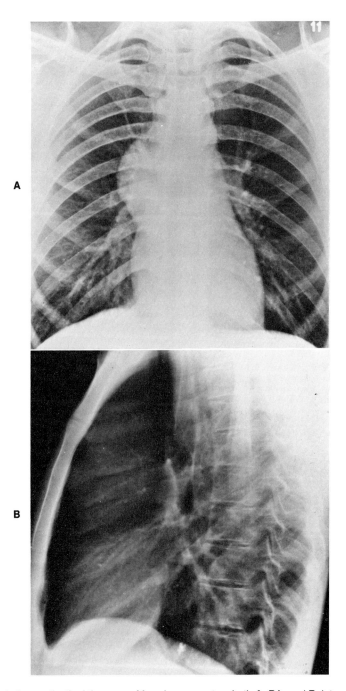

Fig. 4-46. Anterior mediastinal thymoma. Mass is apparent on both **A,** PA, and **B,** lateral, radiographs.

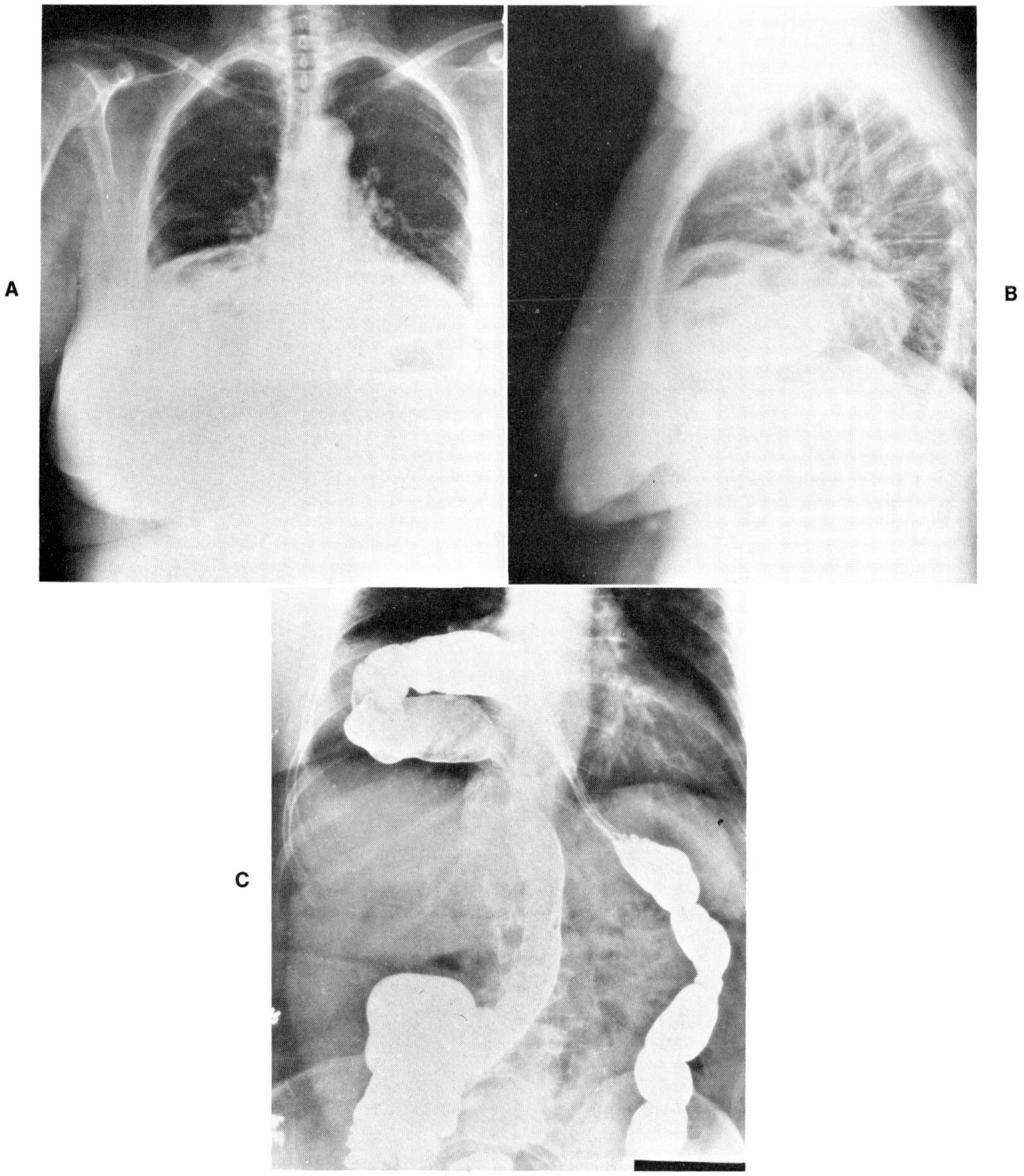

Fig. 4-47. Foramen of Morgagni hernia. **A,** PA chest radiograph shows mass adjacent to heart on right. Mass contains several gaseous densities. **B,** Lateral chest radiograph shows gaseous densities within mass. **C,** Barium enema shows mass to represent hernial sac through foramen of Morgagni. Sac contains loops of colon, which account for gaseous densities. (From Daffner, R. H., Gehweiler, J. A., and Carden, T. S., Jr.: Case studies in radiology, New York, 1975, Appleton-Century-Crofts. Reproduced with permission of the publisher.)

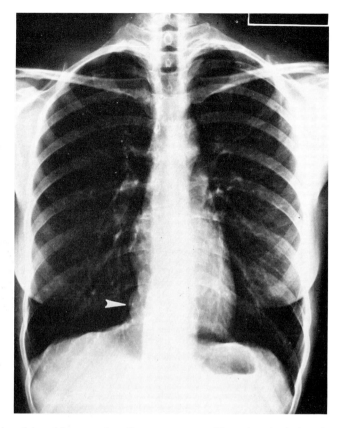

Fig. 4-48. Pericardial cyst in asymptomatic young woman. There is extra bulge along right cardiac border (arrowhead). This is common location for pericardial cyst. (From Daffner, R. H.: New Physician **23:**54, 1974. Reproduced with permission of the publisher.)

The radiographic findings of classic emphysema reflect the overinflation, loss of compliance, and parenchymal destruction that are the pathophysiology of the disease. The most reliable radiographic sign is deceased vascularity. Other signs are hyperlucency; increased retrosternal clear space; increased lung volume; depression, flattening, or reversal of the curvature of the diaphragm; decreased diaphragmatic excursion; presence of prominent central pulmonary arteries with rapid tapering (marker vessels); and vertical cardiac configuration. Bullae may be present to a greater or lesser extent (Fig. 4-54).

Patients with chronic pulmonary disease may not have all the classic findings of emphysema. Some may have prominent interstitial markings, the so-called dirty lung seen particularly in smokers. In some younger individuals the only finding may be hyperlucency, representing early overinflation. Emphysematous changes are often combined with other abnormalities.

Interstitial and acinar disease

Diseases that primarily involve the interlobular connective tissue with or without secondary involvement of the air space are called interstitial diseases. They consti-

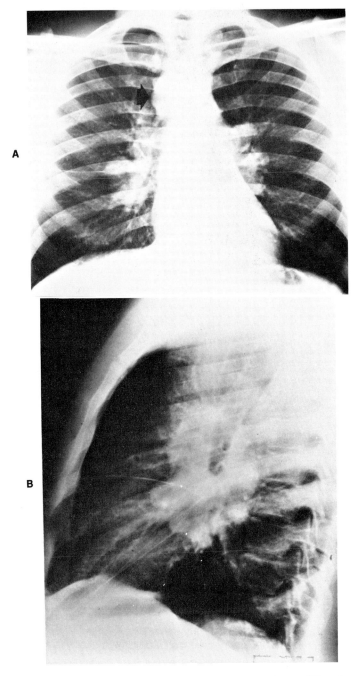

Fig. 4-49. Sarcoidosis. **A,** PA and, **B,** lateral views of chest show massive perihilar adenopathy. In addition, there is enlargement of azygos lymph node on PA radiograph (arrow).

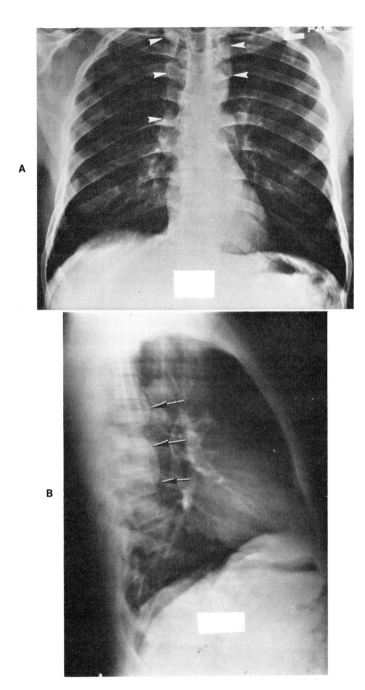

Fig. 4-50. Neurofibromatosis. **A,** Multiple paraspinous lobular densities are seen on this frontal radiograph (arrowheads). **B,** Lateral radiograph clearly shows posterior location of these lesions (arrows). (From Daffner, R. H.: New Physician **21:**80, 1972. Reproduced with permission of the publisher.)

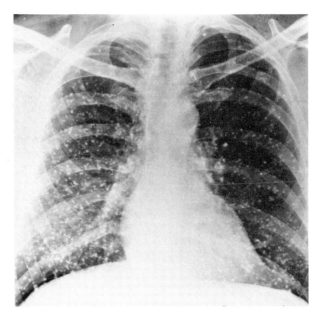

Fig. 4-51. Diffuse histoplasmosis. Note multiple calcified nodules.

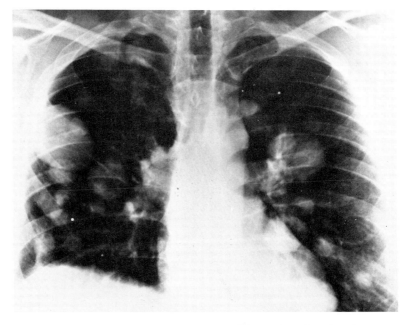

Fig. 4-52. Metastatic carcinoma. Note multiple nodules of varying size.

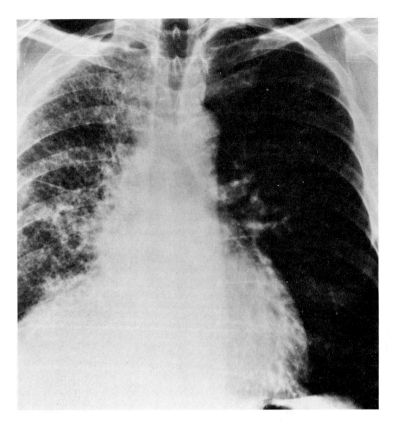

Fig. 4-53. Metastatic carcinoma, lymphangitic pattern. Diffuse interstitial process is apparent on right. Similar changes but to a much less marked degree were present on left.

tute a group of diseases that have recognizable radiographic patterns: linear, nodular, combined lineonodular, and reticular (weblike, "honeycombing"). The etiologies vary and include early heart failure (edema), pneumoconiosis, collagen disease (fibrosis), metastatic neoplastic permeation, and primary inflammatory conditions (early viral pneumonia, interstitial pneumonia). Many of these diseases as they progress produce some degree of air space or acinar pattern.

Pure acinar lesions produce a pattern characterized by fluffy margins, coalescence, a segmental or lobar distribution, a butterfly shadow (radiating out from the hila), air bronchograms, and a rapid sequence of onset and clearing. Conditions that produce acinar patterns include acute alveolar edema (pneumonia, congestive heart failure with pulmonary edema, toxic or chemical reaction), bleeding (idiopathic pulmonary hemorrhage), aspiration of any fluid, and alveolar cell carcinoma. A rare condition that produces this pattern is alveolar proteinosis.

Pure acinar disease may frequently be distinguished from pure interstitial disease by pattern recognition. For demonstration purposes, consider the lung to be analogous to a piece of chicken wire, where the wire hexagons represent the interstitial tissues and the spaces, the air spaces. Under normal circumstances there is a uniform black background with thin interlacing strands of gray (Fig. 4-55, A). In acinar disease the air spaces are filled in. Unless there is total consolidation of a lobe or a

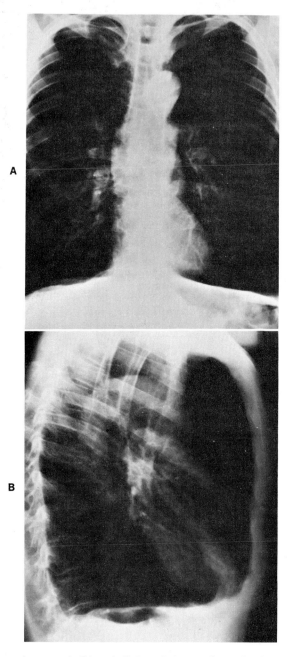

Fig. 4-54. Severe emphysema. **A,** PA and, **B,** lateral chest radiographs demonstrate hyperinflation. Marked blackness of both lungs is caused by this hyperaeration. Note flattening and lobulation of diaphragm, increased AP diameter of chest, and prominent pulmonary arteries.

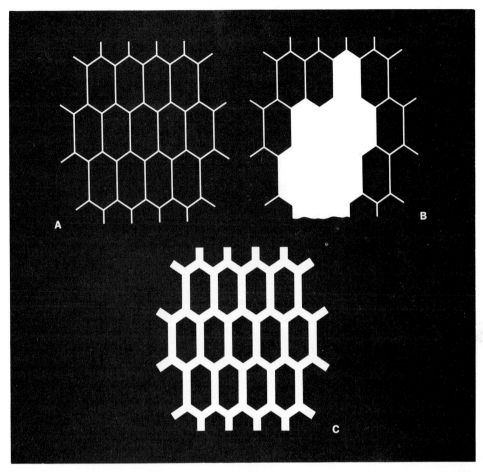

Fig. 4-55. Schematic drawing comparing alveolar with interstitial disease. **A,** Normal. Thin white lines represent interstitial tissues and spaces between, air spaces. **B,** Alveolar, acinar, or air space consolidation pattern. Note confluence of abnormality from one air space to next. This appearance on radiograph is of white dots on black background. **C,** Interstitial pattern. Diffuse interstitial thickening has resulted in honeycombing.

lung, an alveolar infiltrate will appear as white dots (representing the so-called acinar shadows) on a black background of aerated lung (Fig. 4-55, *B*). If, however, the disease is primarily interstitial, there is thickening of the borders around the acini, and the resulting pattern is that of black dots (representing aerated acini) surrounded by a white background of the thickened interstitial tissue (Fig. 4-55, *C*). Combined airway and interstitial disease produce a combined pattern. The following outline lists some of the more common interstitial diseases.

PRIMARY PULMONARY INTERSTITIAL DISEASES
  I. Infectious disorders
    A. Tuberculosis
    B. Histoplasmosis
    C. Coccidioidomycosis

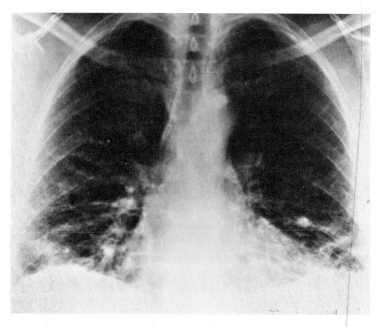

Fig. 4-56. Silicosis. There are prominent pulmonary interstitial markings. In addition, several confluent areas (progressive massive fibrosis) are present in both lung bases. Bases are affected more than apices. Silicosis may be considered a prototype of interstitial lung disease.

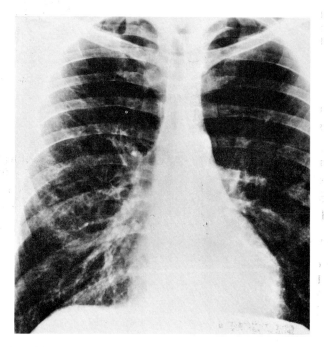

Fig. 4-57. Idiopathic pulmonary fibrosis. Diffuse interstitial pattern is present.

II. Inhalational disorders
  A. Inorganic dust
    1. Silicosis
    2. Asbestosis
    3. Pneumoconiosis (mixed dust)
    4. Siderosis
    5. Other inorganic dust diseases
  B. Organic dust
    1. Farmer's lung
    2. Mushroom workers' disease
    3. Bagassosis
    4. Other organic dust diseases

III. Miscellaneous
  A. Sarcoidosis
  B. Drug-induced disease
  C. Rheumatoid arthritis
  D. Scleroderma
  E. Hemosiderosis
  F. Chronic thromboembolism
  G. Histiocytosis
  H. Desquamative interstitial pneumonia
  I. Idiopathic interstitial fibrosis
    (Hamman-Rich syndrome)

Quite often the presence of ancillary radiologic and clinical findings will be needed to make the correct diagnosis. A good clinical history is also essential, especially if we are entertaining a diagnosis of pneumoconiosis or other industrial exposure. Figs. 4-56 through 4-58 show representative examples of pure interstitial disease.

Pneumothorax

Pneumothorax may result from a variety of causes, including trauma (laceration by fractured rib, stab, or bullet wound) and iatrogenic factors (postthoracocentesis, lung biopsy, or placement of subclavian catheter) or may occur spontaneously. The most common radiographic findings are absence of pulmonary vessels extending to the chest wall, a visible pleural line displaced from the chest wall, and increased lucency of one hemithorax. If the patient has a tension-type pneumothorax, air continuously enters the pleural space and builds up pressure, which compresses the mediastinum toward the opposite lung. This may result in severe respiratory distress unless immediately recognized. The most common sign of tension pneumothorax is a shift of the mediastinum away from the abnormal side (Fig. 4-59). This is a true emergency and requires immediate tube decompression. An ancillary sign in tension pneumothorax is depression of the affected hemidiaphragm. A pneumothorax may be enhanced by an expiratory film (Fig. 4-5).

Pulmonary embolus

It is estimated that pulmonary embolus is the most common disease found in hospitalized patients who are autopsied. Fortunately, in most cases, embolism occurs without infarction because of the double blood supply to the lung. Pulmonary emboli are most likely to occur in severely ill patients who are bedridden, in those with venous disease, and in those with chronic congestive heart failure.

Interestingly, the radiographic findings in pulmonary embolus may be few in any particular patient. Clinicians and radiologists should have a high index of suspicion to make this diagnosis, since the most common radiographic findings are those of a "normal" chest, which is incompatible with a patient in acute cardiopulmonary distress. Radiographic signs that may be seen, however, include pleural effusion, pulmonary infiltrates, focal atelectasis, elevation of the diaphragm, and hypovascular peripheral lung segments. Infiltration and formation of "mass" may occur with in-

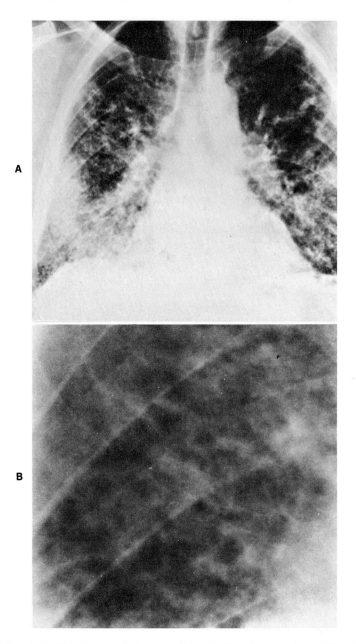

Fig. 4-58. Diffuse interstitial disease with honeycombing. **A,** PA radiograph shows diffuse interstitial disease, more marked in bases. Pattern is that of "black dots on a light background." **B,** Detail film of upper lobe disease shows honeycomb pattern.

farction. With healing, these areas of consolidation shrink in the same pattern as a melting ice cube, retaining its original outline, only becoming smaller.

The radioisotope lung scan is a useful diagnostic procedure in patients strongly suspected of having pulmonary embolus. As mentioned in Chapter 1, the lung scan depends on the trapping of radioactive particles in the capillary bed and thus is an

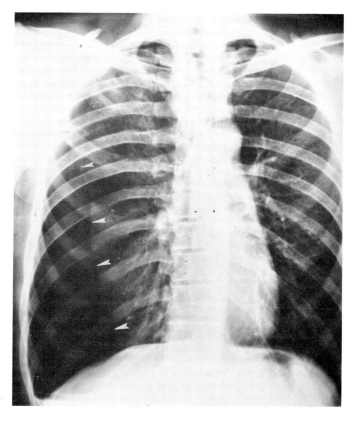

Fig. 4-59. Tension pneumothorax. Large tension pneumothorax is present on right. Aerated lung is clearly seen delineated against pneumothorax (arrowheads). Heart and mediastinum, however, are shifted to left.

index of pulmonary arterial perfusion. Patients with emphysema, pneumonia, pulmonary fibrosis, or pleural effusions may demonstrate abnormal lung scans because of displaced vessels, shunting, and attenuation of the isotope emission, respectively. However, the scan is indeed useful in patients with these conditions if there are areas of decreased perfusion in an otherwise normal area of lung on the radiograph (Fig. 4-60). If a patient who is highly suspected of having a pulmonary embolus can be shown to have perfusion defects in previously normal-appearing areas, the diagnosis is certain. Furthermore, if a patient is shown to have normal perfusion despite the radiographic appearance, you can exclude embolus as a cause for that appearance.

If the isotope scan is equivocal, pulmonary arteriography may be used to confirm the diagnosis of pulmonary emboli. Radiographic findings include filling defects, delayed flow, and a disparity of flow as indicated by the venous phase being present on one side whereas the arterial phase is still seen on the abnormal side. Pulmonary arteriography does carry considerable hazard, however, and may result in severe arrhythmia or death. It should be reserved for situations where the diagnosis cannot be made by any other means. Fig. 4-61 shows a patient with pulmonary embolus diagnosed by arteriography.

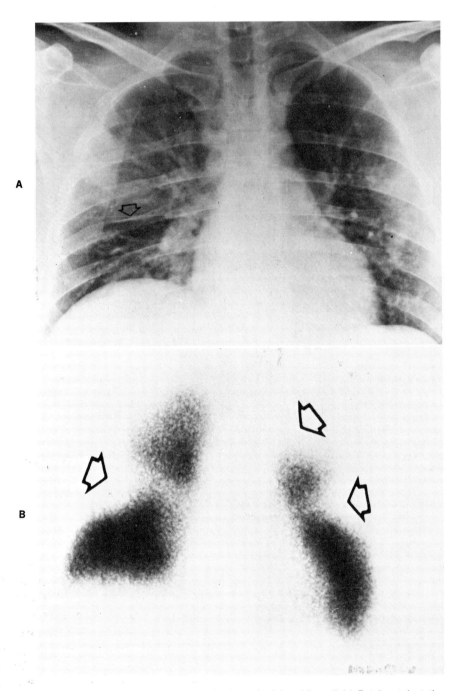

Fig. 4-60. A, PA radiograph of chest shows haziness in right midlung field. Patchy atelectatic area is present as well (arrow). Left lung is essentially normal. **B,** Lung scan shows multiple bilateral defects (arrows). In view of normal-appearing left lung on radiograph, this is highly suggestive of pulmonary embolism.

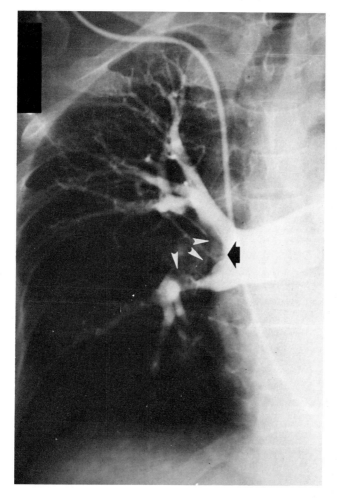

Fig. 4-61. Pulmonary arteriogram demonstrates saddle embolus (arrow) at bifurcation of right pulmonary artery. Arrowheads outline normal lumen on that side.

SUMMARY

This chapter has briefly described techniques involved in chest radiography. The normal anatomy was described in macroscopic and microscopic terms. The unit of structure and function in the lung is the pulmonary lobule. The mediastinum, its compartments, and its contents were also described in detail.

Pathologic alterations seen in the lung include consolidation, atelectasis, pleural fluid, masses, emphysema, pneumothorax, and pulmonary embolus. Each of these abnormalities produces clearly recognizable patterns. In addition, the concepts of the silhouette sign and air bronchogram were described. The concept of acinar versus interstitial disease was briefly described. Specific disease entities were not discussed in this chapter. You are now invited to test yourself on the case studies that follow.

Selected case studies

Case 4-1: COUGH AND MALAISE

A 50-year-old black man consulted his physician because of 6 weeks of persistent cough and malaise. He admitted to frequent night sweats. He lost 30 pounds over the 6-week period. He has smoked one pack of cigarettes a day for 35 years. Physical examination revealed a cachectic man who appeared chronically ill. Temperature was 39° C, pulse 120, and respirations 32. Pertinent physical findings include small nodules within the choroid of the eye. The lungs were clear. Mild splenomegaly was present. A chest radiograph (Case 4-1, A) was obtained. *What are the radiographic findings? What is your differential diagnosis? What additional studies would you perform to confirm the diagnosis?*

ROENTGEN DIAGNOSIS AND DISCUSSION

The PA (Case 4-1, A) view of the chest shows a diffuse, fine miliary pattern throughout both lungs. The distribution is uniform. The heart is of normal size and shape. The findings are those of miliary tuberculosis.

A tuberculin skin test was positive within 24 hours, which, when combined with the radiographic and eye findings, confirmed a diagnosis of miliary tuberculosis.

Miliary tuberculosis results from hematogenous dissemination of tubercle bacilli. Although more common in children, the incidence of miliary tuberculosis in adults is sufficiently high for it to be considered in any patient with a history similar to this patient's accompanied by a diffuse or miliary roentgenographic pattern on the chest film. Unless properly diagnosed and vigorously treated, miliary tuberculosis may be fatal.

Infection with *Mycobacterium tuberculosis* is a worldwide problem, with the greatest incidence in areas of heavy poverty. In the United States in 1965, it was estimated that less than 20% of the total population had positive tuberculin skin tests. However, in the same period of time in India, positive skin tests were found in 20% of the children under age 5 years and in 90% of the population over age 40 years!

Tuberculosis does not respect age or social status. Although it is primarily a disease of the very young and the very old, any age group may be affected. Although people in the lower socioeconomic classes tend to have a greater incidence, the disease is also seen in "high society."

Primary pulmonary tuberculosis usually occurs in children. The disease begins as a nonspecific pulmonary infection that generally involves the hilar lymph nodes and tracheobronchial tree. The typical radiographic picture is one of air space consolidation associated with hilar lymph node enlargement. Compression of airways may result in atelectasis. As the dis-

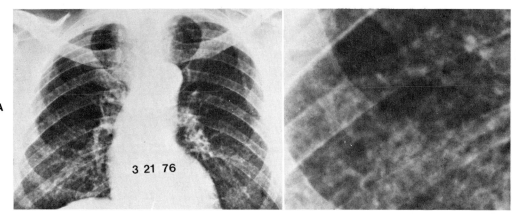

A

3 21 76

Case 4-1. A, PA chest radiograph, March 1976. **B,** Close-up of right midlung field.

ease is treated or resolved, a focal scar is left in the periphery, sometimes accompanied by calcified hilar nodes. This appearance is the *Ranke complex*. The *Ghon lesion* is the parenchymal scar.

Reinfection, or secondary, tuberculosis is a term applied to a clinical and radiographic pattern of tuberculosis seen in adults. Although the exact terminology has been questioned, reactivation of a previously dormant tuberculous lesion in the adult patient is implied. Radiographically, reinfection tuberculosis is generally localized to the apical and posterior segments of the upper lobes. The lesions are often seen as stringy, fibronodular densities with patchy parenchymal consolidation (Case 4-1, *C* and *D*). Cavitation may occur in this form of the disease (Case 4-1, *E*).

Miliary tuberculosis may result, as previously mentioned, from hematogenous dissemination of tubercular bacilli from a previous focus of the disease. Once diagnosed and properly treated the improvement may be extremely rapid (Case 4-1, *F*).

Other forms of tuberculosis manifest in the chest include tuberculous bronchiectasis, bronchostenosis, and tuberculoma. The reader is referred to the bibliography for further information on these entities.

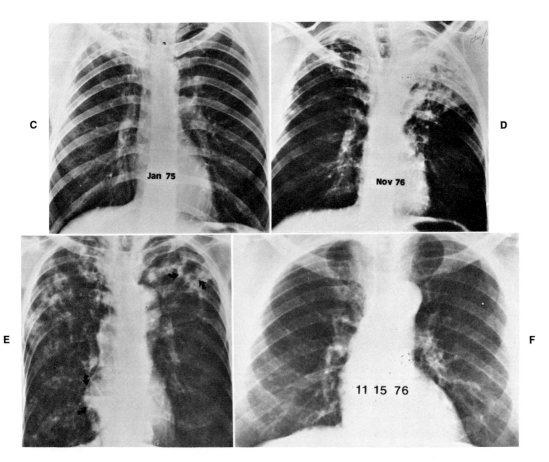

Case 4-1. C, Another patient, January 1975. There are patchy infiltrates in right apex. This is an unusual location for nontubercular pneumonia. **D,** Same patient, November 1976. Fibronodular scarring is present in right upper lobe. Patient has developed extensive tubercular disease in left upper lobe. **E,** Another patient with cavitary tuberculosis. There is extensive pulmonary fibronodular infiltration bilaterally. Cavities are present in left upper and right lower lobes (arrows). **F,** Same patient as in **A.** Following adequate treatment with antitubercular agents, patient's chest returned to normal.

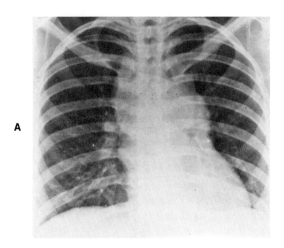

Case 4-2. A, Routine chest radiograph of 25-year-old nurse.

Case 4-2: ROUTINE CHEST EXAMINATION

A 25-year-old black nurse had a routine chest examination performed prior to employment at a local hospital (Case 4-2, A). She claimed good health and is asymptomatic at the time of this examination. The only positive finding on physical examination is palpable cervical adenopathy. *What are the main radiographic findings? What is the differential diagnosis? How would you go about establishing the correct diagnosis?*

ROENTGEN DIAGNOSIS AND DISCUSSION

PA and lateral views of the chest show a normal cardiac silhouette. There is enlargement of the hilar and paratracheal nodes. In particular there is enlargement of the azygos node. The lungs are clear. In this age group the differential diagnosis includes sarcoidosis, tuberculosis, and Hodgkin disease/lymphoma.

A tuberculin skin test was normal. The patient underwent biopsy of the liver and of one of the enlarged cervical lymph nodes. Both of these showed noncaseating granulomas, which, when combined with the findings on the chest radiograph, confirmed a diagnosis of sarcoidosis.

Sarcoidosis, a disease of unknown etiology, is characterized by the presence of noncaseating granulomas in many organs. Nodal enlargements, particularly in the hilar and paratracheal region on the chest radiograph, and evidence of noncaseating granulomas elsewhere in the body generally confirm the diagnosis.

The greatest incidence of sarcoidosis appears to be concentrated in the United States, Scandinavia, and England. In the United States the Southeast region seems to be "endemic." The disease is more prevalent in rural areas. The disease was thought to be more common in blacks than in whites. However, recent evidence suggests an equal racial incidence. The incidence with regard to sex is equal.

Clinically, many of these patients are asymptomatic, their disease suggested by the finding of an abnormal "routine" chest radiograph. Symptoms, when present, are often associated with multisystem disease. They may be quite nonspecific: fatigue, malaise, weakness, weight loss, and fever. Some patients have a skin rash (erythema nodosum). Pulmonary symptoms, if present, include dyspnea and a dry, nonproductive cough. Peripheral lymph node involvement is a common finding, occurring in approximately 75% of cases. A minority of patients have eye involvement characterized by uveitis. Bony manifestations include a migratory polyarthritis and erosive changes, particularly of the phalanges.

Radiographically, Fraser and Paré group the findings in four categories: (1) lymph node involvement without pulmonary abnormality, (2) diffuse pulmonary disease without lymph-

Case 4-2. B, Unilateral paratracheal node enlargement in patient with lymphoma. Compare this with **A.** Parenchymal involvement is present in lingula. **C,** Same patient as in **A.** There has been marked reduction in size of mediastinal lymph nodes. With further treatment, appearance of chest returned to normal.

adenopathy, (3) combined diffuse pulmonary disease and lymphadenopathy, and (4) pulmonary fibrosis. Most patients fall into the first and third categories.

Lymph node involvement without pulmonary abnormality occurs in up to 90% of patients with sarcoidosis. The nodes involved are generally the paratracheal, tracheobronchial, and bronchopulmonary groups. The distribution is almost always bilateral and symmetric. The configuration is bulbous or rounded. Calcification may occur in lymph nodes, but this is unusual. Characteristic involvement of the paratracheal nodes almost always occurs in combination with perihilar nodal involvement. The symmetry and paratracheal enlargement in sarcoidosis contrast sharply with nodal patterns in primary tuberculosis and in the lymphomas. In the first instances, enlargement tends to be unilateral unless sharply demarcated; in the latter, enlargement tends to be in the paratracheal group and often is unilateral (Case 4-2, *B*). Another contrast between sarcoidosis and lymphoma is seen when the patient develops pulmonary parenchymal disease. In sarcoidosis the onset of diffuse lung disease commonly occurs with a diminution of the lymph node size. This is not observed in lymphoma.

Pulmonary disease, when it occurs, is generally of a reticulonodular interstitial pattern. It is often combined with nodal enlargement.

Pulmonary fibrosis occurs in long-standing disease that has not been successfully treated. Scarring is coarse, consisting of irregular linear strands extending from the hila toward the periphery. The distribution is not as even as that seen in the parenchymal pattern alone.

The diagnosis generally may be made by lymph node biopsy; presence of a scalene node is usually a positive sign, even if the node is not enlarged. Pathologic examination shows non-caseating granulomas. This picture, combined with the radiographic pattern, is rather characteristic of the disease.

Traditional treatment of the disease has been with steroids. Following successful treatment the nodes return to normal size (Case 4-2, *C*). The majority of the patients recover completely or have only minimal residual disease. However, up to 25% may have some degree of permanent disability.

Case 4-3: COUGH AND WHEEZE

A 9-year-old boy was brought to his family physician because of sudden onset of wheeze and nonproductive cough. The patient had been well until several hours earlier, when, while eating peanuts, he suddenly began coughing. The cough was accompanied by an audible wheeze. Physical examination revealed an apprehensive child. On percussion of the chest the right side was somewhat hypertympanic. On auscultation, an inspiratory wheeze was heard anteriorly just to the right of the midline. There were diminished breath sounds on the right. *What is your diagnosis? What radiographic examination would you recommend?*

This patient should be suspected of having an intrabronchial foreign body. Inspiratory and expiratory PA chest films were ordered (Case 4-3, A and B). *What are the radiographic findings?*

ROENTGEN DIAGNOSIS AND DISCUSSION

The PA chest film in inspiration is normal. On the expiratory film the right lung remains inflated at inspiratory level. There is a shift of the heart and mediastinum to the left side. These findings suggest a "ball valve" type of obstruction in the right main stem bronchus.

Bronchoscopy was performed, and a peanut was removed from the patient's right main stem bronchus.

The aspiration of foreign material into a main stem bronchus in a child is not uncommon. This occurs especially in young children, who are prone to swallow food whole without proper chewing or who walk around with a toy or other piece of foreign material in their mouths.

The main clinical presentation is the sudden onset of cough and wheeze in a previously healthy child. The child may appear quite apprehensive. Often he will tell you that he had something in his mouth at the time he began coughing. A peanut is the classic offender because it is just the right size to wedge in a bronchus. Because of the slope of the tracheobronchial tree, the right main stem bronchus is more affected than the left.

Once this entity is suspected, the easiest radiographic examination to perform is inspiratory and expiratory chest films. In patients with a ball valve type of obstruction, air enters the lung but cannot leave. Consequently, on expiration the affected lung remains at full inspiratory size while the normal side diminishes in volume. Because of the decrease in volume on the normal side the heart and mediastinum shift toward that side.

Once the foreign body has been removed, there are seldom any residual problems. However, aspiration of oily peanuts may be accompanied by a chemical pneumonia because of the oil present. These patients should be followed carefully clinically, and if signs of pneumonia develop, a follow-up radiograph should be obtained. If your child insists on eating peanuts, give him the dry-roasted kind. They are less likely to produce a chemical pneumonia if they are aspirated.

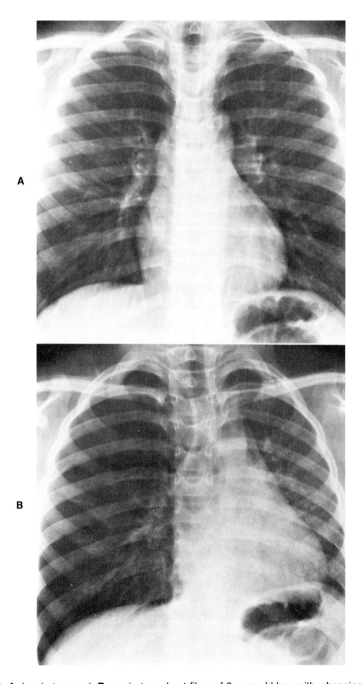

Case 4-3. A, Inspiratory and, **B,** expiratory chest films of 9-year-old boy with wheezing. Can you account for the difference in the appearance?

Case 4-4: COUGH AND WEIGHT LOSS

A 55-year-old white man consulted his family physician because of a persistent cough over a 6-month period. Concomitant with this was a 40-pound weight loss, more marked in the past 2 months. The patient has been a heavy cigarette smoker, consuming two to three packs a day for the past 30 years. He noted having productive, blood-streaked sputum, especially in the morning. Physical examination, aside from showing evidence of weight loss, was unremarkable. A chest radiograph (Case 4-4, A) was obtained. *What are the radiographic findings? What is the diagnosis?*

ROENTGEN DIAGNOSIS AND DISCUSSION

PA and lateral views of the chest show a decrease in the radiability of the left lung compared to the right. In addition, there is an abnormal soft tissue density adjacent to the mediastinum on the left. There is slight tracheal deviation to the left. The left hilum is elevated and appears full; the left hemidiaphragm is elevated. The right lung is clear. On the lateral film there is a zone of increased density in the substernal region (arrows, Case 4-4, B). These arrows represent the oblique fissure on the left, which has shifted anteriorly. The findings are those of classic left upper lobe collapse, which most likely has resulted from an endobronchial occlusion by a carcinoma. *What additional studies would you order?*

Chest tomography of the left hilum and mediastinal region was performed (not shown). This confirmed the presence of a mass within the hilum and demonstrated encroachment of the left upper lobe bronchus. Bronchoscopy revealed an endobronchial mass occluding the lumen. Biopsy of the mass showed squamous cell carcinoma.

A CT scan of the hilum (not shown) was also performed and showed evidence of mediastinal nodal invasion. This was confirmed surgically. A biopsy was performed, and the patient was referred for radiation therapy.

Statistics show that bronchogenic carcinoma is the leading cause of death from cancer in men. The initial presenting complaints may be very nonspecific, with cough the most prominent. Ten percent of patients, however, are asymptomatic, and the lesion is detected on a "routine" chest film (Case 4-4, C). Other patients with apparently normal-appearing chest films may have hemoptysis or positive sputum cytologies.

Pulmonary symptoms are produced by airway obstruction that results in wheezing, obstructive pneumonitis, and dyspnea. Peripheral lesions are usually asymptomatic unless the pleura or chest wall is involved. A classic example of this is the superior sulcus (Pancoast) tumor (Case 4-4, D).

Radiographically, we evaluate these lesions by plain chest radiography, fluoroscopy, tomography, and CT. The radiographic findings reflect the pathologic findings and illustrate pneumonia, atelectasis, and evidence of lobar segmental collapse. Occasionally, cavitation will occur in an area of pneumonia distal to an obstructed segment.

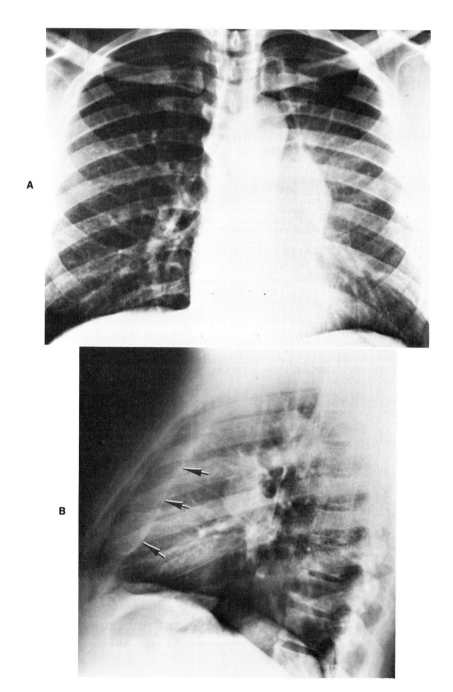

Case 4-4. A, PA and, **B,** lateral films in 55-year-old man with persistent cough. What are the arrows in the lateral film pointing to?

Continued.

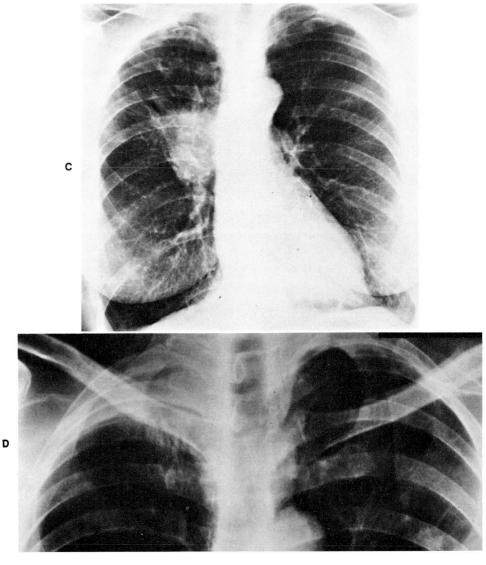

Case 4-4, cont'd. C, Preoperative chest film of woman who was to undergo hysterectomy. There is large carcinoma in right perihilar region. **D,** Superior sulcus (Pancoast) tumor in patient with shoulder pain. Tomography (not shown) revealed erosion of first two ribs.

Case 4-5: RECURRENT PLEURAL EFFUSION

A 65-year-old man was admitted to the hospital for evaluation of recurrent pleural effusion. He was first noted to have a pleural effusion when he consulted his family physician 3 months previously for a "cold." A chest radiograph at that time (Case 4-5, *A*) revealed a large right pleural effusion. The patient was given antibiotics and told to return for a repeat examination in 10 days. This showed no change. Follow-up examinations over the next 2 months similarly showed no change. The admission chest film was similar to that of Case 4-5, *A. What studies can be performed to evaluate patients with persistent recurrent pleural effusion?*

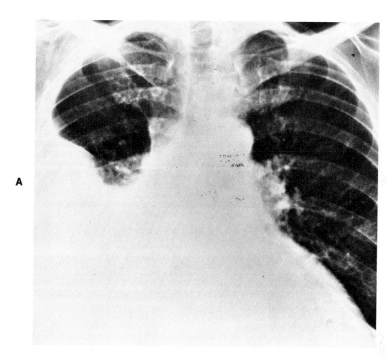

A

Case 4-5. A, PA radiograph in man with cough. There is massive right pleural effusion.

Continued.

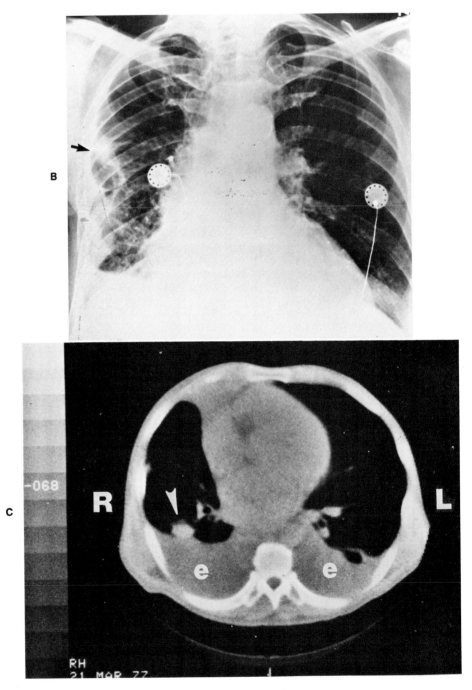

Case 4-5, cont'd. B, Following thoracocentesis, during which 1500 ml of fluid was removed. There is nodular density in right upper lobe (arrow). **C,** CT scan of chest. One of three peripheral nodules is shown (arrowhead). Bilateral effusions *(e)* are present.

ROENTGEN DIAGNOSIS AND DISCUSSION

Pleural effusion is a sign rather than a disease. The effusion may be a transudate, an exudate, pus, blood, chyle, or a combination of these. Until the advent of CT scanning, it was impossible to tell the approximate composition of the effusion by plain radiography. Standard evaluation of recurrent effusion necessitates aspiration of the fluid and cytologic and bacteriologic examination. A thoracocentesis was performed on our patient, and 1500 ml of straw-colored fluid containing malignant cells was removed. A follow-up chest radiograph (Case 4-5, *B*) revealed a nodular density at the margin of the minor fissure. *What additional radiographic studies could be performed to aid in the diagnosis?*

Decubitus films may be performed to determine whether or not the fluid is free flowing. In addition, if the fluid can be made to flow away from an area of lung parenchyma, better visualization of that area may be obtained.

CT is of value in evaluating these lesions, as illustrated in Case 4-5, *C*. The study was performed on this patient and demonstrated three peripheral pulmonary nodules. The pleural effusion is seen as a separate density surrounding the lung. The fluid had a density measurement (CT number) near that of water (0). If the fluid was pus, it would have a CT number higher than water (8 to 12); if it were blood, the number would be higher still. Chyle, which contains fat, would have a CT number below that of water (-10 to -40).

This patient subsequently underwent surgery. The nodules were shown to represent metastatic foci of squamous cell carcinoma from a central endobronchial lesion.

References

Armstrong, J. D., and Bragg, D. G.: Radiology in lung cancer: problems and prospects, CA **25**:242, 1975.

Berkmen, Y. M., and Javors, B. R.: Anterior mediastinal lymphadenopathy in sarcoidosis, Am. J. Roentgenol. **127**:983, 1976.

Daffner, R. H., Gehweiler, J. A., and Carden, T. S., Jr.: Case studies in radiology, New York, 1975, Appleton-Century-Crofts.

Felson, B.: Chest roentgenology, Philadelphia, 1973, W. B. Saunders Co.

Fraser, R. G., and Paré, J. A. P.: Diagnosis of diseases of the chest, vol. 1-4, ed. 2, Philadelphia, vol. 1, 1977, vol. 2-4, 1978, W. B. Saunders Co.

Heitzman, E. R.: The lung: radiologic-pathologic correlations, St. Louis, 1973, The C. V. Mosby Co.

Heitzman, E. R.: The mediastinum: radiologic correlations with anatomy and pathology, St. Louis, 1977, The C. V. Mosby Co.

Higgins, G. A., Shields, T. W., and Keehn, R. J.: The solitary pulmonary nodule. Ten year follow-up of Veterans Administration–Armed Forces cooperative study, Arch. Surg. **110**:570, 1975.

Janower, M. L., and Blennerhassett, J. B.: Lymphangitic spread of metastatic cancer to the lung. A radiologic-pathologic classification, Radiology **110**:267, 1971.

Johnson, T. H., Jr., Gajaraj, A., and Feist, J. H.: Patterns of pulmonary interstitial disease, Am. J. Roentgenol. **109**:516, 1970.

Jost, R. G., Sagel, S. S., Stanley, R. J., and Levitt, R. G.: Computed tomography of the thorax, Radiology **126**:125, 1978.

Kelley, M. J., and Elliott, L. P.: Radiologic evaluation of the patient with suspected pulmonary thromboembolic disease, Primary Care **3**:145, 1976.

McCreary, C. B.: Tuberculosis control in India, Dis. Chest **53**:699, 1968.

Moser, K. M.: Pulmonary embolism, Am. Rev. Respir. Dis. **115**:829, 1977.

Nathan, M. H.: Management of solitary pulmonary nodules. An organized approach based on growth rate and statistics, J.A.M.A. **227**:1141, 1974.

Neifeld, J. P., Michaelis, L. L., and Doppman, J. L.: Suspected pulmonary metastases. Correlation of chest x-ray, whole lung tomograms, and operative findings, Cancer **39**:383, 1977.

Ray, J. F. III, Lawton, B. R., Magnin, G. E., Doverbarger, W. V., Smullen, W. A., Reyes, C. N., Myers, W. O., Wenzel, F. J., and Sautter, R. D.: The coin lesion story: update 1976. Twenty years experience with early thoracotomy for 179 suspected malignant coin lesions, Chest **70**:332, 1976.

Reed, M. H.: Radiology of airway foreign bodies in children, J. Can. Assoc. Radiol. **28**:111, 1977.

Reeder, M. M., and Hochholzer, L.: Large (>4 cm) solitary pulmonary mass, J.A.M.A. **229**:1493, 1974.

Reeder, M. M., and Reed, J. C.: Solitary pulmonary nodule (<4 cm in diameter), J.A.M.A. **231**:1080, 1975.

Reid, L.: The lung: its growth and remodelling in health and disease, Am. J. Roentgenol. **129:**777, 1977.

Reimann, H. A.: Problems in the control of tuberculosis, Dis. Chest **53:**670, 1968.

Rigler, L. G.: An overview of cancer of the lung, Semin. Roentgenol. **12:**161, 1977.

Sagel, S. S.: Special procedures in chest roentgenology, Philadelphia, 1976, W. B. Saunders Co.

Stead, W. W.: The iceberg of medicine: tuberculosis. Radiol. Clin. North Am. **3:**299, 1965.

Stead, W. W., Kirby, G. R., Schleuter, E. P., and Jordahl, C. W.: The clinical spectrum of primary tuberculosis in adults: confusion with reinfection in the pathogenesis of chronic tuberculosis, Ann. Intern. Med. **68:**731, 1968.

Theros, E. G.: Varying manifestations of peripheral pulmonary neoplasms: radiologic-pathologic correlative study, Am. J. Roentgenol. **128:**893, 1977.

Thurlbeck, W. M., and Simon, G.: Radiographic appearance of the chest in emphysema, Am. J. Roentgenol. **130:**429, 1978.

5 Cardiac radiology

Cardiovascular radiology is a subspecialty shared by radiologists and cardiologists. Too often the clinician is content to merely have made a diagnosis of "large heart," "congestive heart failure," or "congenital heart disease." It is possible, however, for you as the clinician to recognize certain patterns of disease based on the alterations those diseases produce in the pulmonary vascularity and in specific chambers of the heart. This chapter, then, will examine the criteria for certain *categories* of diseases rather than discuss specific entities. For a complete discussion of those entities, you are referred to a comprehensive text on cardiology.

TECHNICAL CONSIDERATIONS

The same technical considerations that were discussed for pulmonary disease apply to evaluation of the cardiovascular system. You should first decide if the film was a PA or AP view, if the patient is lordotic, and if rotation is present. The degree of penetration on the film, the presence of motion, and the degree of inspiration are all important factors to consider. A film made with the patient in a slightly lordotic position will falsely distort and magnify the cardiac size. A film that is too light will accentuate the pulmonary vessels; a film with the patient not in maximum inspiration may result in further accentuation of pulmonary vessels and cause an appearance of cardiac enlargement and/or an erroneous diagnosis of congestive heart failure (Fig. 5-1).

It is also necessary to pay close attention to the patient's body habitus. A narrow AP diameter of the chest or a pectus excavatum deformity may result in posterior compression of the heart and a spurious appearance of cardiac enlargement (Fig. 5-2).

In the bony thorax, particular attention should be given to the undersurfaces of the ribs for any evidence of rib notching. Although the most common cause of rib notching is coarctation of the aorta, the reader should keep in mind that many other conditions produce this abnormality. The following outline lists causes of rib notching.

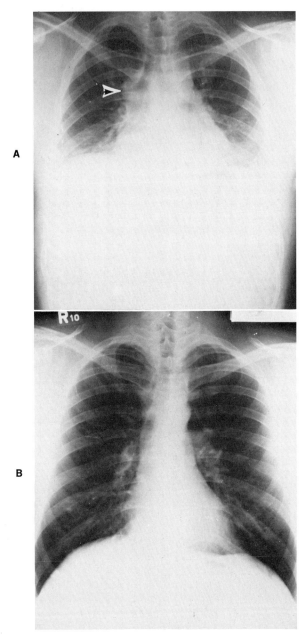

Fig. 5-1. A, Expiratory chest film. Heart appears enlarged. There is prominence of azygos vein (arrowhead). Pulmonary vasculature is prominent as well. This patient could easily be misdiagnosed as being in congestive heart failure. **B,** Full inspiratory film in same patient. (From Daffner, R. H., Gehweiler, J. A., and Carden, T. S., Jr.: Case studies in radiology, New York, 1975, Appleton-Century-Crofts. Reproduced with permission of the publisher.)

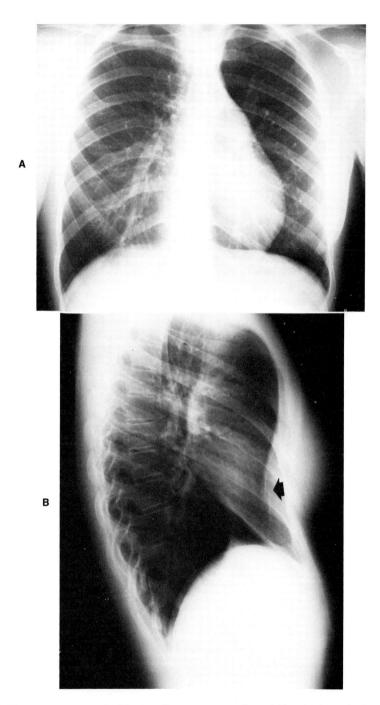

Fig. 5-2. Pectus excavatum. **A,** PA view. Heart appears enlarged. Note horizontal orientation of ribs in posterior portion and more vertical orientation anteriorly. **B,** Lateral view shows narrow PA diameter of chest. Arrow points to pectus deformity.

CAUSES OF RIB NOTCHING

I. Arterial factors
  A. High aortic obstruction
    1. Coarctation of the aorta
  B. Low aortic obstruction
    1. Aortic thrombosis
  C. Subclavian or brachiocephalic
    obstruction
    1. Blalock-Taussig operation
    2. Pulseless (Takayashu) disease
  D. Bronchial flow to lungs in pulmo-
    nary oligemia
    1. Tetralogy of Fallot
    2. Absent pulmonary artery
    3. Pulmonary valvular stenosis
    4. Pseudotruncus arteriosus
    5. Emphysema
    6. Pulmonary hypertension
    7. Pulmonary sequestration

II. Venous factors
  A. Superior vena cava obstruction
  B. Obstruction of brachiocephalic or
    subclavian veins
III. Arteriovenous communication
  A. AV fistula of chest wall
  B. Pulmonary AV fistula
IV. Neurogenic factors
  A. Neurofibromatosis
V. Miscellaneous
  A. Extramedullary hematopoiesis
  B. Idiopathic disease
  C. Normal

There are six basic imaging techniques used for evaluation of the heart: (1) plain film radiography, (2) cardiac fluoroscopy, (3) cardiac series, (4) cardiac catheterization and coronary arteriography (angiocardiography), (5) echocardiography, and (6) radioisotope studies.

Plain film radiography is a standard screening examination in patients with suspected cardiac disease. By knowing the normal anatomy portrayed on the PA and lateral films and by analyzing the pulmonary arteries and veins, you may be able to make a correct diagnosis in the majority of cases.

A popular method used to determine cardiac size is the cardiothoracic ratio: the maximum width of the cardiac shadow on the PA chest film divided by the maximum width of the thorax. This method has received criticism, since a true determination of cardiac enlargement necessitates evaluation of the cardiac silhouette on *both* the PA and lateral views. As a rule of thumb, however, the cardiac width should never exceed half the width of the thorax on the PA film.

Fluoroscopic examination of the heart and pulmonary vessels is used for (1) an assessment of cardiac motion and dynamics (useful for evaluation of cardiac aneurysms), (2) investigation of intracardiac calcifications (valvular, coronary artery, or pericardial), and (3) assessment of patients with suspected pericardial effusion (dampened pulsations and displaced subepicardial fat line).

The *cardiac series* is a four-view examination consisting of PA, lateral, and right anterior oblique views with the patient drinking barium and a left anterior oblique view without barium. Barium is used to determine whether or not specific chamber enlargement impinges on the esophagus. The anatomic relationships will be discussed in the next section.

Cardiac catheterization and coronary arteriography are sophisticated procedures performed almost exclusively by cardiologists or cardiac radiologists. These procedures allow accurate evaluation of the size and configuration of the cardiac chambers, the great vessels, and the coronary arteries. They are also used to evaluate patients with suspected shunt lesions.

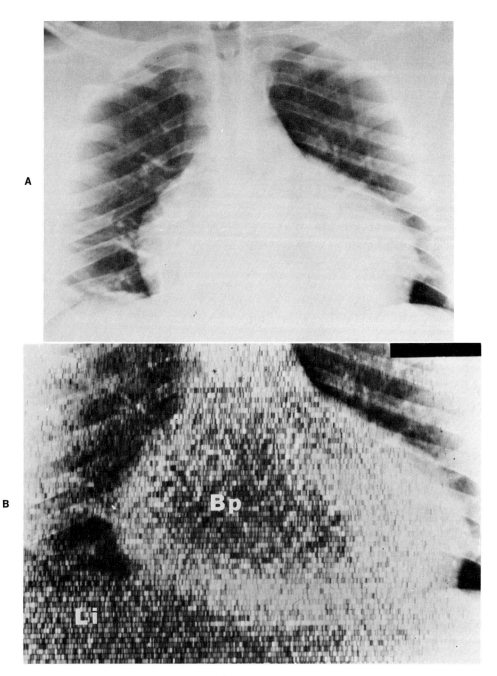

Fig. 5-3. Pericardial effusion. **A,** Chest film shows enlargement of cardiac silhouette. **B,** Liver/lung scan superimposed over chest radiograph. Cardiac blood pool *(Bp)* shows actual cardiac size to be smaller than cardiac silhouette. Clear area surrounding blood pool is pericardial effusion. *Li,* Liver.

Echocardiography is an ultrasound examination of the heart using the M mode. The most common indications are abnormalities of the valves, abnormalities of contractility, and suspected pericardial effusion. The study is performed primarily by cardiologists.

Radioisotope studies are also used to evaluate patients suspected of having a pericardial effusion. They are performed by injecting an isotope tagged to serum albumin, which acts as a blood pool agent. The patient is scanned on a rectilinear scanner, and the scan is superimposed on a radiograph made with the patient in the same position. If the scan picture completely fills the cardiac silhouette on the radiograph, the patient has no effusion. If, however, the scan shows a smaller blood pool in the cardiac silhouette, an enlarged pericardial space is indicated (Fig. 5-3). Myocardial scanning for localization of infarcts is another type of radioisotopic study that is being investigated for clinical application.

At the time of this writing, investigators are studying imaging the heart with CT scans. This promises to be a valuable adjunct in the future.

ANATOMIC CONSIDERATIONS

For an appreciation for the anatomic relationships of the heart and its chambers, it is necessary to think in three-dimensional terms. Let us examine the position of the cardiac chambers, the great vessels, and the aortic and mitral valves as seen in the four-view cardiac series (Fig. 5-4).

On the PA view the bulk of the cardiac silhouette is made up almost exclusively of the right side of the heart; the left ventricle forms the left cardiac border. The position of the anterior interventricular sulcus may be determined on an angiocardiogram by following the course of the anterior descending branch of the left coronary artery. The right atrium forms the right border of the heart, merging imperceptibly into the shadow of the superior vena cava. The left atrium is not seen under normal circumstances in this view. However, a small portion of the left border of the heart just beneath the pulmonary trunk is represented by the left atrial appendage. In this view the aortic valve is positioned obliquely, with its lower end pointing to the right, approximately in the midline just below the waist of the cardiovascular silhouette (Fig. 5-4, *A*). The mitral valve, which is oriented on a similar plane in this view, lies just below the aortic valve area and to the left.

In the normal lateral view (Fig. 5-4, *B*) the anterior border of the cardiac silhouette consists of the right ventricle. The posterior and inferior cardiac border is that of the left ventricle. The shadow of the inferior vena cava superimposes on the posteroinferior border of the left ventricle, occasionally extending just posterior to the left ventricular outline. The left atrium forms the superoposterior border of the heart. The barium-filled esophagus courses almost immediately posterior to the cardiac silhouette. It should not be indented by the heart under normal circumstances. Occasionally the shadow of the pulmonary artery may be seen arcing up from the right ventricle and passing inferiorly to the arch of the aorta, which is also visible on the lateral film. In this view the aortic valve lies almost horizontally just below the narrow waist of the cardiovascular pedicle. The mitral valve ring lies in an oblique plane, as indicated in Fig. 5-4, *B*, inferiorly and posterior to that of the aortic valve.

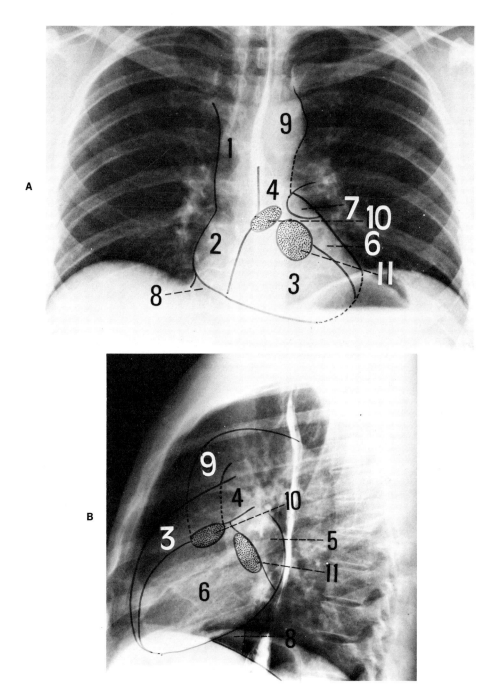

Fig. 5-4. Normal cardiac series. **A,** PA view. **B,** Lateral view.

Continued.

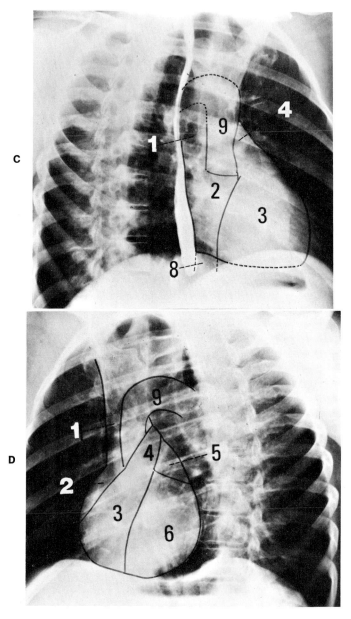

Fig. 5-4, cont'd. C, RAO view. **D,** LAO view. *1,* Superior vena cava; *2,* right atrium; *3,* right ventricle; *4,* pulmonary outflow tract; *5,* left atrium; *6,* left ventricle; *7,* left atrial appendage; *8,* inferior vena cava; *9,* aorta; *10,* aortic valve; *11,* mitral valve.

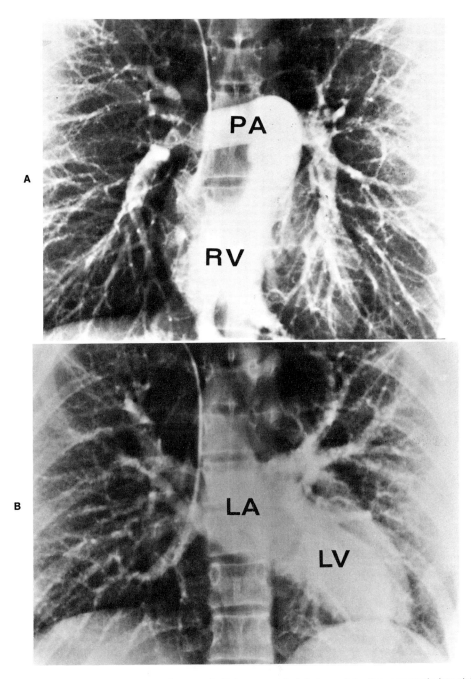

Fig. 5-5. Normal pulmonary arteriogram. **A,** Pulmonary arterial phase. Injection was made into right ventricle *(RV)*. Contrast material passes through pulmonary outflow tract into pulmonary arteries *(PA)*. **B,** Venous phase. Contrast material passes from pulmonary veins into left atrium *(LA)* and then into left ventricle *(LV)*. Note difference in orientation between pulmonary arteries and pulmonary veins.

In the right anterior oblique (RAO) view (Fig. 5-4, C) the bulk of the cardiac silhouette consists of the right ventricle. The left ventricle contributes a small portion to the cardiac silhouette over the apex anteriorly. The right cardiac border consists of the right atrium inferiorly and the left atrium superiorly. In this view the barium-filled esophagus is intimately associated with the posterior aspect of the cardiac silhouette. Once again the esophagus should not be indented in any way; if this occurs, it indicates an enlarged left atrium.

In the left anterior oblique (LAO) position (Fig. 5-4, D), all the cardiac chambers contribute to the cardiac silhouette. Only a small segment of the upper portion of the right heart border is formed by the right atrial appendage; the rest are delineated by the right ventricle. On the left side the lower border is exclusively left ventricle. The left atrium forms the upper portion of the left silhouette. Under normal circumstances the shadow of the left ventricle should not overlap that of the thoracic spine by more than 1 cm. Any overlap greater than this indicates left ventricular enlargement. A small "clear" aerated area may be seen just above the border of the left atrium. In patients with left atrial enlargement, this area "fills in." Barium is not used in the LAO view.

One additional useful anatomic relationship is that of the main stem bronchi to the heart. The trachea bifurcates below the aortic arch. The bronchi continue downward and branch from this point. The left main stem bronchus, however, has a close relationship with the left atrium. Consequently, enlargements of the left atrium may result in elevation of the left main stem bronchus, widening the normal carinal angle above 75 degrees in adults; greater angulation is allowed for infants and children.

The pulmonary arteries and veins constitute the lung markings seen on a chest

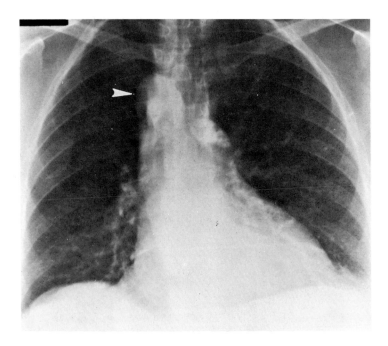

Fig. 5-6. Right aortic arch (arrowhead).

radiograph. It is sometimes difficult to differentiate between arteries and veins on the radiograph. However, a useful method is by analyzing the direction of the vessels to determine whether or not they are arterial or venous. Under normal circumstances the pulmonary arteries radiate out from the hilar region in a fairly uniform fanlike appearance (Fig. 5-5, *A*). The veins, on the other hand, follow a different course because of the lower location of the left atrium, into which they must terminate. The upper lobe veins assume an obliquely downward course, in some instances almost vertical, as they "dive" for the left atrium; the lower lobe veins assume a more horizontal course, located almost directly opposite the level of the left atrium (Fig. 5-5, *B*). It is important to be able to differentiate arteries from veins, since the proposed approach for diagnosis is based on analysis of the pulmonary vasculature.

Under normal circumstances the vascularity of the lower lobes is more prominent than that of the upper lobes. In normal individuals, this relationship is altered in the recumbent position, where gravity would allow a greater flow to the cephalic regions.

Finally, it is important to note on which side the aortic arch is located and the position of the gastric bubble. Under normal circumstances the aortic arch is on the left. However, there are anomalies of this vessel in which the arch is on the right (Fig. 5-6). Under ordinary circumstances the gastric air bubble is on the left. However, in patients with certain forms of situs inversus and dextrocardia the gastric bubble may be seen on the right.

PATHOLOGIC CONSIDERATIONS

There are many ways to classify cardiac disease. A popular classification uses two large categories: congenital and acquired cardiac disease. Congenital cardiac disease is further subdivided into cyanotic and acyanotic types. Most books on cardiology prefer this method. For the noncardiologist, a *physiologic* approach affords an understandable and useful basis for dealing with congenital and acquired heart disease. In addition to this physiologic approach, it is preferable to evaluate patients with cardiac disease on the basis of their age, that is, adult or pediatric.

Adult patients

From a physiologic standpoint, all types of cardiac disease may be categorized into the following:
  I. Obstruction
 II. Volume overload
     A. Shunt (right-to-left, left-to-right)
     B. Admixture
     C. Valvar insufficiency
III. Disorders of contraction or relazation
     A. Myocardial disease
     B. Conduction disorders (arrhythmias)
 IV. Combination of the preceding

Evaluation of the pulmonary vascularity is an important step that enables exclusion of many diseases. The *physiologic* type of disease may be inferred from the pattern of pulmonary blood flow. Pulmonary vascularity may be normal, decreased, or increased. Fig. 5-7 illustrates the varying forms of pulmonary blood flow and lists some important disease processes that accompany those patterns. The normal size of pulmonary vessels should be about the same as the size of an accompanying airway. Any significant disparity in size is abnormal (Fig. 5-8).

	PATTERN			
DISTRIBUTION	Normal	Decreased	Increased	
	Arterial and venous	Arterial and venous	Predominantly arterial	Predominantly venous
Normal 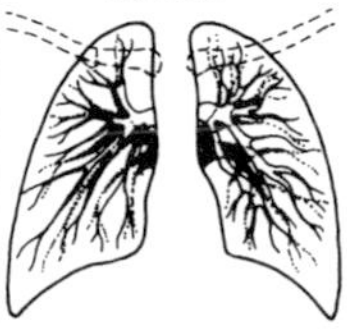 — Apex less than base	Normal	Tetralogy of Fallot or other right-sided obstructive lesion	Left-to-right shunts Systemic AV shunts Hyperkinetic circulatory state Transposition of great vessels without pulmonary stenosis Truncus arteriosus type	
Cephalization 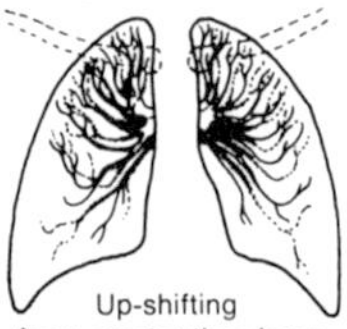 — Up-shifting Apex greater than base		Same as above with prominent bronchial collateral circulation	Same as above with left ventricular failure (PVO)	Left ventricular failure of any cause (PVO)
Centralization 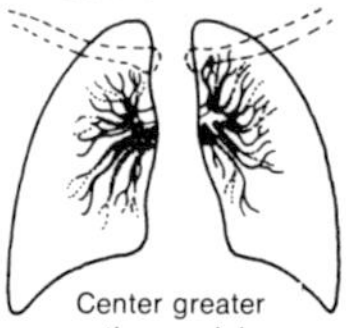 — Center greater than periphery	Pulmonary hypertension	Severe pulmonary emphysema Chronic (diffuse) pulmonary thromboembolic disease Eisenmenger syndrome	Left-to-right shunt with pulmonary hypertension Cor pulmonale with high cardiac output	Acute pulmonary edema of any etiology
Lateralization 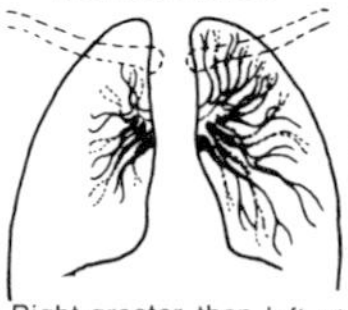 — Right greater than left or right less than left	Pulmonic stenosis with intact ventricular septum Proximal interruption of one pulmonary artery without shunt Swyer-James syndrome	Pulmonary hypoplasia Tetralogy of Fallot after palliative shunting precedure (Blalock, Potts, Glenn, Waterston)	Multiple congenital anomalies produce this pattern	Left atrial myxoma or mural thrombi causing local pulmonary edema
Localization 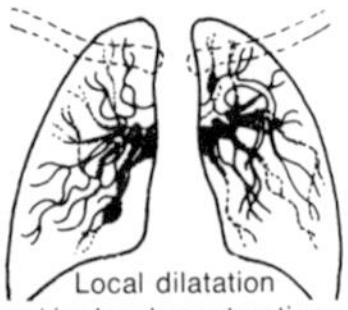 — Local dilatation and/or local construction or abnormal course of vessel	Pulmonary emboli Pulmonary stenosis of peripheral vessels	Same as normal and decreased flow	Anomalous pulmonary drainage Also multiple other types of congenital heart disease	Same as normal Severe tetralogy with bronchial flow to one area

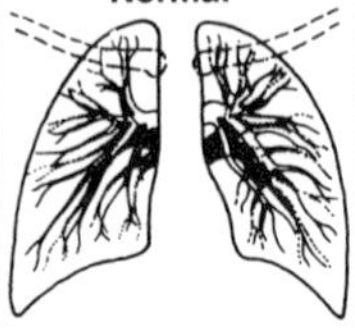

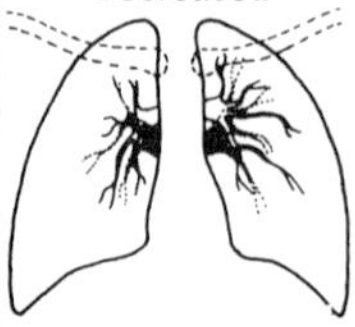

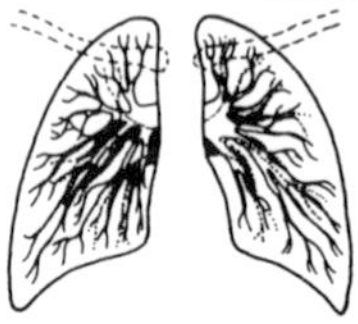

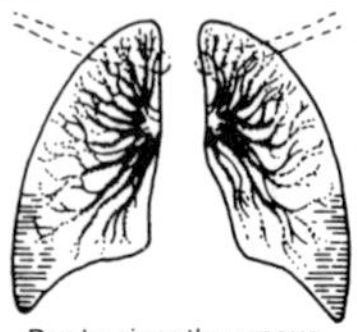

Fig. 5-7. Correlation of pulmonary vascular patterns, distribution, and diseases that produce these patterns.

Surprising as it may seem, patients with normal pulmonary vascularity may have significant cardiac disease. In these patients the heart has compensated for the abnormality by enlarging. The pulmonary vascularity remains normal until the heart decompensates. Diseases that produce cardiac chamber enlargement without appreciable change in the pulmonary vascularity until decompensation occurs include cardiomyopathy, coronary artery disease, hypertensive cardiovascular disease, aortic stenosis, and coarctation of the aorta. All these conditions except coarctation and a form of aortic stenosis are acquired.

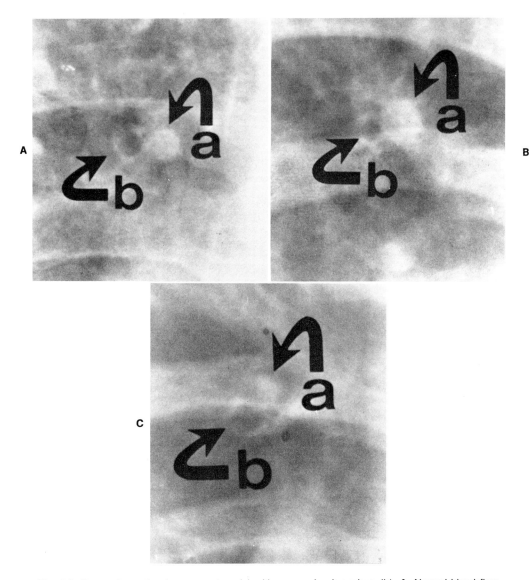

Fig. 5-8. Comparison of pulmonary artery *(a)* with companion bronchus *(b)*. **A,** Normal blood flow. Artery and bronchus are approximately equal in size. **B,** Shunt vascularity (increased arterial flow). Artery is larger than bronchus in this patient with atrial septal defect. **C,** Diminished pulmonary arterial flow. Artery is smaller than bronchus in this patient with tetralogy of Fallot.

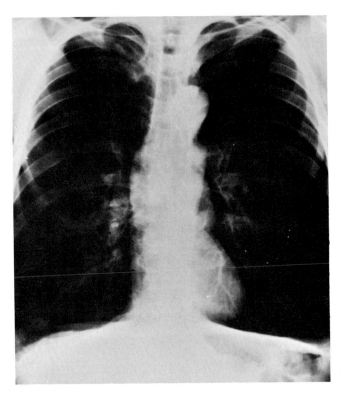

Fig. 5-9. Generalized decreased pulmonary vascularity in patient with severe bullous emphysema. This is not overpenetrated film. Large amount of air within emphysematous lungs has resulted in extremely black-appearing lung fields.

Decreased vascularity indicates a severe obstruction to the outflow of blood from the right ventricle, usually at the pulmonic valve or subvalvar level. These patients are often visibly cyanotic. If the decreased vascularity is of a diffuse nature, a congenital anomaly is most likely. This pattern is seldom seen in the adult, since the abnormalities that produce this pattern will result in the patient's death unless corrective surgery is performed during childhood.

Decreased vascularity may be apparent locally or unilaterally. A local decrease in vascularity may be the result of pulmonary embolism (Westermark sign), emphysema (Fig. 5-9), or scarring with rearrangement of vessels in a lung. A unilateral decrease in vascularity without changes in the cardiac size may result from either hypoplasia of a lung or the Swyer-James syndrome (Fig. 5-10).

Increased vascularity is of four types: (1) shunts, (2) pulmonary venous obstruction, (3) precapillary hypertension, and (4) high output state.

Shunts represent an increased flow through the pulmonary bed. They are characterized by large vessels in the upper and lower lobes. In patients with shunt who are not in congestive heart failure the redistribution of blood will be in the same proportion as that occurring normally: greater to the lung bases than to the upper lobes. This vascular pattern is most commonly seen in a left-to-right shunt at the cardiac or great vessel level (septal defect or patent ductus arteriosus). This pattern

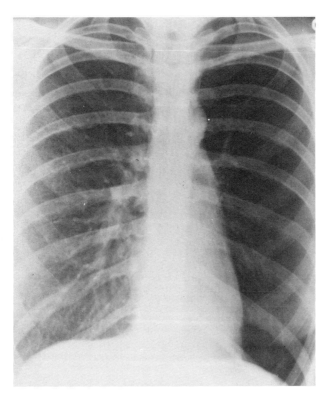

Fig. 5-10. Diffuse decrease in pulmonary vasculature in patient with unilateral hyperlucent lung (Swyer-James syndrome). Compare vessels in this patient's normal right side and abnormal left side.

is uncommon in adults, since the condition is usually diagnosed and treated in childhood (Fig. 5-11).

Patients with pulmonary venous obstruction (PVO) demonstrate large veins in the upper lobe as a reflection of reversal of the normal flow pattern. This indicates increased left atrial pressure. Severe PVO is manifest by pulmonary edema and prominent interlobular septal (Kerley) lines (Fig. 5-12).

Patients with precapillary hypertension (pulmonary arterial hypertension) have large central vessels that taper rapidly into small vessels peripherally. This is referred to as centralized flow and occurs in patients with severe pulmonary disease, recurrent pulmonary embolism (Fig. 5-13), and Eisenmenger phenomenon.

Once the pulmonary vascular pattern is decided on, look at the heart to determine if specific chamber enlargements are present. If there is evidence of left atrial enlargement (with or without PVO), rheumatic heart disease (mitral stenosis) or an obstruction at or proximal to the mitral valve is present (Fig. 5-14). If there is evidence of left ventricular enlargement with a "concavity" in the area of the main pulmonary artery, the disease is one of left ventricular stress (Fig. 5-15): hypertensive cardiovascular disease, coronary artery disease, aortic stenosis, and coarctation of the aorta.

PVO plus left ventricular configuration (LVC) equals left ventricular stress with

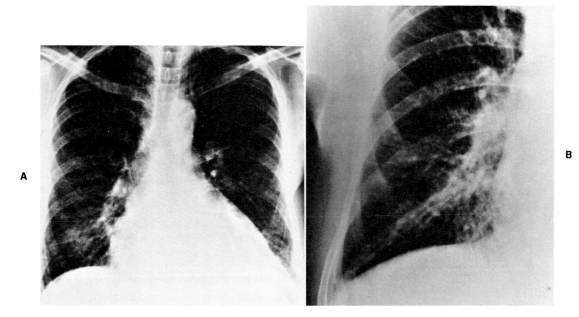

Fig. 5-11. Shunt vascularity in patient with atrial septal defect. **A,** PA view shows prominent pulmonary vessels. **B,** Lateral view shows right ventricular prominence in substernal region.

Fig. 5-12. Congestive heart failure with septal (Kerley) lines. **A,** PA view of chest shows cardiac enlargement. Pulmonary venous engorgement is present. Interstitial edema causing fine haze, best seen in lung bases, is present. **B,** Detail view of lower lung fields in another patient with congestive heart failure demonstrates septal lines, which are seen as fine linear striations near periphery.

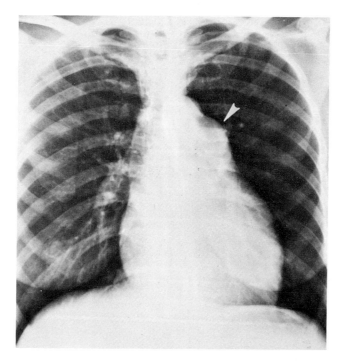

Fig. 5-13. Pulmonary arterial hypertension in patient with recurrent pulmonary emboli. There is prominence of main pulmonary artery near outflow tract on left (arrowhead). Right main stem pulmonary artery is enlarged and tapers rapidly in periphery, a sign of pulmonary arterial hypertension.

failure. All the preceding conditions occur with this pattern. It is possible to further narrow the list of causes in this situation by scanning the film for evidence of rib notching and/or decreased size of the aortic knob, as in aortic coarctation (Fig. 5-16), or for calcification in or about the aortic valve region (Fig. 5-17), as in calcific aortic stenosis.

A high output state, such as severe anemia or thyrotoxicosis, may have increased vascularity with a normal distribution as a result of the increased volume being pumped through the heart. The heart itself may be normal or slightly enlarged as a result of this increased activity.

Pediatric patients

Cardiac disease in pediatric patients is usually congenital. However, rheumatic heart disease is an important form of acquired disease that may be seen in this age group.

Before beginning an analysis of the pulmonary vascularity in pediatric patients, it is important to know whether or not they are visibly cyanotic. The presence of visible cyanosis changes the physiologic state of the patient and the category of disease. It is also important to know whether the cyanosis was present at birth (as in transposition of great vessels) or developed later (as in tetralogy of Fallot). Plain film analysis will be considered in both circumstances: the acyanotic patient and the cyanotic patient.

• • •

Text continued on p. 147.

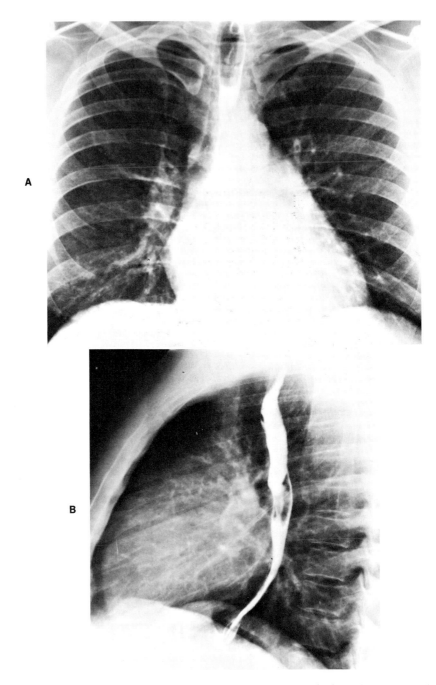

Fig. 5-14. Mitral stenosis. Cardiac series showing typical changes of left atrial enlargement in mitral stenosis. See text for description of changes. **A,** PA view. **B,** Lateral view.

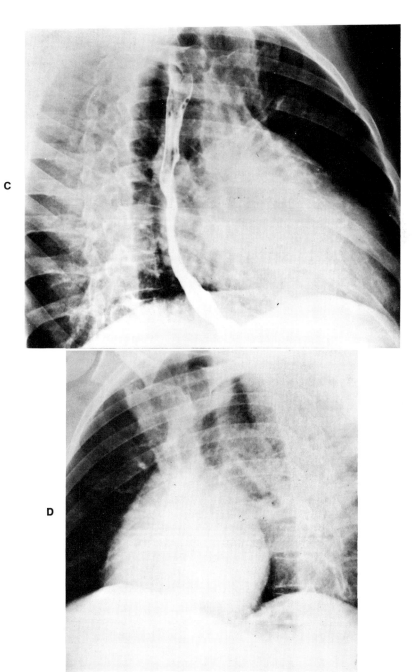

Fig. 5-14, cont'd. C, RAO view. **D,** LAO view.

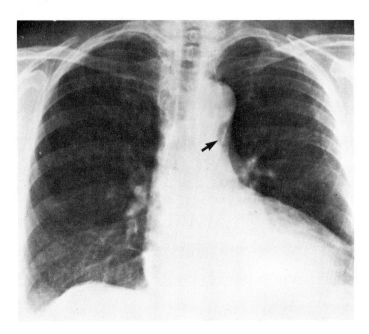

Fig. 5-15. Hypertensive cardiovascular disease. There is left ventricular prominence and slight increase in tortuosity of aorta at its arch. Note calcification within descending aorta (arrow).

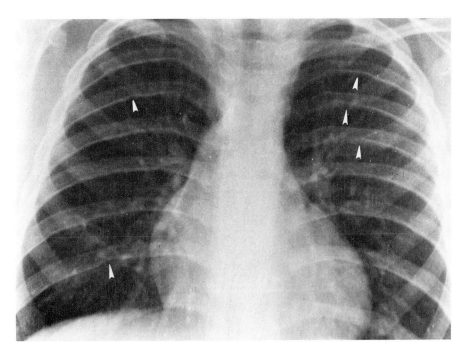

Fig. 5-16. Coarctation of aorta in 9-year-old child. There is definite left ventricular configuration of heart. Aortic knob is small. Rib notching (arrowheads) is present on undersurfaces of multiple ribs.

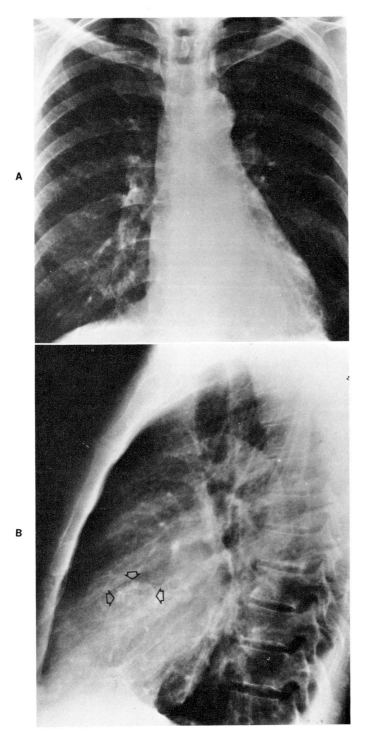

Fig. 5-17. Calcific aortic stenosis. **A,** PA view shows left ventricular configuration. **B,** Calcification in aortic ring is present (open arrows).

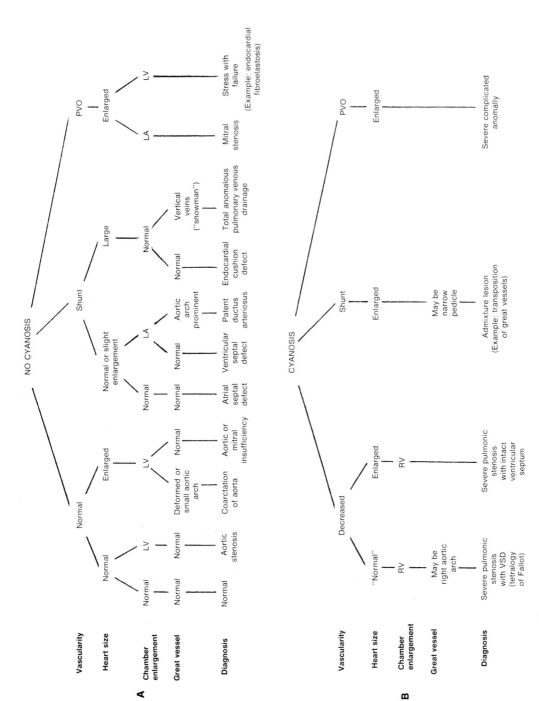

Fig. 5-18. Flow charts for radiographic diagnosis of cardiac disease. **A,** Acyanotic patient. **B,** Cyanotic patient.

Fig. 5-18 is a flow sheet that summarizes the analyses necessary in the diagnosis of cardiac disease.

Acyanotic patients

If the vascularity is normal, it is necessary to rely on the heart size and configuration and the appearance of the great vessels to provide clues to the etiology of the suspected cardiac disease. A normal heart size does not rule out a heart lesion. A mild or compensated lesion may be accompanied by a normal-appearing heart on plain radiographs. Furthermore, an obstructive lesion may cause hypertrophy but not enlarge the heart enough to be detectable on the chest roentgenogram. A diagnosis of left or right ventricular *hypertrophy* is an electrocardiographic and not a radiographic diagnosis. Radiography identifies chamber *enlargements*, not hypertrophy.

Left ventricular configuration in a child indicates a left-sided obstructive lesion such as aortic stenosis or coarctation of the aorta (Fig. 5-19). The left ventricular configuration may be normal in adults but is always abnormal in children.

A prominent main pulmonary artery or proximal left pulmonary artery segment suggests a right-sided obstructive lesion: pulmonic valvar stenosis with poststenotic dilatation (Fig. 5-20). If the peripheral vascularity is normal, the degree of stenosis is not severe.

In patients with enlarged hearts but normal vascularity, volume overload most likely caused by valvar insufficiency may be inferred. Volume overload dilates the involved cardiac chambers without causing increased pressure until cardiac failure

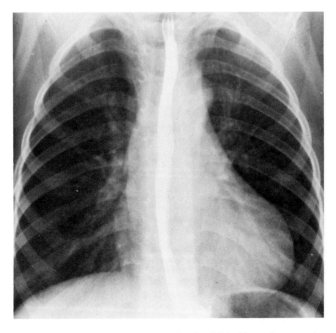

Fig. 5-19. Left ventricular configuration in child with aortic stenosis.

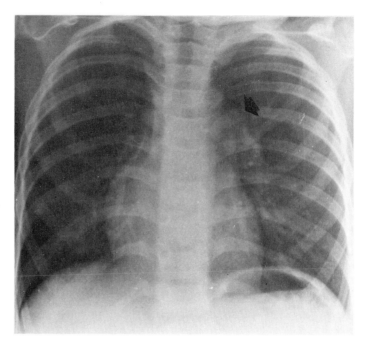

Fig. 5-20. Pulmonic stenosis in child. There is prominence of left main pulmonary artery near outflow tract caused by "jet phenomenon" (arrow).

occurs. A left ventricular configuration (indicating left ventricular stress) with an enlarged heart suggests aortic or mitral insufficiency (Fig. 5-21). In mitral insufficiency, volume overload occurs in the left atrium as well, and this may be detected on plain films or on the cardiac series as a bulge along the left cardiac border (indicating displacement of the left atrial appendage); a double density seen on the PA film, representing the enlarged left atrium itself; splaying of the carinal angle greater than 75 degrees; and impingement on the barium-filled esophagus. These findings are illustrated in Fig. 5-22, a patient with mitral stenosis and insufficiency.

The preceding findings are summarized as follows:

1. Normal vascularity + Normal size heart = Normal or "mild anything"
2. Normal vascularity + Left ventricular configuration (overall heart size normal) = Left ventricular obstructive lesion without heart failure
3. Normal vascularity + Prominent main pulmonary artery = Right ventricular obstructive lesion
4. Normal vascularity + Big heart = Volume overload lesion, valvar insufficiency type

As mentioned previously, a generalized increase in the size of the pulmonary arteries throughout the lungs indicates either a left-to-right shunt or a hyperdynamic state such as thyrotoxicosis or large systemic arteriovenous (AV) fistula. In the pediatric age group the most common lesion to produce this pattern is a shunt, the most common type of congenital lesion.

Once shunt vascularity is identified, the size of the left atrium is used to determine the level of the shunt. An enlarged left atrium (LAE) indicates that the atrial septum is intact (LAE results from the increased pulmonary venous return). In this situation the shunt must be distal to the AV valves, as in a ventricular septal defect (VSD) (Fig. 5-23) or patent ductus arteriosus (PDA).

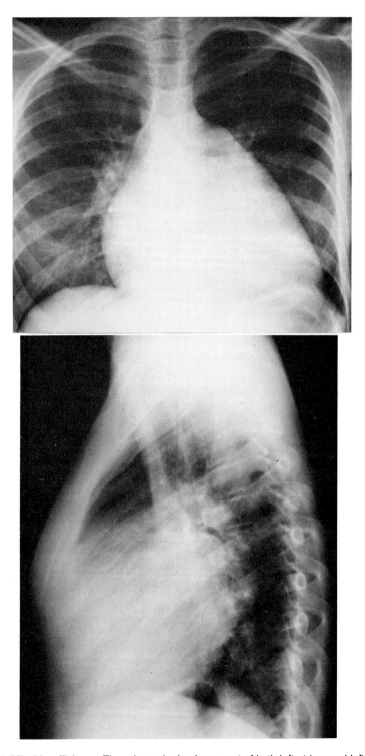

Fig. 5-21. Mitral insufficiency. There is marked enlargement of both left atrium and left ventricle.

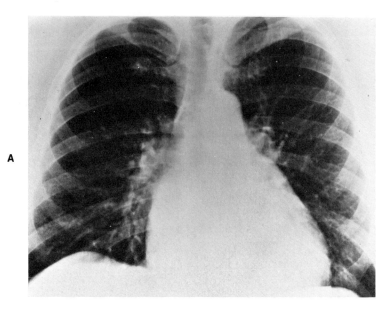

Fig. 5-22. Mitral stenosis and insufficiency. When these two lesions are combined, there is greater cardiomegaly than in isolated lesion. **A,** PA view.

Shunt vascularity without atrial enlargement indicates an atrial septal defect (ASD) (Fig. 5-11). In this situation the excess blood flows immediately into the lower pressure right atrium, resulting in no net volume overload of the left atrium. In a patient with an isolated ASD the heart is either normal in size or mildly enlarged. Shunt vascularity coupled with marked cardiomegaly indicates a complicated ASD.

These findings are summarized as follows:

1. Shunt vascularity + Left atrial enlargement = Shunt distal to AV valves
2. Shunt vascularity + Normal-sized left atrium = ASD
3. Shunt vascularity + Normal-sized left atrium + Big heart = Complicated ASD

Severe pulmonary venous obstruction in the newborn usually occurs in patients with cyanotic congenital heart disease. However, cardiac failure may occur in very young children in the presence of large systemic AV fistulae. Interestingly enough, because infants spend most of their hours in a recumbent position, the pulmonary blood flow is equally distributed throughout the lungs and the adult pattern of PVO —a redistribution to the upper lobes—is therefore not seen. The older a child becomes, however, the closer the picture is to the adult pattern of PVO.

As in the adult, once a pattern of PVO is recognized, attention should be directed to the cardiac configuration to determine the level of the obstruction. If the heart is triangular in shape, that is, having a prominent bulge along the left cardiac border, and there is evidence of LAE, the obstruction is at or proximal to the mitral valve. The most common etiology of this situation is rheumatic heart disease. Remember,

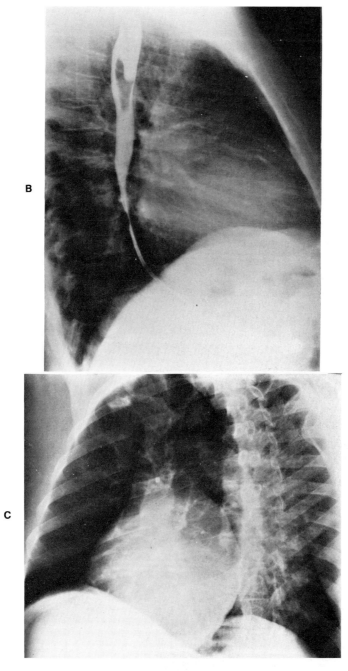

Fig. 5-22, cont'd. B, Lateral view. **C,** LAO view.

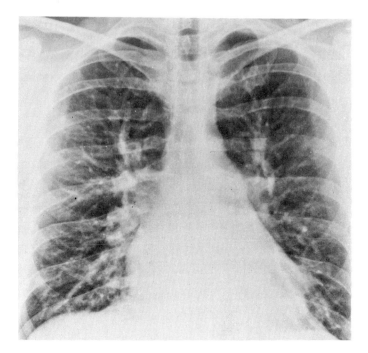

Fig. 5-23. Ventricular septal defect. Note shunt vascularity.

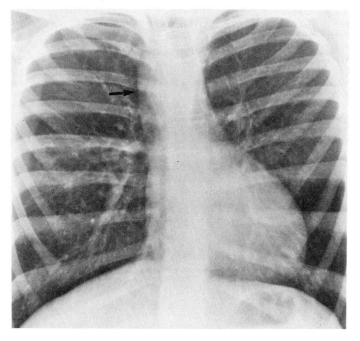

Fig. 5-24. Tetralogy of Fallot. Overall heart size is normal. Pulmonary vascularity, however, is diminished. Right aortic arch (arrow) is present.

however, that the failure pattern may also be seen in patients with mitral insufficiency or aortic valve disease as well. These patients will have an LVC. If, however, the heart is of a pure LVC without any evidence of LAE, a primary left ventricular stress situation is present. This is similar to the case of the adult patient and results from a variety of causes.

There findings are summarized as follows:

1. PVO + LAE = Obstruction at or proximal to the mitral valve (usually rheumatic)
2. PVO + LVC = Primary left ventricular stress (of any cause) with failure

Cyanotic patients

In a cyanotic patient the vascularity is never normal. It must be either decreased or increased. In this discussion, no attempt will be made to describe specific intracardiac lesions. The physiologic alterations produced by the lesions as manifest in the pulmonary vascularity will be stressed.

Cyanosis in the presence of decreased vascularity generally indicates the severe form of pulmonic stenosis. Once the observation of cyanosis and decreased vascularity is made, you must decide whether or not the heart size is normal. If the overall cardiac size is normal, even in the presence of evidence of specific chamber enlargement, the most likely abnormality is severe pulmonic stenosis plus VSD (tetralogy of Fallot) (Fig. 5-24).

A cyanotic patient with decreased vascularity and an enlarged heart is suffering from a complicated type of cardiac abnormality, usually severe pulmonic stenosis with an intact intraventricular septum. A shunt must be present to allow oxygenated blood to enter the circulation to permit survival.

If cyanosis is combined with shunt vascularity, an admixture lesion is present. In this situation, arterial and venous blood is mixed, so that the aortic blood is oxygen desaturated. This occurs in persistent truncus arteriosus and complete transposition of the great vessels.

A cyanotic patient with a PVO pattern, particularly an infant, constitutes a medical emergency. The patient should be referred for immediate cardiac catheterization to determine whether or not a correctable lesion is present. Most of the abnormalities found in this group of patients are complex.

The cyanotic patient is summarized as follows:

1. Cyanosis + Decreased vascularity + "Normal" heart size = Severe pulmonic stenosis + VSD (tetralogy of Fallot)
2. Cyanosis + Decreased vascularity + Enlarged heart = Severe pulmonic stenosis + Intact ventricular septum
3. Cyanosis + Shunt vascularity = Admixture lesion
4. Cyanosis + Severe PVO = Severe complex abnormality—patient to be referred for emergency catheterization

Chamber and vessel enlargements

The preceding sections considered the analysis of vascular patterns to be the key to diagnosing congenital and acquired cardiac disease. At this point the radiographic appearance of specific chamber enlargements will be briefly discussed.

Left ventricular enlargement produces a downward and left bulge of the cardiac

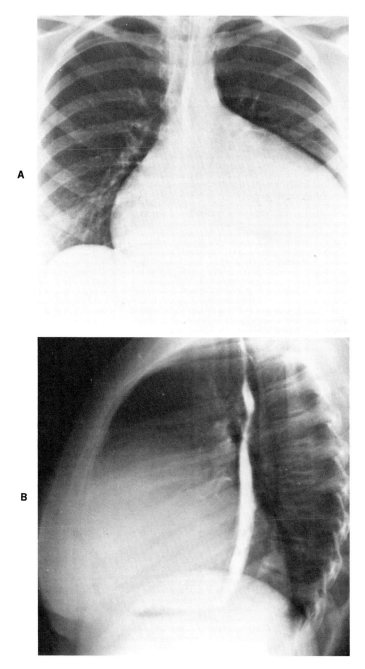

Fig. 5-25. Ebstein anomaly. Extreme cardiac enlargement is all right sided in this patient.

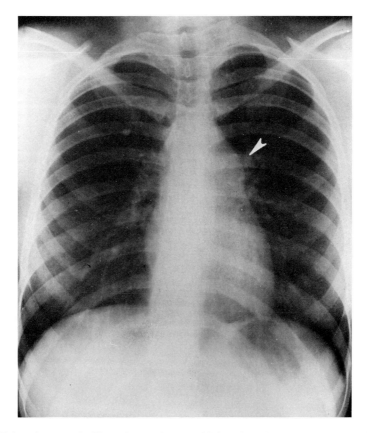

Fig. 5-26. Pulmonic stenosis. There is prominence of left main pulmonary artery (arrowhead) near outflow tract secondary to "jet phenomenon."

apex on the frontal film. In the lateral view of the shadow of the enlarged left ventricle is seen posterior to that of the inferior vena cava. Conditions that produce pure left ventricular enlargement were discussed in the previous section (Figs. 5-15 to 5-17).

Enlarged left atrium was discussed previously (Figs. 5-14, 5-21, and 5-22).

Right ventricular enlargement, when marked, may elevate the apex of the left ventricle. This produces the so-called "boot-shaped" heart (Fig. 5-24) on the frontal radiograph. On the lateral film there is a prominent or full retrosternal space.

Right atrial enlargement as an isolated finding is rare. It usually accompanies enlargement of the right ventricle and pulmonary arteries. Right atrial enlargement is suggested by prominence of the right cardiac border. Often the heart has a boxlike appearance (Fig. 5-25).

Main pulmonary artery enlargement produces bulging of the main pulmonary artery segment along the left cardiac border (Fig. 5-26). In addition, prominent right and left main pulmonary arteries may also be seen. Peripheral enlargements were discussed in the previous section.

Various portions of the aorta may enlarge, producing a prominence of that par-

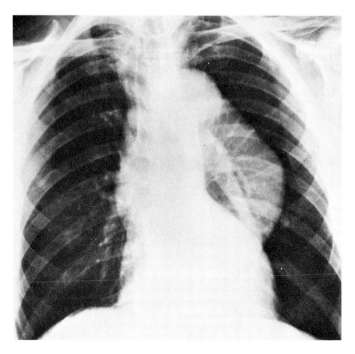

Fig. 5-27. Severe tortuosity of descending aorta. Arteriogram proved this patient did not have aneurysm.

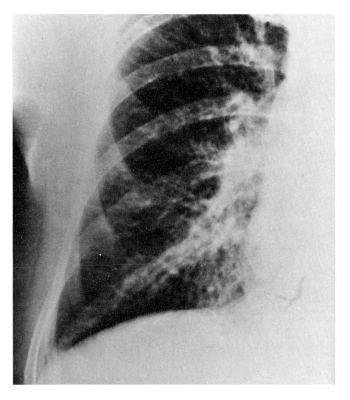

Fig. 5-28. Septal (Kerley) lines.

ticular shadow. In addition, considerable tortuosity may be seen in the descending aorta (Fig. 5-27).

Congestive heart failure

The vascular changes in congestive heart failure have been discussed. To reiterate, these include dilatation of the upper lobe vessels with contraction of the lower lobe vessels. In addition, there is enlargement of the cardiac silhouette in a poorly defined pattern. Although you may presume left ventricular enlargement, it is hard to specifically identify this in view of the "flabbiness" and poor contractility of cardiac muscles.

Associated findings of heart failure include interstitial and intra-alveolar edema. Interstitial edema occurs when the left atrial pressure increases and fluid transudes into the interstitial tissues, resulting in thickening of the interlobular septa. Kerley originally described these multiple linear densities and designated them according to their orientation:

1. *Kerley A lines* are long, thin, nonbranching linear densities obliquely directed toward the hilum.
2. *Kerley B lines*, the best known and most often seen, are thin, short, transverse lines best seen near the lung bases laterally at the costophrenic angle (Fig. 5-28).
3. *Kerley C lines* are in reality A and B lines oriented in an AP direction. On the frontal films, they appear as a fine reticular network.

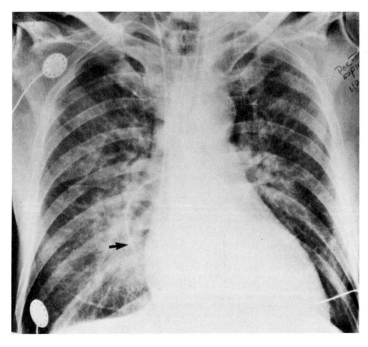

Fig. 5-29. Pulmonary edema. Note diffuse haziness emanating from central regions. Swann-Ganz catheter is present, with tip of catheter in right lower lobe pulmonary artery (arrow).

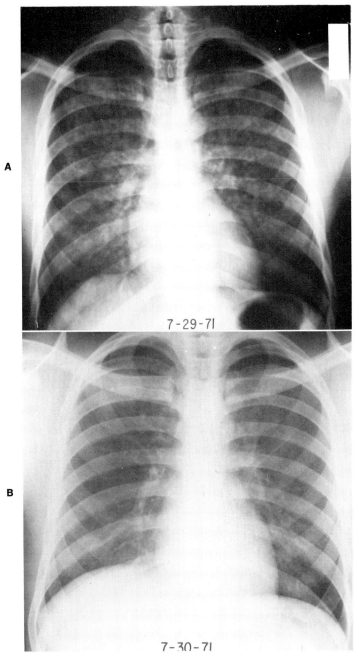

Fig. 5-30. Noncardiac pulmonary edema in heroin addict. **A,** There is diffuse pulmonary edema. Heart is normal. **B,** One day later, edema has cleared. Study is normal. (From Daffner, R. H.: New Physician **22:**315, 1973. Reproduced with permission of the publisher.)

Remember all three types of lines represent edematous *interlobular septa* and not dilated lymphatic vessels.

Intra-alveolar pulmonary edema results from further transudation of fluid into the air spaces, producing patchy, ill-defined, coalescent densities that radiate outward from the hilum. Sometimes this may have a batwing or butterfly distribution (Fig. 5-29). Air bronchograms are often seen in this pattern. As with any alveolar

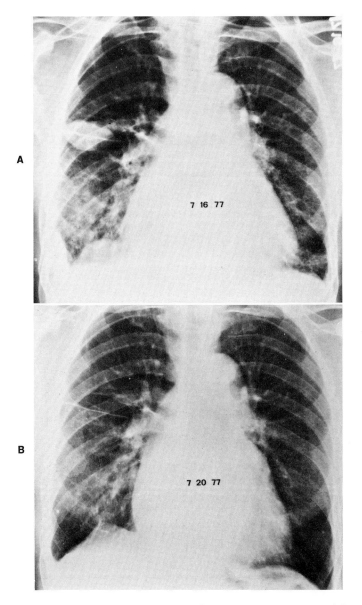

Fig. 5-31. Pulmonary pseudotumor. **A,** July 16, 1977. Patient is in congestive heart failure. Oval density is seen in right midlung field spanning minor fissure. Bilateral pleural effusions, more marked on right, are present. **B,** July 20, 1977. There has been improvement in patient's cardiac status. Pseudotumor has cleared, as has considerable amount of pleural fluid. Note change in cardiac silhouette.

process, the onset and clearing may be dramatic within a short period of time. Alveolar pulmonary edema may be asymmetric if the patient has been lying on one side before the filming. The edema may also be mistaken for other causes of alveolar density such as pneumonia and hemorrhage. You should be careful to analyze the pulmonary vessels, if visible, and the cardiac size before making a diagnosis of alveolar pulmonary edema. Furthermore, edema may be present from another (noncardiac) etiology such as heroin intoxication (Fig. 5-30), inhalation of noxious fumes, or drowning. In these conditions the heart is usually normal size.

Pleural fluid is another nonspecific finding that may be present in patients with congestive heart failure. If the fluid collects along a fissure, a pseudotumor (Fig. 5-31) may be seen. In the lateral view the borders are generally tapering, and the collection of fluid is oriented in a slanted configuration. These densities disappear after successful therapy.

Pericardial effusion

Pericardial effusion must always be considered when evaluating a patient with an enlarged heart. The diagnosis may be made by one or a combination of imaging studies. In general a large heart of nonspecific configuration, particularly in the absence of pulmonary venous engorgement, should suggest a pericardial effusion. Occasionally the pericardium will be seen as a thin dense line separated by layers of subepicardial and mediastinal fat under normal circumstances. In patients with pericardial effusion, this line, which never should measure more than 2 mm, is thickened.

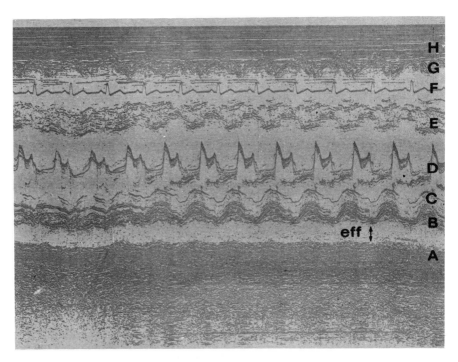

Fig. 5-32. Echocardiogram in patient with pericardial effusion *(eff)*. *A,* Pericardium; *B,* left ventricular wall; *C,* chorda tendinae; *D,* mitral valve; *E,* septal wall; *F,* ECG; *G,* right ventricular wall; *H,* chest wall.

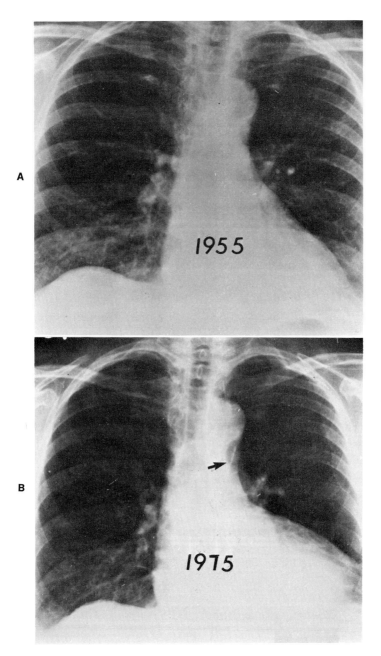

Fig. 5-33. Changes in patient with aging. This patient was known to have hypertension. **A,** 1955. Only significant abnormality is slight left ventricular prominence. **B,** 1975. There has been an increase in size of left ventricle. There is increased tortuosity of descending aorta. Calcification is now present in aorta (arrow).

Cardiac fluoroscopy is a useful procedure for the diagnosis of pericardial effusion. A dampened cardiac pulse in the presence of an enlarged heart and no congestive heart failure suggests the diagnosis. However, this is by no means pathognomonic, since a poorly contracting heart in a patient with a cardiac arrhythmia, a scarred myocardium, or an infiltrated myocardium will produce poor pulsations. A pulsating subepicardial fat line within the immobile fluid band is, however, diagnostic of pericardial effusion.

Echocardiography is probably the most useful study with the least risk to the patient. Ultrasonic shadows reflected off the pericardial and myocardial surfaces will demonstrate an abnormal collection of fluid in the pericardial sac (Fig. 5-32).

CT scanning may be used to diagnose pericardial effusion. A CT number near the density of water surrounding the heart ensures the diagnosis.

As previously mentioned, a blood pool scan may also be used to diagnose pericardial effusion. This has been illustrated previously (Fig. 5-3).

The most invasive technique for making the diagnosis is angiography. Carbon dioxide or positive contrast material may be injected directly into the right atrium and rapid sequence filming performed to show discrepancy between the contrast-filled chamber and the outer border of the cardiac silhouette. This technique is seldom used since the advent of echocardiography and CT scanning.

Changes in the chest with age

The normal aging process produces visible changes on serial chest radiographs, including a change from a more horizontal to a vertical position of the heart from youth into adulthood, tortuosity of the aorta and brachiocephalic vessels, calcification within the aortic arch, and, occasionally, increasing tortuosity of the descending aorta. These findings are illustrated in Fig. 5-33. In addition, degenerative changes may be seen in the dorsal spine. Postmenopausal women often demonstrate osteoporosis and may, on occasion, show evidence of collapse of one or more thoracic vertebrae. The lungs themselves may show little change with age. Occasionally, hyperinflation, so-called senile emphysema, may be seen. Scarring from subclinical pulmonary infections may be seen over both apices.

SUMMARY

This chapter has attempted to analyze cardiac diseases based on the physiologic alterations they produce on chest radiographs. A logical analysis may be made by first observing the pulmonary vasculature. Combining the vascular findings with those of specific chamber enlargements allows the diagnosis of specific diseases. Specific attention was directed to chamber enlargement, congestive heart failure, pericardial effusion, and changes in the chest with age.

Selected case studies

Cases 5-1 to 5-4: HEART MURMUR

We will consider the following four cases to demonstrate the application of the principles of cardiac roentgen diagnosis. All four patients were referred for examination because of a heart murmur.

Patient 1 is 2 years old. He has had a heart murmur since birth. There is a history of cyanosis when the patient cries or eats. He is slightly undersized in weight for his age. Case 5-1 is a PA radiograph of his chest.

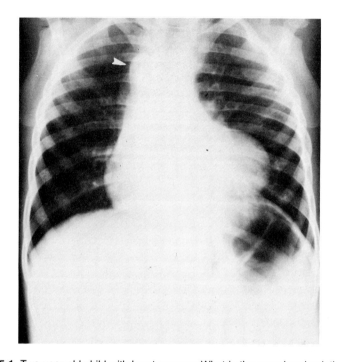

Case 5-1. Two-year-old child with heart murmur. What is the arrowhead pointing to?

Patient 2 is an 18-year-old woman who has had a known heart murmur since early childhood. She has been in otherwise good health. She was referred to her family physician because of an abnormal chest radiograph taken as part of a college entrance physical examination (Case 5-2).

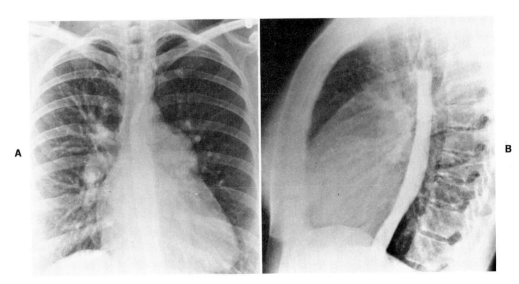

A

B

Case 5-2. A, PA and, **B,** lateral chest films of young woman with heart murmur. What is the main radiographic finding? How does this compare with Case 5-1?

Patient 3 is a 27-year-old man who has had a heart murmur since age 12 years, at which time he had a febrile illness. On exertion he complains of dyspnea that has progressed over the past few months. His cardiac series is shown in Case 5-3.

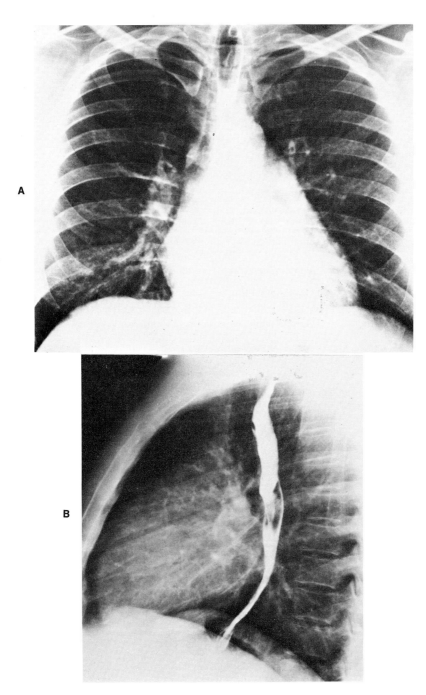

Case 5-3. Cardiac series in patient 3. **A,** PA view. **B,** Lateral view.

Continued.

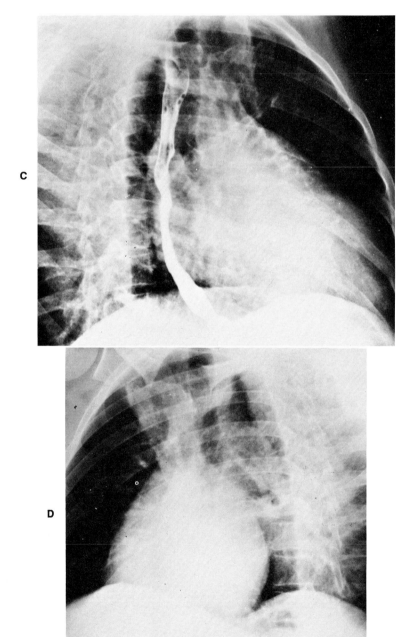

Case 5-3, cont'd. C, RAO view. **D,** LAO view.

Patient 4 is a 60-year-old woman who has had a recent onset of dyspnea on exertion, peripheral edema, and occasional nocturnal dyspnea. A pertinent physical finding is a widened pulse pressure. Her admission chest film is shown in Case 5-4.

What are the radiographic findings in each of these patients? What is your clinical diagnosis? What additional studies would you perform on these patients?

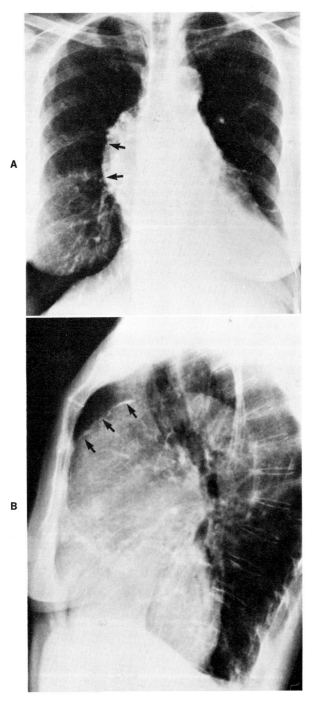

Case 5-4. A, PA and, **B,** lateral views. What are the arrows pointing to?

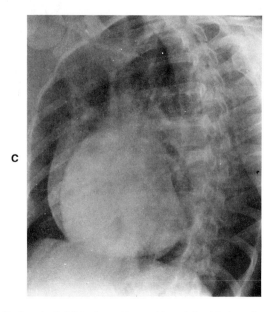

C

Case 5-2. Patient 2. **C,** LAO view of heart. Note right-sided cardiac enlargement.

ROENTGEN DIAGNOSIS

Patient 1. The most striking feature about this chest radiograph is that the pulmonary vascularity is *decreased.* The overall heart size is normal; however, there is prominence of the left border, giving the heart the overall appearance of a wooden shoe *(coeur en sabot).* A right aortic arch is present. This combination of findings in a young child with a history of intermittent cyanosis is characteristic of an obstructive lesion at or about the pulmonic valve with ventricular septal defect (tetralogy of Fallot). The patient was referred for cardiac catheterization, which confirmed the diagnosis.

Patient 2. The main abnormality on this patient's radiograph is the *prominence* of the pulmonary vessels, the direct opposite of that seen in patient 1. These vessels are predominantly arterial and are typical of shunt vascularity. The overall heart size is normal. On the lateral view there is convex bowing of the upper third of the sternum. Chest fluoroscopy showed prominent hilar vascular pulsations ("hilar dance"). A cardiac series was performed and showed right-sided cardiac enlargement on the LAO view (Case 5-2, *C*). These findings are characteristic of an atrial septal defect. Subsequent cardiac catheterization confirmed this.

Patient 3. There is prominence of the pulmonary vasculature. However, analysis of these vessels shows that they are *veins.* The overall heart size is normal. However, there is a bulge along the left cardiac border. Furthermore, a double density is seen in the frontal view, as with left atrial enlargement. The cardiac series shows evidence of left atrial enlargement on the other views. These findings are characteristic of an obstructing lesion at the mitral valve. This patient was known to have had rheumatic fever at age 12 years. Cardiac catheterization confirmed the findings of mitral stenosis.

Patient 4. The pulmonary vascularity is normal at this time. There is massive left ventricular enlargement as well as dilatation of the ascending aorta and aortic arch. Chest fluoroscopy denoted prominent pulsation of the aorta. Because of the findings, serologic examination for syphilis was performed. This was positive. The combination of findings suggest aortic insufficiency in a borderline compensated patient of which the most likely etiology is luetic. Cardiac catheterization confirmed the radiographic findings.

DISCUSSION

Each of these patients demonstrates a different type of cardiac disease. Two patients have congenital lesions; two have acquired. Although plain film radiography of the chest may be sufficient to suggest a diagnosis, it is necessary to perform other studies, including cardiac catheterization, for definitive diagnosis.

In the first patient the clinical history plus the finding of a normal-sized heart in the presence of diminished pulmonary vascularity is strongly suggestive of tetralogy of Fallot. This, in combination with a *right aortic arch*, which is found in approximately 25% of patients with tetralogy, virtually confirms the diagnosis. Right aortic arch may occur in patients without evidence of cardiac disease. In these patients the right aortic arch occurs without mirror-image branching, and the arch descends posterior to the esophagus in a normal relationship. In patients with severe cyanotic congenital heart disease a right aortic arch is usually of the mirror-image branching type, demonstrating a right subclavian, right carotid, and left brachiocephalic artery. This arch descends anterior to the esophagus.

The second patient has an uncomplicated atrial septal defect. This type was shown to be the so-called ostium secundum defect occurring at the fossa ovalis. There are essentially two other types of atrial septal defect: the first occurs inferior to the fossa ovalis (ostium primum defect) and is seen as part of a complex deformity known as an endocardial cushion defect. The other form is the sinus venosus type, where the defect lies superior to the fossa ovalis. The characteristic radiographic findings in atrial septal defect are prominent shunt vascularity and an overall normal cardiac size. Electrocardiographic evidence of right ventricular hypertrophy is almost always present. A prominent right cardiac border may be seen on the LAO view of a cardiac series. Fluoroscopic examination shows the characteristic "hilar dance" of the engorged pulmonary arteries. If the defect remains untreated until adulthood, a prominent outward convexity of the upper portion of the sternum secondary to right-sided cardiac enlargement may be seen.

We discussed the findings of mitral valve disease in the previous section. Mitral stenosis almost always results from rheumatic heart disease. If there is left ventricular enlargement in the presence of findings suggesting mitral stenosis, a combination of stenosis and insufficiency may exist. In uncomplicated mitral stenosis the left ventricle remains normal.

Syphilitic aortitis was one of the leading causes of death in patients with lues. With the introduction of antibiotics, this disease is now uncommon in patients under the age of 50 years. The characteristic lesion is aortic insufficiency secondary to dilatation of the diseased ascending aorta. Massive left ventricular enlargement is present, often combined with congestive heart failure. Secondary mitral insufficiency may occur when the degree of left ventricular enlargement becomes great.

Occasionally a curvilinear calcification (arrows, Case 5-4) of the ascending aorta may be seen. This finding is considered pathognomonic of syphilis, especially in patients under the age of 50 years. The chief differential diagnosis is with rheumatic aortic insufficiency, in which the aortic valve may be calcified. However, the ascending aorta (which often shows poststenotic dilatation) is not calcified. Furthermore, calcification of the aortic valve does not occur in luetic disease.

References

Chen, J. T. T., Capp, M. P., Johnsrude, I. S., Goodrich, J. K., and Lester, R. G.: Roentgen appearance of pulmonary vascularity in the diagnosis of heart disease, Am. J. Roentgenol. **112:**559, 1971.

Daffner, R. H., and Deal, P.: A logical approach to cardiac radiology. Part II, the pediatric patient, New Physician **23:**35, 1974.

Daffner, R. H., Gehweiler, J. A., and Carden, T. S., Jr.: Case studies in radiology, New York, 1975, Appleton-Century-Crofts.

Deal, P., and Daffner, R. H.: A logical approach to cardiac radiology. Part I, the adult patient, New Physician **23:**39, 1974.

Elliott, L. P., and Schiebler, G. L.: X-ray diagnosis of congenital cardiac disease, Springfield, Ill., 1968, Charles C Thomas, Publisher.

Feigenbaum, H.: Principles of echocardiography, Am. J. Med. **62:**805, 1977.

Gedgaudas, E., and Knight, L.: Plain-film diagnosis of heart disease. A physiologic approach, J.A.M.A. **232:**63, 1975.

Johnson, M. L., and Kisslo, J. A.: Basic diagnostic echocardiography, DM **23:**1, Dec., 1976.

Meszaros, W. T.: Cardiac roentgenology, Springfield, Ill., 1969, Charles C Thomas, Publisher.

6 Appearance of the chest after surgery

Chapters 4 and 5 dealt with patients who have not had any surgery performed on their heart or lungs. Thoracic surgery has made monumental advances in the past 25 years in developing new techniques for cardiopulmonary bypass, lung surgery, coronary revascularization procedures, development of new prosthetic heart valves, and perfection of new techniques for esophageal bypass surgery. These advances have reduced the morbidity and mortality in patients who were formerly subjected to cardiothoracic surgery. This chapter will outline the appearance of the "normal" chest postoperatively following a variety of procedures. Very brief mention will be made of the chest in the immediate postoperative period.

Although the appearance of the chest in a patient who has undergone cardiac, thoracic, or esophageal surgery may be quite characteristic of the procedure following recovery from surgery, the chest in the immediate postoperative period has many findings common to all procedures. Operative manipulation of lung may result in areas of patchy consolidation. Pleural effusion is a common finding in both cardiac and pulmonary surgery. Patients who have undergone cardiac surgery often show enlargement of the cardiac silhouette. Congestive heart failure, pneumonia, atelectasis, and pneumothorax are frequent findings in the immediate postoperative period.

Following heart or lung surgery a variety of foreign objects may be seen within the chest. These include chest tubes placed anteriorly in the supine patient for drainage of air and posteriorly for drainage of fluid, wire staples representing lines of resection of lung, metal clips placed across vessels or at the site of dissection around vessels, wire sutures in the sternum, mediastinal drains, a variety of intravascular catheters, and prosthetic heart valves. Furthermore, pacemaker leads may be seen either intraventricularly or epicardially. Electrocardiographic leads may also be seen on the chest wall. Some of these "foreign bodies" are illustrated in Figs. 6-1 through 6-3.

We can divide the discussion of the chest during the postoperative period into three categories:

1. Primary lung surgery
2. Primary cardiac surgery
3. Primary esophageal surgery

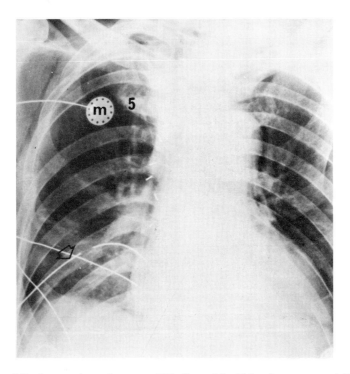

Fig. 6-1. Chest following esophageal surgery. Fifth rib on right *(5)* has been removed. Electrocardiographic monitor lead *(m)* is present. Note chest tube (open arrow) and multiple metallic clips.

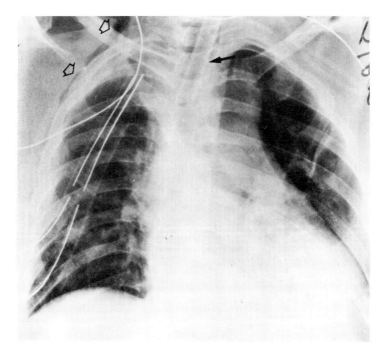

Fig. 6-2. Postoperative film in patient who underwent right upper lobectomy. There are two chest tubes on right. Endotracheal tube (solid arrow) is present. Electrocardiographic monitoring wires are visible as well. Note subcutaneous emphysema in right axilla and neck (open arrows).

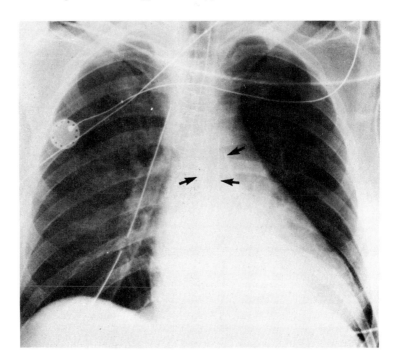

Fig. 6-3. Chest film of patient who underwent heart valve replacement. Chest tubes are present in right pleural cavity as well as mediastinum (arrows). Wire sutures, electrocardiographic leads, and endotracheal tube are also in evidence.

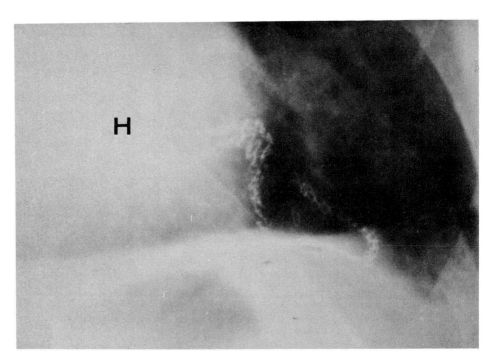

Fig. 6-4. Detail view of lung in patient who underwent wedge resection of nodule adjacent to heart *(H)*. Note wire staples marking excision site.

Patients undergo *lung* surgery for basically five types of procedures: biopsies, pneumonectomy, lobectomy, thoracoplasty, and plombage.

The most common radiographic manifestation of excisional biopsy or wedge resection of a lesion is a line of wire staples across the lung (Fig. 6-4). Often this is accompanied by the absence of a portion of a rib, generally the fifth rib posteriorly.

Following pneumonectomy the affected hemithorax fills with fluid. Air within the affected side gradually resorbs, leaving an opaque hemithorax. As fibrosis ensues, the heart and mediastinum are drawn toward the side of surgery. Quite often the cardiac silhouette will not be seen. The remaining lung hyperinflates to fill the space vacated by the shifted heart and mediastinum. These findings are illustrated in Fig. 6-5.

In patients who have undergone a lobectomy, wire staples representing the line of resection across the bronchus are seen. Metal clips may be present across the vessels. There is a shift of fissures as with atelectasis, the directions being the same as in atelectasis of the affected lobe. Hyperinflation of the remaining lobes on the side of a lobectomy is also seen. These findings are illustrated in Fig. 6-6.

Thoracoplasty and plombage are procedures that were performed in the past to eliminate dead space within the chest. They are seldom used at this time. A patient who has undergone thoracoplasty exhibits deformity of the upper chest wall on the affected side (Fig. 6-7, *A*). Patients who have undergone plombage will exhibit foreign material, as in Fig. 6-7, *B*.

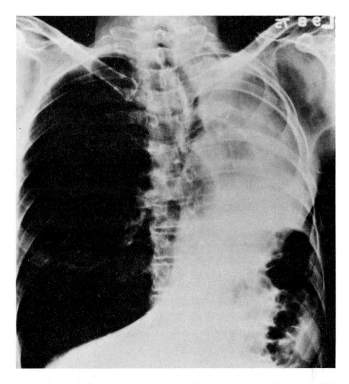

Fig. 6-5. Appearance of chest after pneumonectomy. Heart and mediastinum are shifted to left. Bowel gas shadows are elevated on left secondary to elevation of left hemidiaphragm.

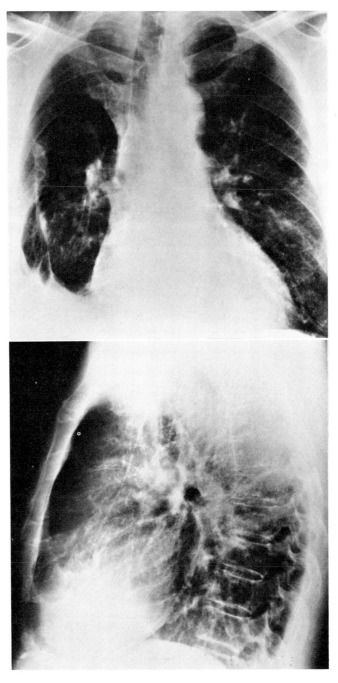

Fig. 6-6. Appearance of chest following right upper lobectomy. Note shift of hilar structures, elevation of right hemidiaphragm, and line of wire staples.

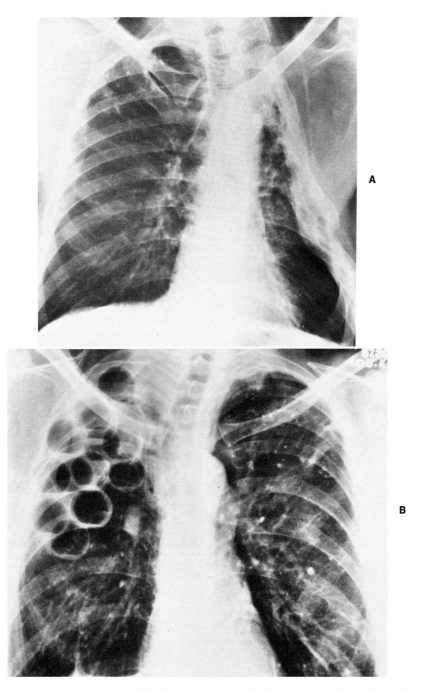

Fig. 6-7. A, Appearance of chest after left-sided thoracoplasty. **B,** Appearance of chest after plombage. Multiple lucencies represent table tennis balls that were used to fill "dead space."

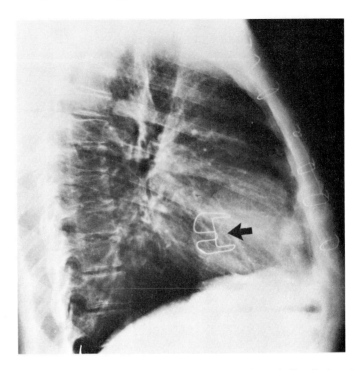

Fig. 6-8. Lateral chest film demonstrates prosthetic mitral valve (arrow). Prosthetic valves are often best seen on lateral film.

Cardiac surgery is performed most often to replace damaged heart valves, to bypass stenotic coronary arteries, and to palliate congenital heart disease. The majority of the patients who have been operated on for acquired disease will demonstrate wire sutures in the sternum, the common exposure of the surgical field.

Prosthetic valves are of several varieties. One of the most popular valves used commonly for mitral and aortic valve replacement consists of a metal cage with a plastic ball. When observing these valves, one can easily appreciate the location on plain film of the mitral and aortic rings (Figs. 6-8 and 6-9).

Patients who undergo bypass surgery of the coronary arteries often show multiple metal clips in the epicardial portions of the heart. On occasion, two small metal rings may represent the site of the coronary bypass graft. These findings are illustrated in Fig. 6-10.

Patients who have had palliative surgery for congenital heart disease may exhibit a variety of changes, depending on the surgical procedure. In some instances, as with palliation of a septal defect or ligation of a patent ductus arteriosus, the findings may be perfectly normal if the surgery has been successful.

Pacemakers are of two varieties: intravascular and epicardial. The intravascular leads are generally wedged into the right ventricle. When seen on the routine PA and lateral chest films, there should be a gentle curve to the catheter (Fig. 6-11). Any kinking or odd course of the lead should suggest that the catheter is not in the right position. Epicardial leads are placed along the outside of the heart in the vicinity of the interventricular septum. Generally, these wires go through the diaphragm to the power box, which is in the abdominal wall (Fig. 6-12).

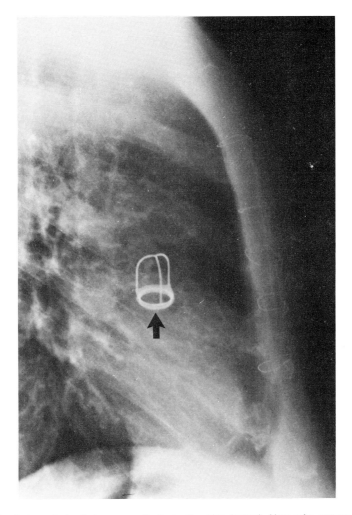

Fig. 6-9. Lateral view of chest shows prosthetic aortic valve (arrow). Note wire sutures in sternum.

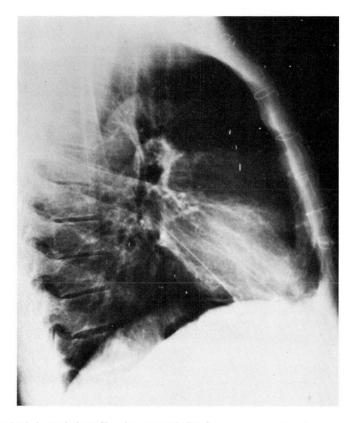

Fig. 6-10. Lateral chest film shows metal clips from coronary artery bypass surgery.

Numerous procedures have been devised for palliation of *esophageal* disease. These are basically of two types: bypass surgery and hiatal hernia repair.

In a bypass procedure the colon or stomach may be used to bypass a stenotic segment of esophagus or a neoplasm. The bypassing tube is often visible on the chest radiograph, as illustrated in Figs. 6-13 through 6-15.

Hiatal hernia repair may on occasion show a mass in the immediate postcardiac region. This represents the fundus of the stomach, which has been plicated around the distal esophagus to create a competent esophageal sphincter. Metal clips may be seen in this region.

You should familiarize yourself with the various appearances of the chest postoperatively. Remember, once the patient has recovered and is free of symptoms of the previous disease, we can consider this chest "normal" for that individual.

One additional postoperative appearance with which you should be familiar is that of the patient following radical mastectomy for carcinoma of the breast. Following mastectomy the affected side appears more lucent. This is because of the absence of the breast shadow and pectoralis muscle. If we follow the soft tissue lines of the axilla on the normal side, we can see that the axillary fold merges imperceptibly with that of the breast shadow. However, on the affected side the axillary fold extends up to and crosses over onto the thorax. These findings are illustrated in Fig.

Text continued on p. 183.

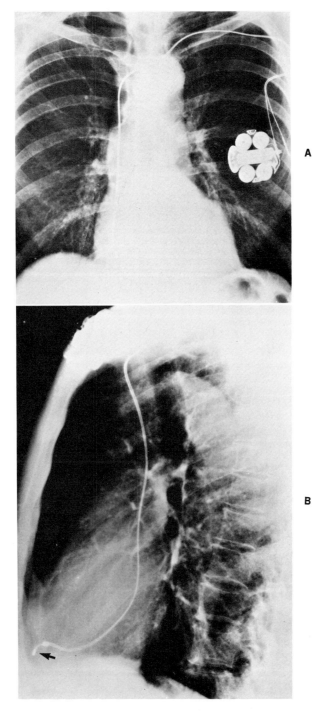

Fig. 6-11. Normal transvenous pacemaker. **A,** PA view shows pacemaker box in subcutaneous tissue of left hemithorax. Box contains four batteries. Pacemaker wires travel from axillary vein into heart. Tip of pacemaker lead should be in right ventricle. **B,** Lateral view shows tip of pacing lead (arrow).

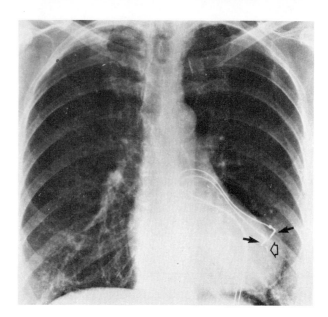

Fig. 6-12. Epicardial pacemaker lead. Battery box is in subcutaneous tissue over abdomen. Electrodes are implanted directly in epicardium (solid arrows). Broken wire is present (open arrow).

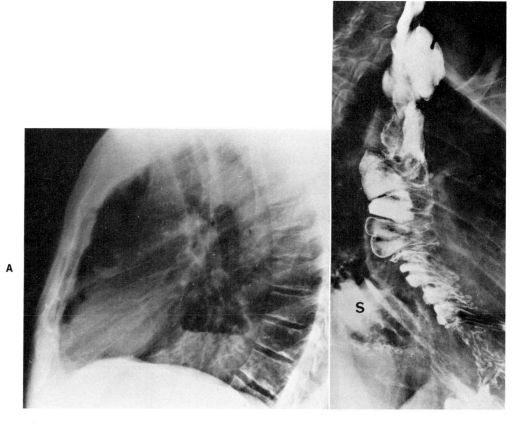

Fig. 6-13. Postoperative colon swing for esophageal carcinoma. **A,** Lateral chest film shows abnormal gaseous densities in substernal region. **B,** "Esophagogram" shows colon in chest. Filling of stomach *(S)* is present.

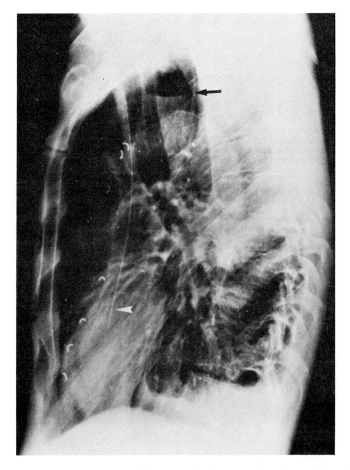

Fig. 6-14. Appearance of chest following Beck gastric tube procedure for esophageal carcinoma. Lateral chest film shows metal clips and staples in substernal region. Note lucency in substernal region. There is a catheter in right atrium (arrowhead). Note retrotracheal air-fluid level (arrow) in obstructed esophagus.

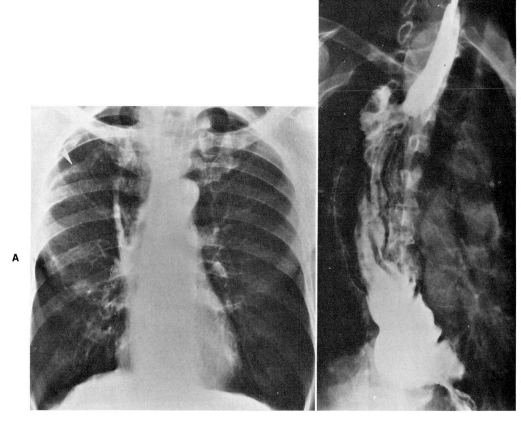

Fig. 6-15. Appearance of chest following esophagogastrectomy. **A,** PA radiograph of chest shows linear density rising vertically on right. Regenerating rib is evidence of previous thoracotomy (arrowhead). **B,** Barium study shows rugal folds typical of stomach.

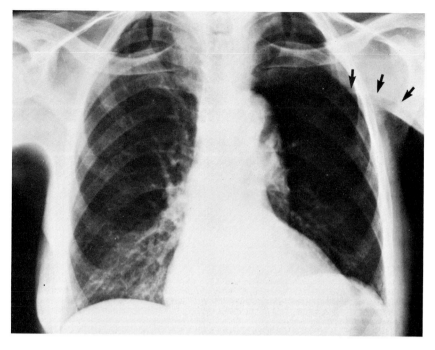

Fig. 6-16. Appearance of chest following radical mastectomy on left. Left lung appears more lucent than right. Note absent breast shadow on left. In addition, note difference in soft tissue lines in left axilla when compared to the right side. Gently curving horizontal line (arrows) represents remnant of amputated soft tissues.

6-16. Occasionally, we may see metal clips that were left at the site of nodal resection within the axilla in patients undergoing radical mastectomy.

References

Chun, P. K. C., and Nelson, W. P.: Common cardiac prosthetic valves. Radiologic identification and associated complications, J.A.M.A. **238**:401, 1977.

McHenry, M. M., and Grayson, C. E.: Roentgenographic diagnosis of pacemaker failure, Am. J. Roentgenol. **109**:94, 1970.

Melamed, M., Hipona, F. A., Reynes, C. J., Barker, W. L., and Paredes, S.: The adult postoperative chest, Springfield, Ill., 1976, Charles C Thomas, Publisher.

Sorkin, R. P., Schuurmann, B. J., and Simon, A. B.: Radiographic aspects of permanent cardiac pacemakers, Radiology **119**:281, 1976.

7 Abdominal plain film

The abdominal plain film is an important examination in the evaluation of patients with suspected intra-abdominal disease. The lack of significant contrast between the abdominal viscera is considered by some to be a disadvantage in diagnosing disease (compared to the natural contrast occurring in the chest). However, there is still a wealth of information that may be obtained from single or multiple abdominal films by knowing the anatomy and applied pathophysiology.

There are certain principles that may help you to make a correct diagnosis in a patient with abdominal disease and/or guide you to perform additional diagnostic studies. You should always consider the diagnostic possibilities before ordering a plain film. For example, numerous abdominal plain films are ordered in patients with known or suspected esophageal varices or bleeding from a peptic ulcer. In these instances there are rarely plain film abnormalities; contrast examination and/or endoscopy is required to make the diagnosis. Plain films will, however, provide diagnostic information concerning gallstones, renal calculi, and appendicoliths.

TECHNICAL CONSIDERATIONS

The type of plain film examination of the abdomen should be tailored to the individual patient. For example, when searching for a missing sponge after surgery, a single supine film of the abdomen will suffice. The single film examination is also satisfactory to determine renal size, to ascertain the presence of foreign bodies, and to detect most intra-abdominal calcifications.

The standard abdominal *plain film* (or KUB*) consists of a supine view, the so-called flat plate. The origin of the latter term is traced to a time when glass plates were used instead of film. At that time, stereoscopic examination was popular. To obtain a single view of the abdomen, not in stereo, a "flat plate" was ordered. This term is obsolete, and *plain film* of the abdomen is the correct modern name.

Most patients suspected to have acute abdominal disease will also have an upright film made. The purpose of this film is twofold: first, to determine the presence of free intraperitoneal air, and second, to detect the presence of intestinal air-fluid levels. This study is made by having the patient stand or sit. The principle involved here is the use of the *horizontal beam.*

---

*A film showing kidneys, ureters, and bladder.

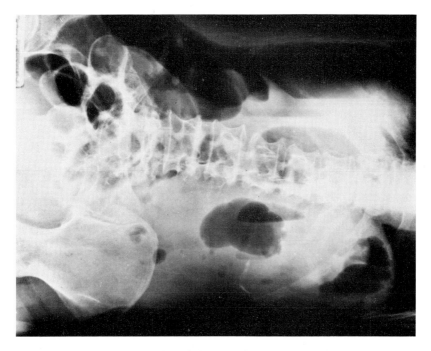

Fig. 7-1. Left lateral decubitus view of abdomen. Large pneumoperitoneum is present.

If the patient is unable to stand, a horizontal beam study may be performed by placing the patient in the left lateral decubitus position (left side down, right side up). This study is especially useful in the severely ill patient who is suspected to have free intraperitoneal air. It is important that the patient be placed on the left side for several minutes to allow any free air to rise over the dome of the liver. Once again, because of the horizontal beam, intestinal air-fluid levels may be detected. Fig. 7-1 shows a patient with a pneumoperitoneum demonstrated in the left lateral decubitus position.

Since most patients with an acute condition of the abdomen will be admitted to the hospital, it is also desirous to obtain a chest radiograph. The order of filming in these patients should be as follows: left lateral decubitus abdominal film, upright PA chest film (this will allow any free air to rise under the diaphragm and be seen on the chest film), and supine abdominal film.

As with any other radiologic study, first examine the film for proper identification and technical quality. A film that is too light or too dark is of little diagnostic value. Motion on the film obscures soft tissue shadows and blurs the outline of gas-filled bowel, calcifications, etc. Furthermore, portable films are helpful in detecting only gross intra-abdominal abnormalities.

Abdominal CT scanning has been one of the best advances in the diagnosis of abdominal disease. As mentioned previously, the lack of sufficient tissue contrast between the different abdominal organs has been a handicap to routine radiographic diagnosis. However, the abdominal CT scan can differentiate organ densities better than radiographs, can outline these organs, and can detect subtle abnormalities that will defy diagnosis on plain films (Fig. 7-2).

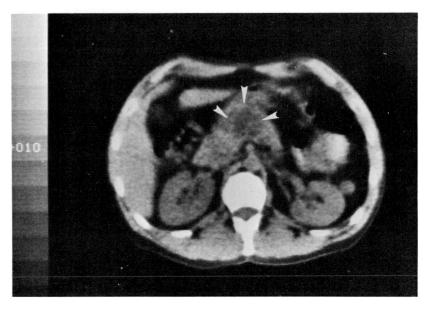

Fig. 7-2. Abdominal CT scan in patient with pseudocyst of pancreas (arrowheads).

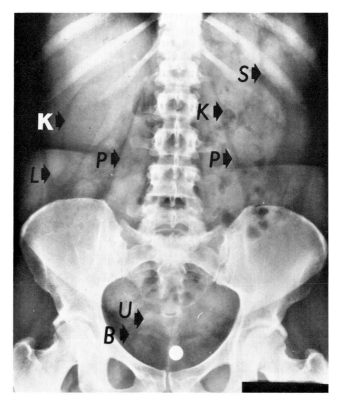

Fig. 7-3. Normal abdomen. There is sparsity of bowel gas. Arrows point to normal soft tissue shadows. *B,* Bladder; *K,* kidney; *L,* liver; *P,* psoas; *S,* spleen; *U,* uterus.

Finally, ultrasonography is an important adjunct in the evaluation of abdominal disease. It is most useful for the evaluation of masses and aortic aneurysms and in the detection of biliary and renal disease.

ANATOMIC CONSIDERATIONS

Fig. 7-3 shows a normal supine abdominal film of a young adult patient. The abdominal gas pattern in this patient is normal. Under normal circumstances, small quantities of gas are present within the stomach and portions of the small bowel and colon. The caliber of these loops is normal. There is no evidence of mucosal thickening. The exact anatomy of these loops is defined by the mucosal pattern (Fig. 7-4).

The shadows of the liver, spleen, kidneys, and psoas muscles should be examined on all abdominal films (Fig. 7-3). These are identifiable because of the small amount of fat surrounding them. In evaluating hepatic size, remember that one is really looking at the posterior margin of the liver as well as that of the spleen because of the indentation the extraperitoneal perivisceral fat makes on these organs.

The peritoneal flank or fat stripe is seen outlining the margins of the abdomen lateral to the ascending and descending colon. This appears as a lucent line separating the soft tissues of the skin from the abdominal cavity. This line is often obliterated in inflammatory conditions of the abdomen (appendicitis, peritonitis, etc.).

Under normal circumstances the gas patterns should change over a period of several minutes if successive films are made. This indicates normal peristaltic activi-

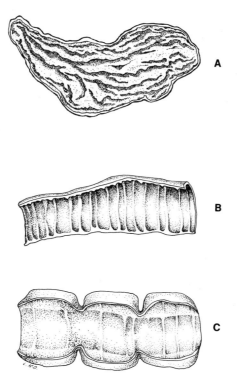

Fig. 7-4. Schematic drawing of normal mucosal folds. **A,** Stomach. **B,** Small intestine. **C,** Colon.

ty. Absence of this activity, particularly when there is absolutely no change in the appearance of the bowel, is strongly suggestive of bowel infarction.

The bony structures commonly seen on an abdominal plain film include the lower thoracolumbosacral spine, lower ribs, pelvis, and hips. Frequently, degenerative changes will be present in the spines of older individuals.

PATHOLOGIC CONSIDERATIONS

Pathologic alterations seen on the plain film include the following:
1. Abnormal gas and mucosal patterns
2. Abnormalities of the soft tissue shadows
3. Abnormal calcifications
4. Abnormal fluid: ascites

The signs of previous surgery must also be recognized.

Abnormal gas and mucosal patterns

Gas seen on abdominal plain films is either intraluminal or extraluminal. The abnormalities produced by intraluminal gas include distention or dilatation of a loop,

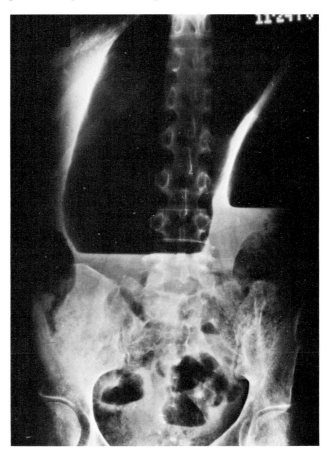

Fig. 7-5. Mechanical bowel obstruction in patient with sigmoid volvulus. Upright film shows air-fluid levels in obstructed loop.

the presence of air-fluid levels (Fig. 7-5), and the presence of mucosal thickening (Fig. 7-6). Distended or dilated bowel may occur under a variety of circumstances. Most often this is of the so-called adynamic ileus type, in which peristalsis is markedly diminished. The typical appearance (Fig. 7-7) shows gaseous distention of colon and small bowel in a rather nonspecific pattern. Interestingly enough, air-fluid levels may be seen in these patients. These occur in both large and small bowel in what has been termed a "balanced" pattern. This pattern is most commonly seen in patients following trauma (including surgery), with peritonitis, as a manifestation of drugs or bowel ischemia, and in chronically ill, bedridden patients.

A localized ileus seen persistently on serial films is highly suggestive of an adjacent area of inflammation. This occurs commonly in pancreatitis (Fig. 7-8) and acute appendicitis.

Distended loops of bowel with air-fluid levels in a localized pattern is highly suggestive of a mechanical obstruction (Fig. 7-5). The typical pattern shows a distended cascade of loops proximal to the obstruction and an essentially gasless distal abdomen. The bowel loops frequently have a stepwise appearance or are of the hairpin type. The presence of gas within the rectum does not rule out a low colonic lesion.

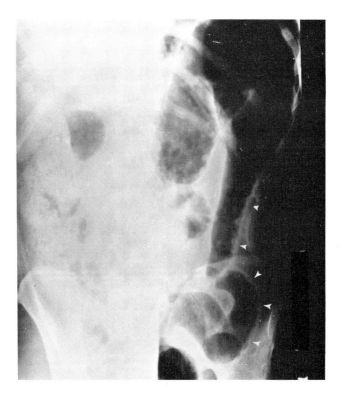

Fig. 7-6. Mucosal thickening in patient with ulcerative colitis. Thickened mucosa (arrowheads) is seen between air contained in bowel and grayness of abdominal cavity. Multiple pseudopolyps are visible within distended bowel.

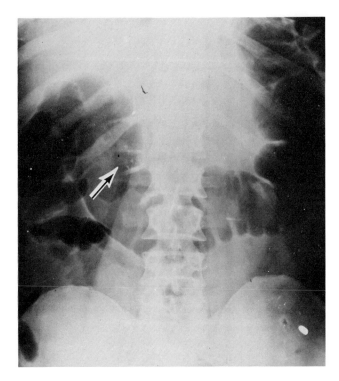

Fig. 7-7. Ileus in patient with pancreatitis. Note gaseous distention of transverse colon. Pancreatic calcifications are present near midline on right (arrow). Incidental finding is bullet in left lower quadrant.

Gas may be introduced into the rectum by digital examination, proctosigmoidoscopy, rectal temperature determination, and enemas. In an early obstruction the characteristic pattern may not be well developed. However, serial films will show the development of the characteristic loops.

The cause of a mechanical obstruction will vary, depending on whether the patient is an adult or child. In the adult, common causes include adhesions, hernia, tumor (Fig. 7-9), and volvulus (Fig. 7-10). In infants and children, intussusception is a common cause of obstruction. In the newborn and very young infant, duodenal atresia and pyloric stenosis should be suspected.

The natural contrast between the soft tissues, the mucosa, and the air within the bowel allows evaluation of that bowel. A thickened bowel wall is abnormal. You cannot determine the exact etiology of the thickening without applying important history and physical examination findings. For example, a patient with a history of sudden onset of abdominal pain accompanied by blood-streaked diarrhea and dilated bowel on plain film is likely to have colitis (Fig. 7-6). Other diseases that produce thickening of the bowel wall include several of the malabsorption syndromes, ischemic disease, intramural hemorrhage, and regional enteritis.

Extraluminal gas may be either free (pneumoperitoneum) or contained within an abscess cavity, the retroperitoneum, the wall of the bowel, or the portal venous or biliary systems of the liver.

Free intraperitoneal air in the absence of immediate previous surgery suggests

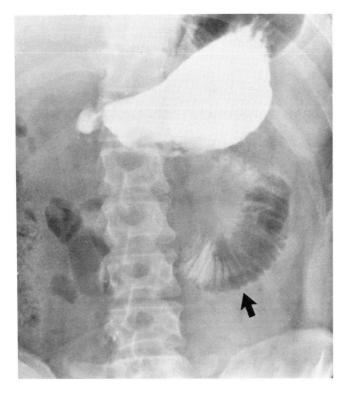

Fig. 7-8. Localized ileus ("sentinel loop") (arrow) of proximal jejunum in patient with pancreatitis.

a ruptured viscus. The most common cause is perforation of a peptic ulcer or of a colonic diverticulum. Trauma is another cause. If the perforation is intraperitoneal, gas will be seen on an upright film collecting under both leaves of the diaphragm (Fig. 7-11, A). Furthermore, decubitus positioning may demonstrate free intraperitoneal air (Fig. 7-1). However, it is possible to make the diagnosis of pneumoperitoneum based on a supine film, because air frequently collects in Morison's pouch. The "double wall sign" results when air on both sides of the bowel wall outlines that structure rather distinctly (Fig. 7-11, B). Under normal circumstances, you do not see the serosal surface of bowel because of its water density. Air within the peritoneal cavity, however, presents a change in radiographic density to outline the bowel wall.

Retroperitoneal air, particularly from a perforated duodenal ulcer or ruptured duodenum secondary to trauma, is often seen as a sharpening or enhancement of the psoas shadow. Occasionally the renal shadow will be highlighted as well. This diagnosis may be difficult to make based on a plain film. However, on CT scan the presence of retroperitoneal air will be easily detected (Fig. 7-12).

Gas loculated within the abdomen generally indicates the presence of an abscess. The air may be confined to a known anatomic space such as Morison's pouch beneath the liver, to an emphysematous gallbladder (Fig. 7-13), to the renal capsule, to the lesser sac, or within an organ (Fig. 7-14) or it may be free within the abdominal cavity. The gas may be a small localized collection or, more commonly, may have a mottled appearance. Frequently, it is necessary to do a contrast examination to deter-

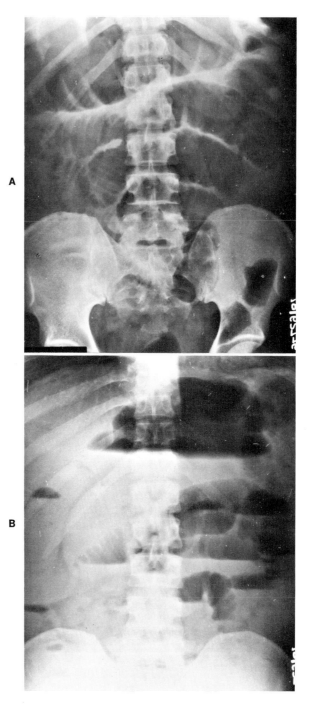

Fig. 7-9. Mechanical small bowel obstruction in patient with metastatic carcinoma. **A,** Supine view shows multiple dilated loops of small bowel. Uppermost loops appear to have colonic configuration. **B,** Upright view shows multiple air-fluid levels.

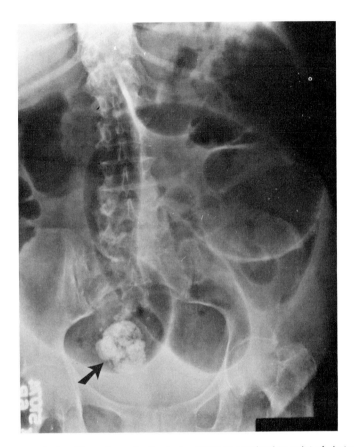

Fig. 7-10. Sigmoid volvulus. There is marked colonic dilatation proximal to point of obstruction. Arrow points to a calcified uterine fibroid.

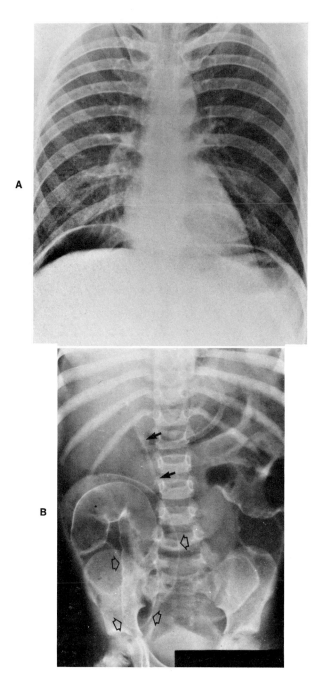

Fig. 7-11. Pneumoperitoneum. **A,** PA upright chest film shows collection of free intraperitoneal air under both leaves of diaphragm. **B,** Supine view demonstrates falciform ligament (solid arrows) and air on both sides of bowel wall, best seen in right lower quadrant (open arrows). (From Daffner, R. H.: New Physician **24:**48, 1975. Reproduced with permission of the publisher.)

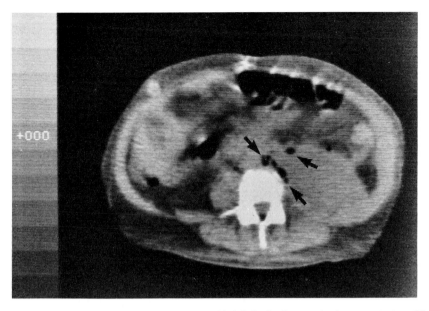

Fig. 7-12. Retroperitoneal air (arrows) in patient with left flank abscess is demonstrated on this CT scan. Note large abscess mass on left as compared to normal right psoas shadow.

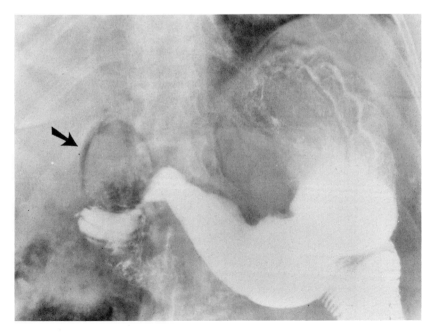

Fig. 7-13. Emphysematous cholecystitis. Gas is present in wall of gallbladder (arrow). Note relationship of gallbladder to duodenum on this upper GI series.

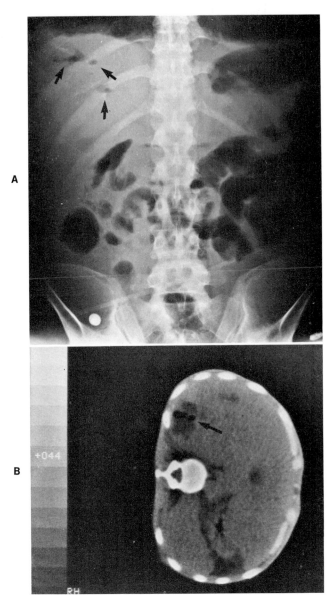

Fig. 7-14. Intrahepatic abscess. **A,** Abdominal plain film shows gaseous densities overlying liver shadow (arrows). **B,** CT scan with patient in lateral decubitus position shows pockets of gas within hepatic abscess (arrow).

mine the location of normal loops of bowel to rule out the presence of an aberrant loop of bowel being responsible for the abnormal shadow. The CT scan has proved quite reliable for the diagnosis of these entities (Figs. 7-12 and 7-14).

Intramural air (pneumatosis intestinalis) may be seen in a variety of benign and pathologic conditions. A common cause of pneumatosis in older adults is microperforation of a diverticulum. Air is seen as streaky densities surrounding the bowel (Fig. 7-15). Occasionally a giant air cyst will occur. Intramural air may also be seen

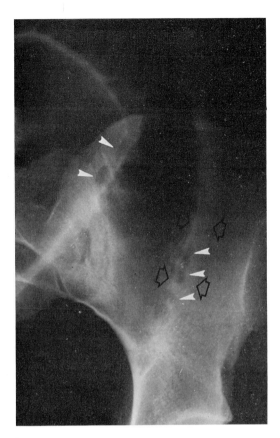

Fig. 7-15. Pneumatosis intestinalis in patient with granulomatous colitis. Detail film shows thickened bowel wall (arrows). Note streaky gaseous densities within wall (arrowheads). (From Daffner, R. H., Gehweiler, J. A., and Carden, T. S., Jr.: Case studies in radiology, New York, 1975, Appleton-Century-Crofts. Reproduced with permission of the publisher.)

in bowel infarction in older patients and particularly in premature newborns with necrotizing enterocolitis (Fig. 7-16). In both these patients, gas may be seen in the liver within the portal system.

Air in the biliary tree may also be seen in infection or following surgery in which the common bile duct is anastomosed to the small bowel. Portal gas is usually located in the periphery, whereas biliary gas is seen more centrally. Corrleation with the clinical findings is necessary for proper interpretation of this observation.

Abnormalities of the soft tissue shadows

Soft tissue abnormalities include displacements or misplacements, enlargement, presence of masses, and loss of margins.

Enlargement of the abdominal organs may cause displacement of the other organs. For example, splenomegaly will displace the gastric air shadow medially (Fig. 7-17). Enlargement of the pancreas will cause anterior displacement of the stomach (demonstrated on an upper GI series). An enlarged adrenal gland or tumor may dis-

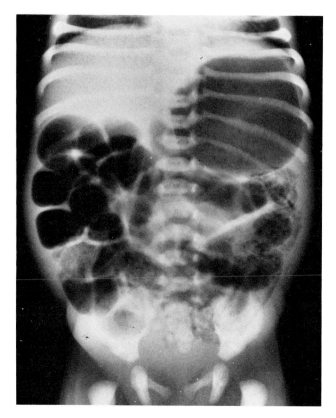

Fig. 7-16. Necrotizing enterocolitis in premature newborn. Note bubbly appearance in left lower quadrant. This represents pneumatosis.

place the renal shadow inferiorly. Enlarged lymph nodes may displace the renal shadows laterally.

Certain congenital anomalies, particularly of the urinary tract, may result in abnormal position of the kidneys. In a patient with a horseshoe kidney the lower poles are oriented toward the midline. A malposition of the kidney may result in the absence of the normal renal outline on the plain film, especially if the kidney is within the pelvis.

Masses within the abdomen may be seen either by themselves or more frequently by the displacements or distortion of normal viscera. The most common mass seen in the pelvis is a distended bladder. If you doubt the diagnosis, a repeat film should be made after the patient has successfully voided.

The loss of the margin of a soft tissue structure is a valuable sign in evaluating patients with abdominal disease. The loss of a renal outline or psoas margin (Fig. 7-18) generally indicates an inflammatory condition in the retroperitoneum. The loss of the psoas margin accompanied by scoliosis is a nonspecific finding that may be seen in acute appendicitis, urinary calculus, or perforated viscus. As mentioned previously, the loss of the properitoneal fat line may also be seen in several inflammatory conditions, particularly appendicitis.

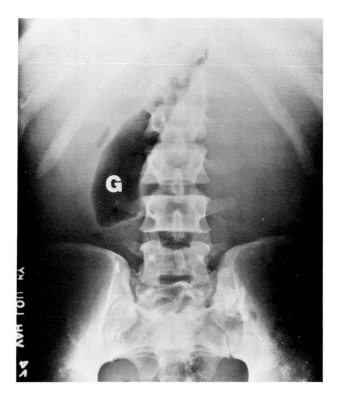

Fig. 7-17. Hepatosplenomegaly in patient with leukemia. Gastric air bubble *(G)* is displaced to right by markedly enlarged spleen. Liver is also enlarged.

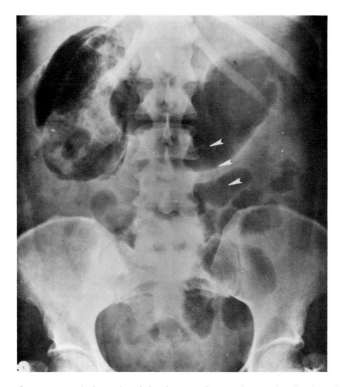

Fig. 7-18. Loss of psoas margin in perinephric abscess. Large abnormal collection of gas is seen in right upper abdomen. This represents gas surrounding right kidney. Psoas margin is not present on right. Compare it with left psoas (arrowheads).

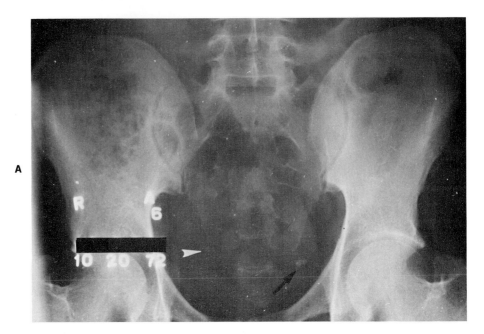

Fig. 7-19. "Physiologic" calcifications within abdomen. **A,** Phleboliths in pelvis (arrow). Calcification just to right of sacrum (arrowhead) represented ureteral calculus.

Abnormal calcifications

The list of calcifications that may be seen on abdominal plain film is quite long and beyond the scope of this text. However, there are certain benign or normal conditions that will produce calcifications frequently seen on abdominal plain films. These include the costal cartilages, vascular calcifications such as phleboliths in the pelvic venous plexus, atherosclerotic plaques of the aortoiliac vessels, prostatic calcifications, and old granulomas of spleen and lymph nodes. These are illustrated in Fig. 7-19. Abnormal calcifications include biliary (Fig. 7-20) and urinary (Fig. 7-21) calculi, calcified aneurysms (Fig. 7-22), pancreatic calcifications (Fig. 7-23), and calcified appendiceal fecaliths (Fig. 7-24). In addition, foreign bodies may often be seen. These may include ingested foreign materials, for example, tablets (Fig. 7-25), or traumatic foreign bodies, for example, bullets, buckshot, or shrapnel. You may, on occasion, see a patient with a self-induced rectal foreign body (Fig. 7-26).

Abnormal fluid: ascites

The classic appearance of ascites has been described as diffuse, ground glass density of the abdomen. Generally by the time this has occurred, ascites is clinically apparent and need not be diagnosed by radiographic means. However, small amounts of peritoneal fluid (ascites or blood) may appear in a subtle manner.

The accumulation of several hundred milliliters of ascitic fluid may be seen on the supine film as a collection of water-density material overlying the sacrum above the bladder. This occurs because the fluid collects posteriorly in the pelvis. With increasing volume, however, the fluid extends superolaterally out of the pelvis, giving the

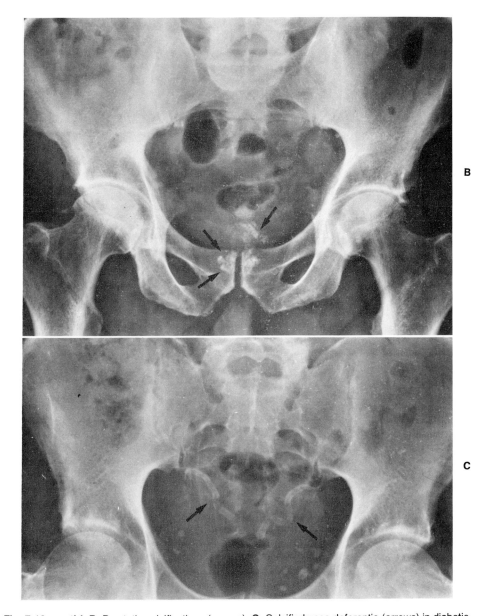

Fig. 7-19, cont'd. B, Prostatic calcifications (arrows). **C,** Calcified vasa deferentia (arrows) in diabetic patient. Note calcified phleboliths as well.

Continued.

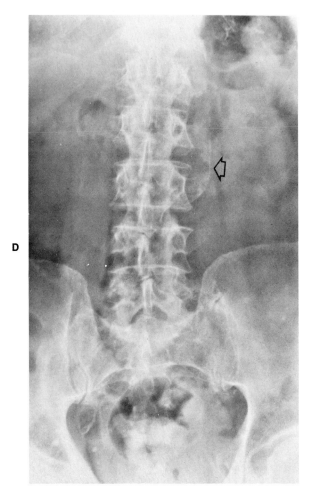

D

Fig. 7-19, cont'd. D, Calcified abdominal aortic aneurysm (arrow). Vascular calcification is quite common in older patients.

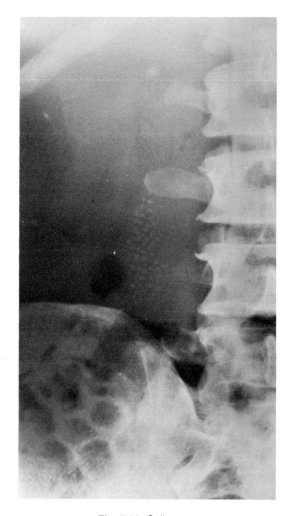

Fig. 7-20. Gallstones.

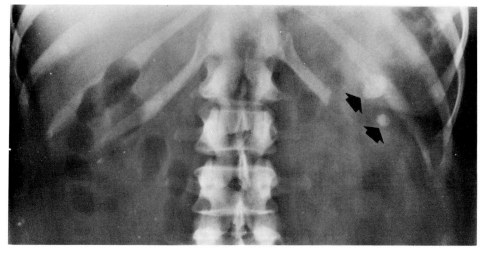

Fig. 7-21. Renal calculi in left kidney (arrows).

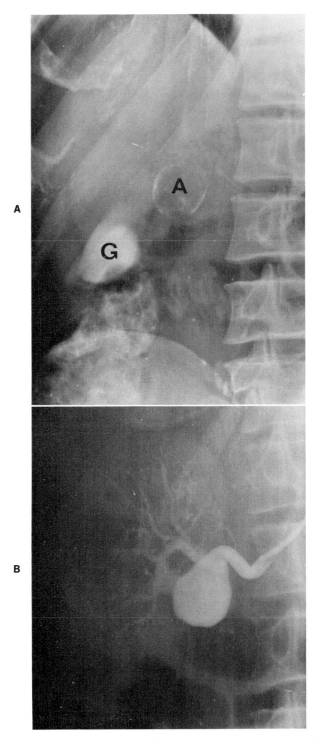

Fig. 7-22. Renal artery aneurysm. **A,** Oblique film of abdomen shows aneurysm *(A)* distinct from gall-bladder *(G).* **B,** Selective arteriogram demonstrates aneurysm.

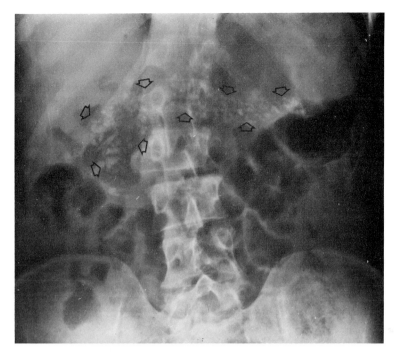

Fig. 7-23. Pancreatic calcifications (arrows) in patient with chronic pancreatitis. Note how calcifications assume shape of pancreas.

so-called dog-ear appearance. Further increase in the amount of fluid (to over 500 ml) will extend up along the lateral gutters, displacing the colon medially from the radiolucent flank stripes (Fig. 7-27). As the amount of fluid increases, there is displacement of liver and spleen from the body wall. Finally, floating loops of bowel may be seen in the "sea of ascites."

It is important to diagnose small collections of fluid in the pelvis in the patient who has had abdominal trauma. This may be the only clue to the presence of a ruptured liver or spleen.

Postoperative appearance of the abdomen

It is important to recognize the signs of previous surgery in the abdomen. Wire sutures in the abdomen indicate previous surgery. The position of the sutures frequently can give an idea of what surgery was performed. For example, wire sutures extending obliquely from the midline toward the right flank may indicate that the patient has had biliary surgery. Other indications of surgery include metallic clips in the region of the esophagogastric junction from previous vagotomy or around blood vessels. If an organ has been removed, its shadow will no longer be present.

Metallic clips in the abdomen or pelvis form valuable landmarks for evaluation of some diseases. In patients with known lymphomas the displacement of clips is an important indication of lymph node enlargement. Furthermore, displacement of clips or of a foreign body such as a bullet may provide important clues to the diagnosis of an intra-abdominal abscess.

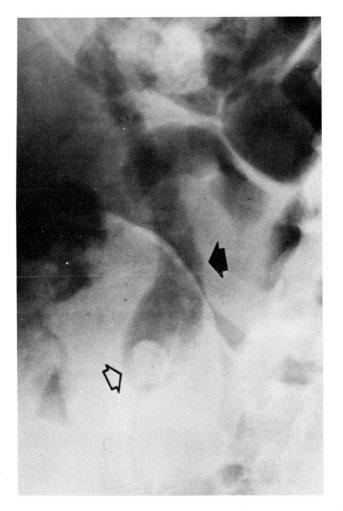

Fig. 7-24. Calcified appendicolith (open arrow) in patient with gangrenous appendicitis. Appendix is filled with gas (solid arrow).

SUMMARY

The analysis of the plain film of the abdomen has been briefly discussed regarding normal appearances and pathologic alterations of those appearances. Alterations in the appearance of the abdominal gas pattern and mucosal changes form a keystone to diagnosis. Common conditions that manifest themselves on the plain film of the abdomen were discussed. The follow-up of suspected lesions with contrast examinations of both the gastrointestinal and urinary tract will be discussed in the following chapters.

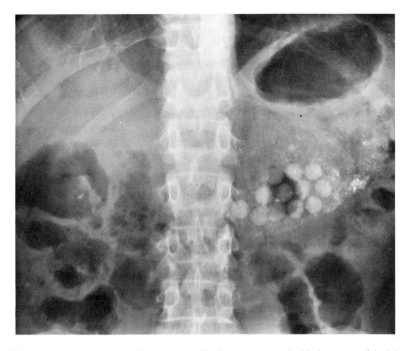

Fig. 7-25. Ferrous sulfate tablets within stomach. Tablets are recognizable because of their increased density caused by iron content.

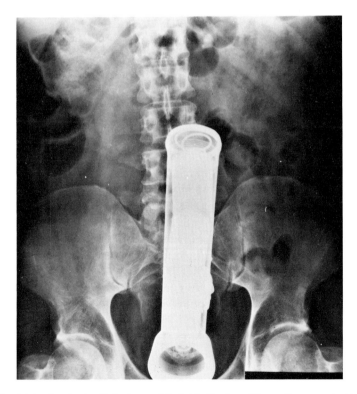

Fig. 7-26. Rectal foreign body. Patient was "de-lighted" when this easily recognizable object was removed.

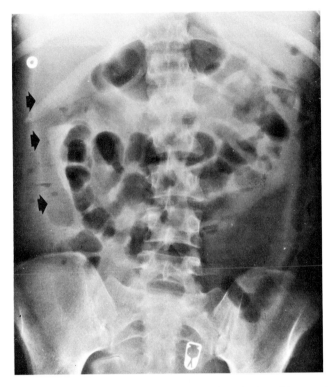

Fig. 7-27. Infected ascites. Colonic gas (arrows) is displaced from body wall by massive effusion. Four thousand milliliters of pus was drained from this patient's abdomen.

References

Daffner, R. H., Gehweiler, J. A., and Carden, T. S., Jr.: Case studies in radiology, New York, 1975, Appleton-Century-Crofts.

Fee, H. J., Jones, P. C., Kadell, B., and O'Connell, T. X.: Radiologic diagnosis of appendicitis, Arch. Surg. **112**:742, 1977.

Felson, B., editor: The acute abdomen, New York, 1974, Grune and Stratton, Inc.

Frimann-Dahl, J.: Roentgen examinations in acute abdominal diseases, ed. 3, Springfield, Ill., 1974, Charles C Thomas, Publisher.

Harris, J. H., Jr., Loh, C. K., Perlman, H. C., and Rotz, C. T., Jr.: The roentgen diagnosis of pelvic extraperitoneal effusion, Radiology **125**:343, 1977.

Menuck, L., and Siemers, P. T.: Pneumoperitoneum: importance of right upper quadrant features, Am. J. Roentgenol. **127**:753, 1976.

Meyers, M. A.: Dynamic radiology of the abdomen: normal and pathologic anatomy, New York, 1976, Springer Verlag New York, Inc.

Miller, R. E.: The radiological evaluation of intraperitoneal gas (pneumoperitoneum), CRC Crit. Rev. Clin. Radiol. Nucl. Med. **4**:61, 1973.

Paster, S. B., and Brogdon, B. G.: Roentgenographic diagnosis of pneumoperitoneum, J.A.M.A. **235**:1264, 1976.

Soter, C. S.: Radiographic findings of acute appendicitis, Med. Radiogr. Photogr. **45**:2, 1969.

Whelan, J. P.: Radiology of the abdomen: an anatomic approach, Philadelphia, 1976, Lea & Febiger.

Wolf, B. S., Khilnani, M. T., and Lautkin, A.: Diagnostic roentgenology of the digestive tract without contrast media, New York, 1960, Grune & Stratton, Inc.

8 Gastrointestinal radiology

Although plain films of the abdomen are a valuable diagnostic study, it is necessary to opacify the gastrointestinal tract with contrast material to determine the presence of intrinsic abnormalities. There are four examinations used for primary evaluation of the gastrointestinal tract: upper gastrointestinal (upper GI) examination, small bowel "follow-through," barium enema, and oral cholecystogram. Ancillary studies such an angiography, CT scanning, ultrasound, and endoscopic retrograde cholangio-pancreatography are particularly useful for examining the liver and pancreas.

TECHNICAL CONSIDERATIONS

The optimal way to study any hollow viscus filled with contrast material is to have that viscus completely empty of any other contents. For examination of the upper GI tract, an overnight fast is usually sufficient to produce this effect. Food within the stomach after a documented overnight fast is a significant finding and usually indicates gastric outlet obstruction (most often secondary to peptic ulcer disease). In this situation the stomach may still be studied after passing a nasogastric tube and suctioning the remaining contents.

Obtaining a clean colon is quite a different matter. Many preparations have been used to cleanse the colon of most of its contents. These include laxatives, enemas, and flushing by ingestion of massive quantities of fluids. In most patients the use of laxatives the night prior to study and a cleansing enema the morning of the study will produce the desired degree of cleansing. These measures may have to be more vigorous during hot summer months when fluid loss through the skin hampers osmotic effects of many types of bowel preparation. Furthermore, any barium left from a previous examination should be removed. The degree of bowel cleanliness can be noted on a scout (plain) film of the abdomen. Patients who are suspected of having toxic megacolon, acute ulcerative colitis, or obstruction *should not have any cleansing enemas.*

There is a logical order in which studies of the GI tract should be performed. Oral cholecystography, barium enema, and upper GI examination may be performed on the same day, in that order. The idea is to do the study that requires the greatest amount of clarity in the abdomen prior to the introduction of any additional contrast material. An upper GI series may be performed immediately after barium enema if the patient has evacuated the colon adequately. If the patient is to have an intravenous urogram performed, it is best done prior to a barium contrast examination.

It is important for the clinician to give as much clinical information as possible to the referring radiologist. The request should always contain pertinent clinical information and a suspected diagnosis. The radiologist should question the patient and ask about symptoms necessitating the examination. It is remarkable, however, that many patients are sent for examination without knowledge of why they are being studied or with minimal or no complaints referrable to the area for which examination has been requested.

The clinician should also inform the patient that the radiologist will send the results of the examination to him and that he (the clinician) will notify the patient of the findings. This removes the radiologist from the position of reporting serious findings to a patient he may not know well. Radiologists should make it a practice to inform patients when a study is normal, since most patients are apprehensive about the condition for which they were studied. Quite often, they will not see their referring physician for several hours or perhaps days or weeks following the examination. To make a patient worry that he may have cancer or some other serious illness when the study is normal is simply not in his best interest.

Under normal circumstances, two modes of radiographic recording are used: fluoroscopy and radiography. Fluoroscopic examination is important to determine the motility of the GI tract (peristalsis) as well as to position the patient so that all parts of the organs being studied are examined. Spot films are usually taken of strategic areas using direct fluoroscopic control: esophagogastric junction, duodenal bulb area, flexures of the colon, ileocecal area, and rectosigmoid colon. The exact number and variety of spot films will vary from examiner to examiner. Furthermore, if an abnormality is found at fluoroscopy, additional spot films are taken. Occasionally the fluoroscopic portion of the examination is recorded on videotape for later playback and evaluation. Following the fluoroscopic portion of the study, overhead films are taken with the patient in various positions for further delineation of whole organs such as the stomach or colon.

One variant of the routine study is to use a thicker preparation of barium and to distend the colon or stomach with gas (air-contrast study). In the first situation, air is introduced through the rectal tube. In the second, a gas-releasing preparation is ingested with the oral barium. The resulting study gives very fine detail, which is often sufficient to reveal subtle abnormalities. Often these studies are performed following pharmacologic enhancement.

Oral cholecystography is performed in much the same way. Spot films are made of the gallbladder with the patient in the upright and recumbent positions to look for the presence of gallstones. This technique is often repeated after the patient has ingested a fatty meal or has been injected with a cholecystokinin-like drug (Sincalide) to produce contraction of the gallbladder.

Ultrasound is used frequently to evaluate patients with suspected biliary and pancreatic disease. The examination is a reliable noninvasive method with a high degree of accuracy.

Similarly, abdominal CT examinations are commonly used in studying patients with jaundice, pancreatic disease, and suspected hepatic metastases. Many studies have shown the complementary nature of CT with ultrasound in evaluating patients suspected to have pancreatic or biliary disease (Fig. 8-1).

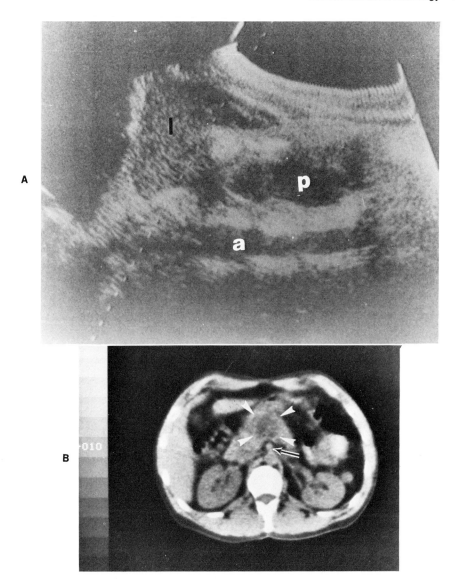

Fig. 8-1. Pancreatic pseudocyst. **A,** Ultrasound shows cystic mass in vicinity of pancreas *(p)*. Aorta *(a)* and liver *(l)* are also clearly seen. **B,** Abdominal CT scan shows pseudocyst in midportion of pancreas (arrowheads). Note relationship of pancreas to superior mesenteric artery (arrow).

Angiography is used to evaluate the gastrointestinal tract for a variety of diseases. The most useful developments in recent years have been the diagnostic and therapeutic applications in patients with acute gastrointestinal hemorrhage wherein a bleeding site may be localized by selective catheterization of celiac or mesenteric branches and vasopressor infused to control or stop the bleeding (Fig. 8-2). Angiography is also used to evaluate patients with portal hypertension prior to contemplated shunt surgery and in diagnosing pancreatic tumors.

Percutaneous cholangiography with the thin-walled (Chiba) needle is used by radiologists and gastroenterologists to study patients with obstructive jaundice. Con-

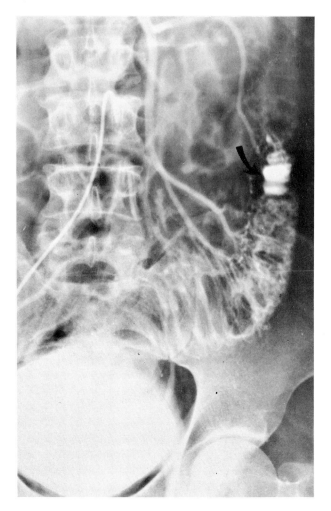

Fig. 8-2. Selective arteriogram in patient with colonic bleeding. Bleeding point may be recognized by pool of contrast material in descending colon (arrow).

trast material injected through the needle, which has been placed in a biliary duct, is used to localize the site of the obstruction (Fig. 8-3).

Endoscopic retrograde cholangiopancreatography (ERCP) is a procedure in which the ampulla of Vater is cannulated under direct endoscopic control. The examination takes a skilled endoscopist and is of some discomfort to the patient. Following cannulation, contrast material is injected into the ductal system, and fluoroscopic spot films and overhead films are made. The study is being replaced in many centers by Chiba needle, ultrasound, and CT examinations of the liver and pancreas.

Before deciding which of these special studies is to be performed, you should thoroughly discuss the case with a diagnostic radiologist to determine the optimal study to do and the order in which the studies should be performed. In this way, you will save time between making the diagnosis and beginning treatment and eliminate more costly and less productive studies.

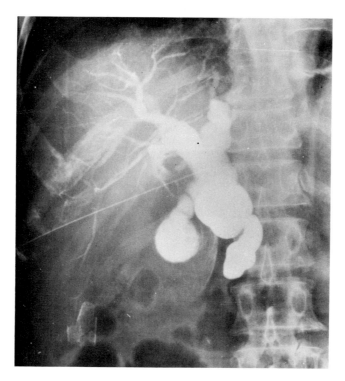

Fig. 8-3. Percutaneous transhepatic cholangiogram using thin-walled (Chiba) needle. There is dilatation of hepatobiliary tree in this patient with carcinoma of pancreas.

ANATOMIC CONSIDERATIONS

It is important for you to recognize the normal anatomy of the gastrointestinal tract and the variations that may occur. For example, six indentations may be seen on the esophagus as it courses from the pharynx into the abdomen. The superiormost is the indentation of the cricopharyngeus muscle posteriorly at the level of C6. Other indentations occur at the thoracic inlet, at the arch of the aorta at the level of T4-5, at the left main stem bronchus, proximal to the diaphragmatic hiatus by the descending aorta, and at the esophagogastric junction (Fig. 8-4).

The stomach may assume a variety of positions, lying either vertically or horizontally within the abdomen. This depends mainly on the patient's body habitus. Radiologic anatomy of the stomach includes fundus, body, antrum, prepyloric region, and pylorus (Fig. 8-5). The gastric mucosa (rugae) appears as linear parallel folds extending along the length of the stomach (Fig. 8-6). There is wide variation in size of the rugae.

The duodenum begins at the pylorus. The first portion is the bulb, which appears as a triangular-shaped structure with the base toward the pylorus. The duodenum then sweeps downward (the second or descending portion), curves medially (third portion), and twists back upward (fourth portion), terminating at the ligament of Treitz. Occasionally, on a normal duodenal examination, a small indentation representing the ampulla of Vater may be seen along the medial border of the descending portion.

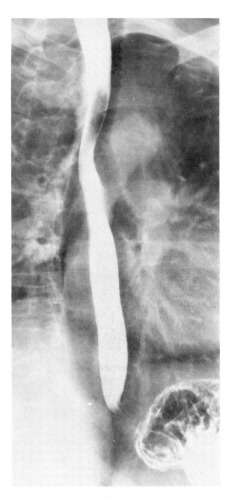

Fig. 8-4. Normal esophagus. Small amount of air is present in upper portion of esophagus.

The jejunum begins at the ligament of Treitz, gradually merging with the ileum, which enters the cecum via the ileocecal valve. Occasionally, it is possible to differentiate jejunum from ileum by the mucosal pattern. In normal individuals the cecum is in the right lower quadrant of the abdomen. The appendix usually projects downward from the cecum. Usually the ileocecal valve is on the medial aspect of the cecum.

The colon ascends, forming two looplike structures in the right and left upper quadrants known as the hepatic and splenic flexures, respectively. The descending colon terminates in the sigmoid colon, which is often quite redundant, particularly in older patients. The sigmoid colon continues on to the rectum. Under normal circumstances the rectum can be distended with barium greater than half the distance between the walls of the pelvis (Fig. 8-7).

In addition to assessing the anatomy of the GI tract, we must also concern ourselves with the physiology, that is, the motility. The causes of motility disorders are

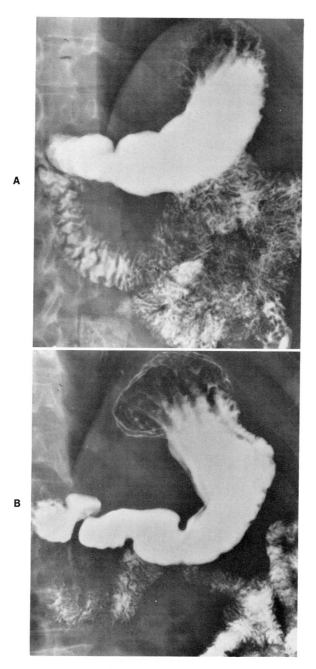

Fig. 8-5. Normal stomach, duodenum, and proximal small bowel. **A** and **B** show normal appearances in two different patients.

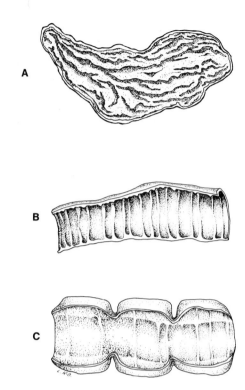

Fig. 8-6. Normal mucosal patterns. From top to bottom, **A,** stomach, **B,** small intestine, and **C,** colon.

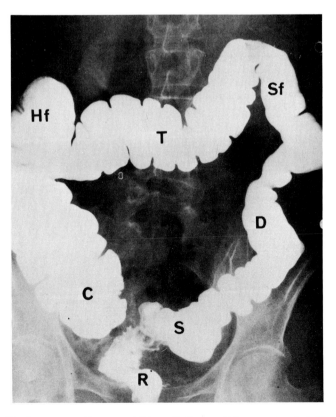

Fig. 8-7. Normal barium enema. *C,* cecum; *Hf,* hepatic flexure; *T,* transverse colon; *Sf,* splenic flexure; *D,* descending colon; *S,* sigmoid colon; *R,* rectum.

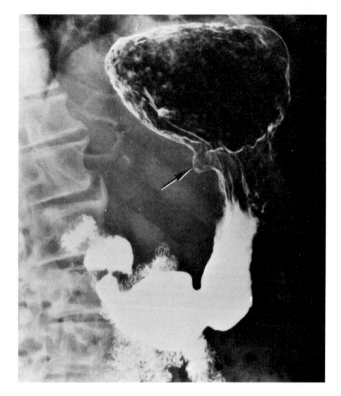

Fig. 8-8. Double contrast upper GI series in patient with healing gastric ulcer (arrow).

varied and complex. It is sufficient to say here that under normal circumstances in the esophagus, we see a stripping wave propagating a bolus of barium in a smooth, progressive motion. Peristalsis continues in the stomach from the fundus extending down to the pylorus. In the duodenum, peristalsis is slightly different. The stripping motion seen in the esophagus and stomach is not present. Instead, we see distention of the duodenal bulb, which opens at its apex and contracts forcibly as a unit moving the bolus through. Propulsive contractions are observed throughout the small intestine and colon.

In the colon there are several areas of normal or physiologic narrowing that may occur with spasm. These are found in the transverse colon near the flexures and in the descending colon.

When encountering spasm of the GI tract, particularly in the colon, it is sometimes useful to perform a pharmacologically enhanced study. Glucagon injected intravenously in 0.5 to 2 mg doses will produce relaxation of the GI tract through its antivagal action. Other drugs that have been used, although with side effects, include atropine, 0.5 to 1 mg, and propantheline (Pro-Banthine), 15 to 60 mg. These agents may also be used to produce relaxation of the GI tract for double contrast examinations, which assist in the delineation of subtle abnormalities (Figs. 8-8 and 8-9).

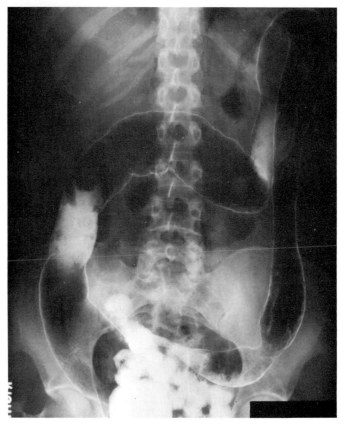

Fig. 8-9. Air-contrast barium enema in patient with ulcerative colitis. Notice absence of haustra.

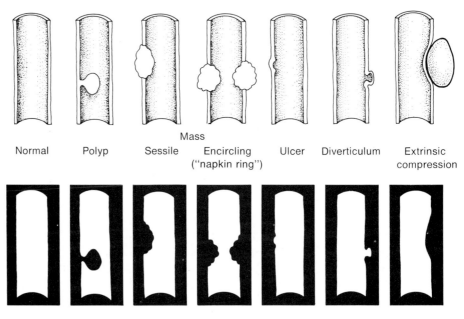

Normal Polyp Sessile Encircling Ulcer Diverticulum Extrinsic
                         Mass   compression
                         ("napkin ring")

Fig. 8-10. Schematic drawing illustrates pathologic alterations affecting gastrointestinal tract. Top row, gross appearance; bottom row, radiographic appearance.

PATHOLOGIC CONSIDERATIONS

Because the GI tract is a tube, pathologic alterations seen in one segment may be seen in any other segment. For example, a mucosal tumor of the esophagus has an appearance identical to a similar-sized tumor of the stomach, small intestine, or colon. The incidence of these lesions will vary from location to location, and you must learn the common locations of these lesions in the particular organs. However, do keep in mind that for practical purposes these lesions all have similar appearances, no matter where they occur. (Using the same concept a broad generalization may be made that similar lesions are also seen in other tubular structures such as the urinary tract, bronchi, and blood vessels.)

There are six basic alterations we can recognize:

1. Polypoid lesions
2. Mucosal mass lesions
3. Ulceration
4. Diverticula
5. Extrinsic compression
6. Benign stricture

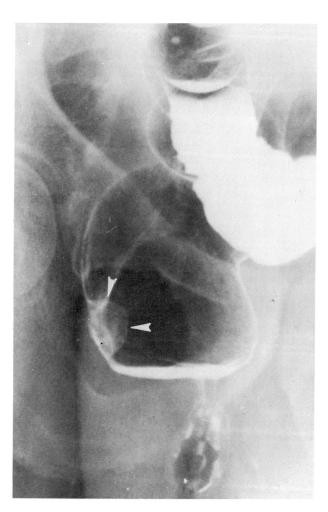

Fig. 8-11. Broad-based (sessile) polyp of rectum (arrowheads).

These are illustrated in Fig. 8-10.

In addition, motility disorders and dilatation may be seen in any portion of the GI tract.

Polypoid lesions appear as small, rounded filling defects in the lumen. They may be broad based (Fig. 8-11) or on a stalk (Fig. 8-12). They are true mucosal lesions, and, when seen end on, their outer margins are indistinct, being obscured by surrounding barium. In contrast, diverticula seen end on have discernible outer margins but indistinct inner margins. This is illustrated in Fig. 8-13.

Mucosal mass lesions frequently begin as small polyps. As the polyp enlarges, its surface may become irregular. Puckering may be seen near the base of the lesion. There is an abrupt change of the mucosa from normal to tumor. Further growth will produce encasement as the tumor grows completely around the lumen, producing the classic apple-core appearance (Figs. 8-14 and 8-15).

There are two other varieties of "filling defects" that may be seen in the GI tract:

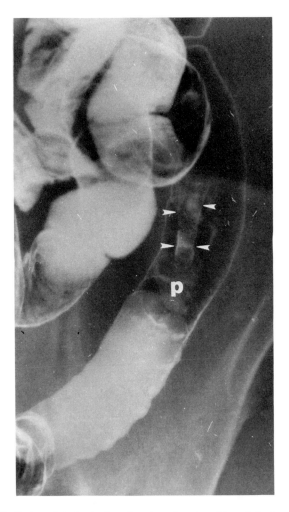

Fig. 8-12. Pedunculated colonic polyp. Arrowheads outline stalk of polyp *(p)*.

mucosal hypertrophy (Fig. 8-16) and varices (Fig. 8-17). With both these entities, it is important not to misinterpret them as tumor.

Ulceration of the GI tract results in a collection of barium being seen outside the normal lumen. Quite frequently the ulcer is surrounded by an edematous ulcer collar or mound. In benign ulcers, particularly of the stomach, mucosal folds may be seen radiating into the ulcer crater. The mass leading up to the ulcer is smooth with gradually sloping margins. Penetration of the ulcer beyond the normal lumen is a sign of a benign lesion. Ulceration may also occur within mass lesions. You should remember that there are no *malignant ulcers;* there are *ulcerating malignancies.* Several ulcers are illustrated in Figs. 8-18 through 8-20. Table 5 lists the radiologic differential features between benign gastric ulcers and ulcerating malignancies.

Diverticula are benign outpouchings of the wall of the GI tract. Diverticula are covered by all layers of the bowel wall. They may be relatively small, as in the colon (Fig. 8-21), or quite large, as a Zenker diverticulum of the esophagus (Fig. 8-22).

Text continued on p. 231.

Table 5. Comparative features of benign gastric ulcers and ulcerating malignancies

Benign gastric ulcers	Ulcerating malignancies
Penetration beyond lumen	Intraluminal crater located between abrupt points of transition (in contrast to intraluminal crater in mound of even edematous surrounding tissue)
Mucosal folds radiate to crater edge	Crater shallow, width exceeds depth
Hampton's line	Absent Hampton's line
Ulcer collar	Ulcer irregularly shaped
Ulcer mound, gradual tapering to normal mucosa	Eccentric location of ulcer in mass
Normal distensibility and pliability	Fixation of affected area
Peristalsis transmitted through area	Peristalsis not transmitted through area
Single, centrally located blood clot in crater base	Irregular base to crater

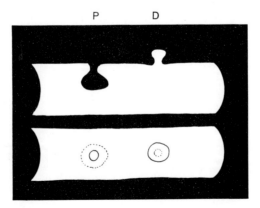

Fig. 8-13. Drawing illustrates difference between radiographic appearance of polyp *(P)* and diverticulum *(D).* Top, profile view; bottom, end-on view. Mnemonic in distinguishing these two lesions when seen on end is *"fuzzy outside—polyp (FOP); fuzzy inside—tic (FIT)."*

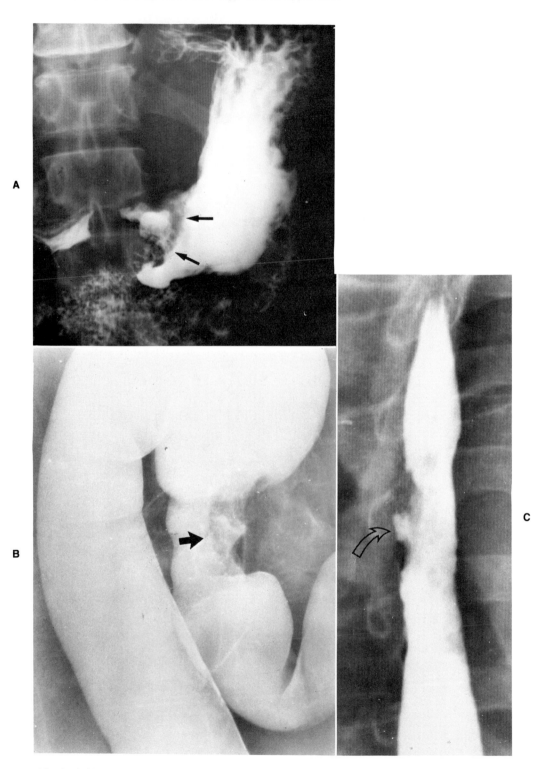

Fig. 8-14. Mucosal mass lesions. **A,** Ulcerating malignancy of antrum. Arrows point to mass. **B,** Carcinoma of colon. Note abrupt margins in lesion (arrow). **C,** Esophageal carcinoma. There is raised mucosal lesion. Central ulcer is present (arrow).

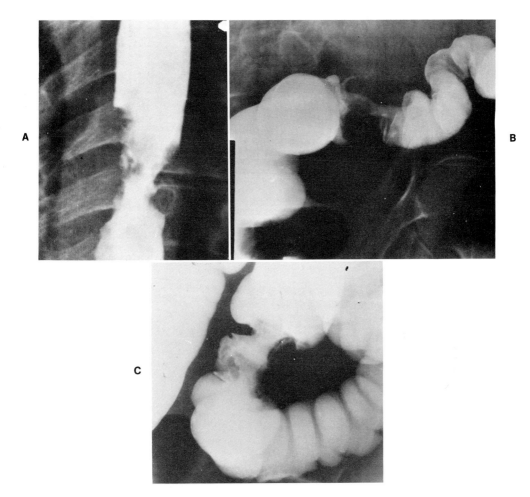

Fig. 8-15. "Napkin ring" ("apple core") mucosal lesions. Note similarity of these lesions. **A,** Esophageal carcinoma. **B** and **C,** Colonic carcinoma.

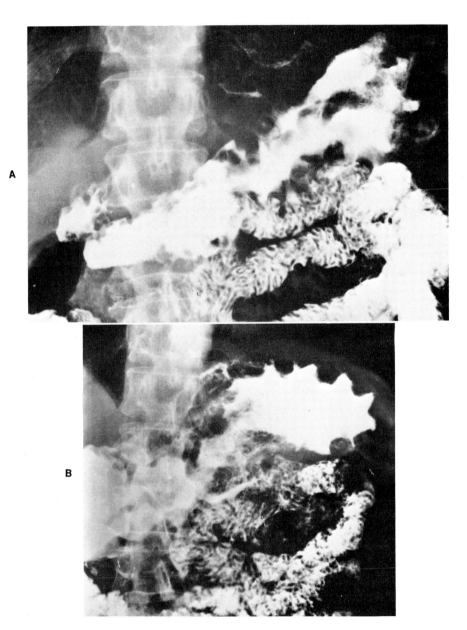

Fig. 8-16. Gastric mucosal hypertrophy. Multiple filling defects in stomach represent hypertrophic gastric folds. Endoscopy was required for confirmation.

Fig. 8-17. Esophageal varices. Multiple wormlike filling defects in esophagus represent esophageal varices in these patients with chronic alcoholism. (From Daffner, R. H., Gehweiler, J. A., and Carden, T. S., Jr.: Case studies in radiology, New York, 1975, Appleton-Century-Crofts. Reproduced with permission of the publisher.)

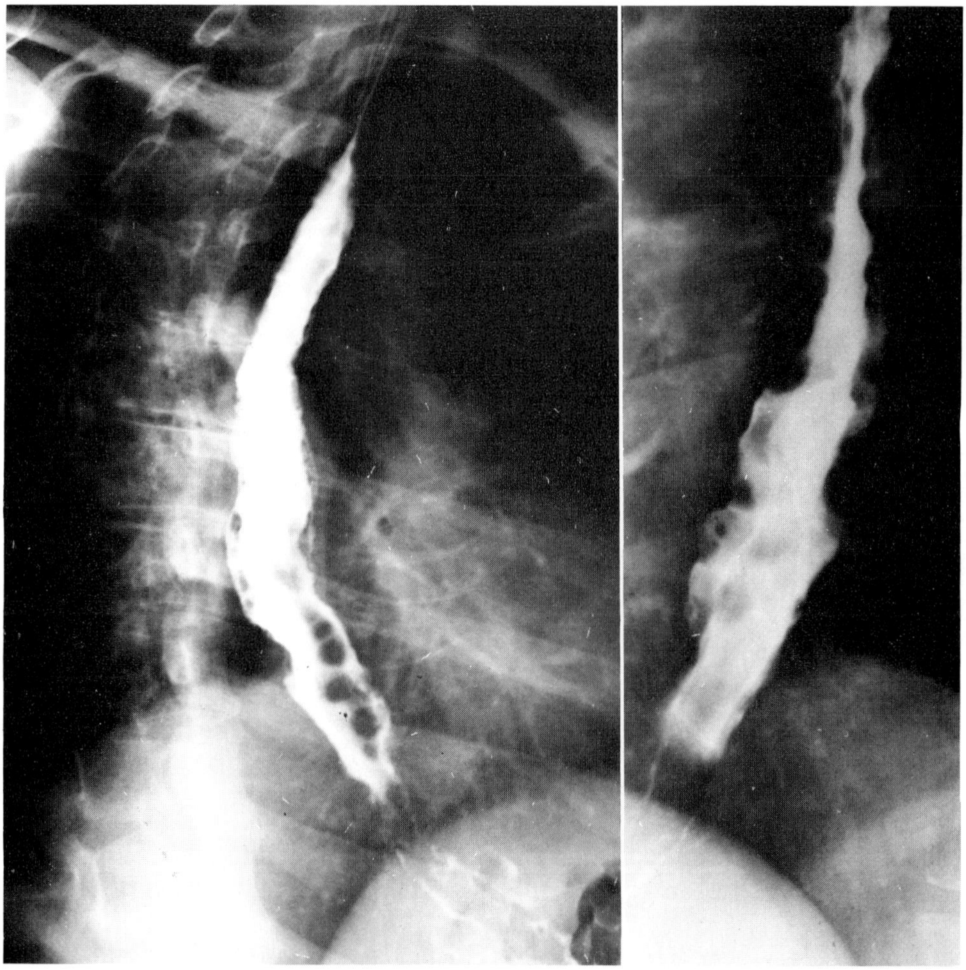

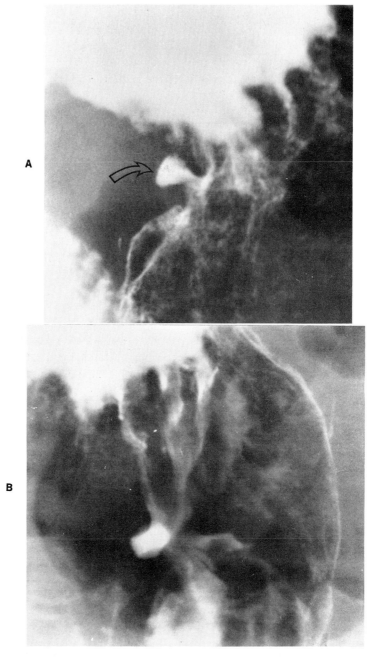

Fig. 8-18. Benign gastric ulcers on lesser curvature side. **A,** Note penetration of ulcer beyond wall of stomach (arrow). **B.** Note radiation of folds toward ulcer crater.

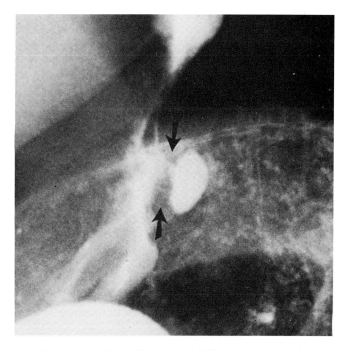

Fig. 8-19. Esophageal ulcer. Note ulcer collar (arrows). This appearance is similar to that of ulcer in stomach.

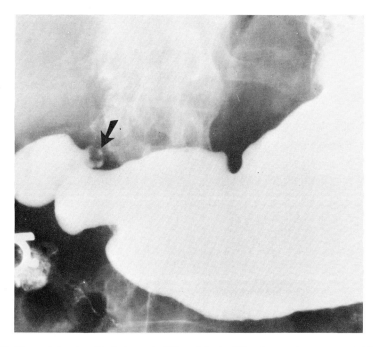

Fig. 8-20. Ulcer of duodenal bulb (arrow). Filling defect within ulcer crater represents blood clot.

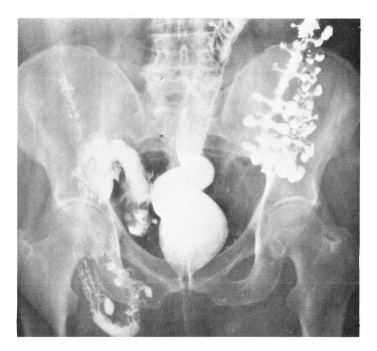

Fig. 8-21. Multiple colonic diverticula. Note inguinal hernia on right.

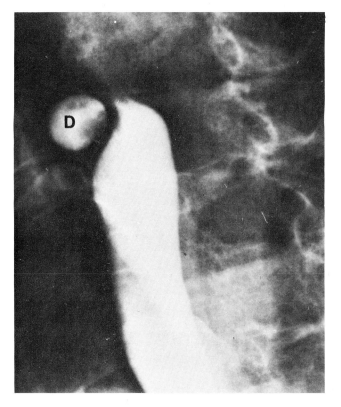

Fig. 8-22. Zenker diverticulum *(D)* of esophagus.

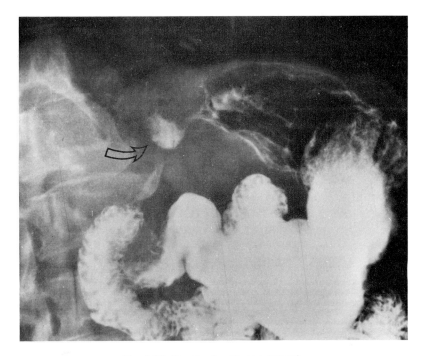

Fig. 8-23. Gastric diverticulum (arrow).

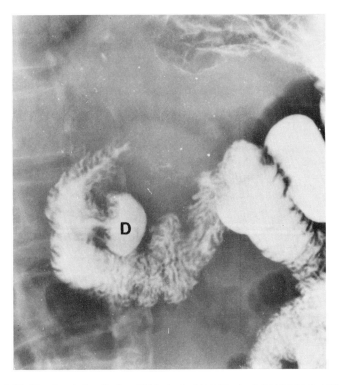

Fig. 8-24. Duodenal diverticulum *(D)* in typical location in descending duodenum.

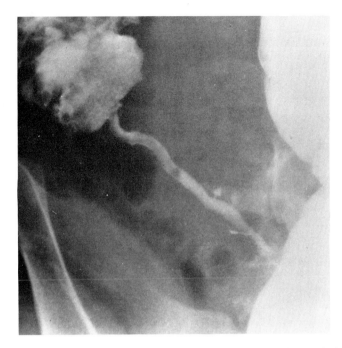

Fig. 8-25. Appendiceal diverticula. Small lucency within appendix is air bubble.

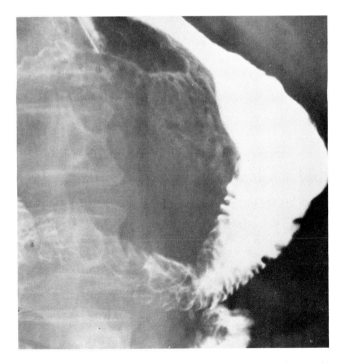

Fig. 8-26. Extrinsic compression of stomach by large pancreatic pseudocyst. Note stretching of mucosal folds on lesser curvature side.

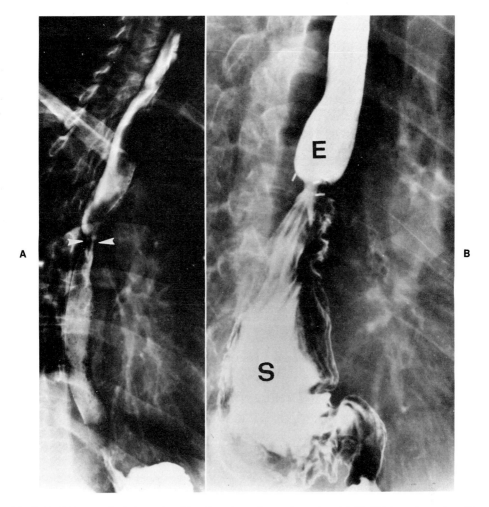

Fig. 8-27. Strictures. **A,** Stricture in midportion of esophagus (arrowheads). **B,** Stricture at anastomotic site in patient who has undergone esophagogastrectomy. *E,* Esophagus; *S,* stomach.

Occasionally, they will contain foreign material. Figs. 8-23 through 8-25 show various diverticula.

Extrinsic compression appears as a smooth indentation of the bowel wall with gradually tapering margins. On palpation during fluoroscopy the mucosa can be seen to be intact. It may be difficult to differentiate this from an intramural lesion causing compression (Fig. 8-26).

Benign stricture formation appears as concentric or eccentric narrowing of the lumen. The margins should be smooth and tapering. The mucosa generally should be intact. They are often difficult to differentiate from carcinoma (Fig. 8-27).

Cholecystography

As previously mentioned, the biliary system may be visualized by either oral or intravenously injected contrast material. The physiology of these substances was dis-

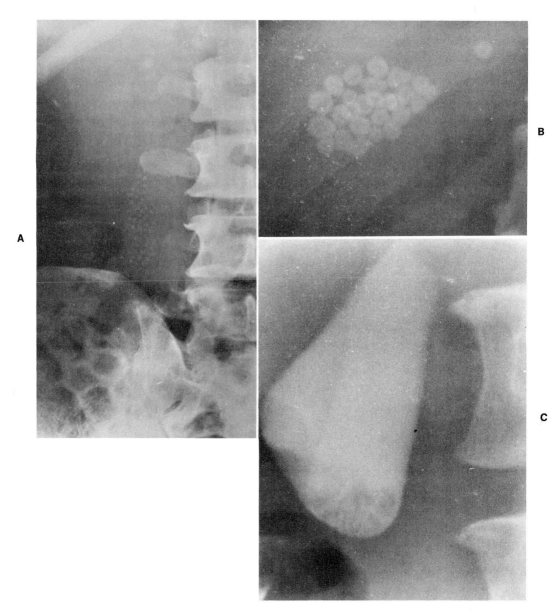

Fig. 8-28. Gallstones. Note variety of shapes stones may take. **A** and **B**, Radiopaque gallstones. **C**, Radiolucent stones seen on oral cholecystogram.

cussed in Chapter 3. The most common abnormalities encountered in the biliary tract are nonvisualization and calculous disease (Fig. 8-28).

Postoperative appearance of GI tract

There are a number of alterations surgical procedures make on the appearance of the barium-filled GI tract. These will be briefly described and illustrated.

Esophageal bypass surgery for carcinoma or stricture may be done in three ways:

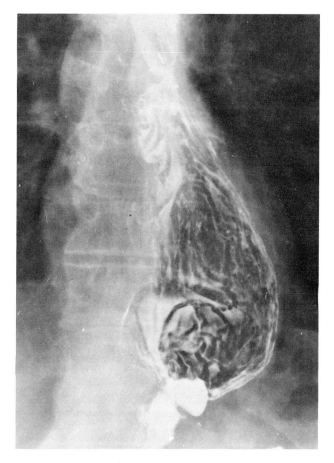

Fig. 8-29. Postoperative esophagogastrectomy. Note gastric rugae that identify stomach.

gastroesophagotomy, gastric (Beck) tube, and colon swing. In a *gastroesophagotomy* (sometimes called esophagogastrectomy) the stomach is mobilized, preserving its blood supply, and is brought into the chest where it is anastomosed with the resected end of the esophagus in its midportion. This is usually done for a distal carcinoma or stricture. On a chest radiograph or esophagogram, this appears as a soft tissue density that may contain air or mottled fluid just to the right of the cardiac silhouette. Frequently the gastric rugae identify this structure. On the lateral film the transposed stomach is in an anterior position (Fig. 8-29).

The *gastric (Beck) tube* procedure was designed as a palliative procedure for a patient with carcinoma of the esophagus and is occasionally used in patients with esophageal stricture. In this procedure a gastric tube is fabricated using the greater curvature of the stomach, preserving the blood supply. The tube is then pulled substernally, where it is anastomosed with the cervical esophagus. The appearance of the Beck tube is shown in Fig. 8-30.

The *colon swing* was a popular procedure that has largely been abandoned at the

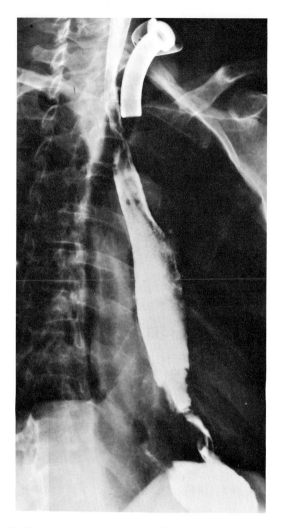

Fig. 8-30. Postoperative appearance of Beck gastric tube interposition.

present time. In this technique a section of transverse colon is mobilized along with its mesentery and pulled substernally to be anastomosed with the upper esophagus (Fig. 8-31).

A number of procedures have been designed for palliation of hiatal hernia. Most of these (Belsey, Thal, Nissen) involve fundoplication, in which the fundus is sutured around the lower esophagus to create a tighter sphincter. This results in the radiographic appearance of a mass with smooth, intact mucosa near the gastroesophageal junction. This finding should alert the fluoroscopist to the type of procedure performed.

Surgery for peptic ulcer disease may take several forms. One popular procedure is vagotomy and pyloroplasty. Previous vagotomy may be recognized by the presence of midline clips at the level of the diaphragm. A pyloroplasty performed at the same

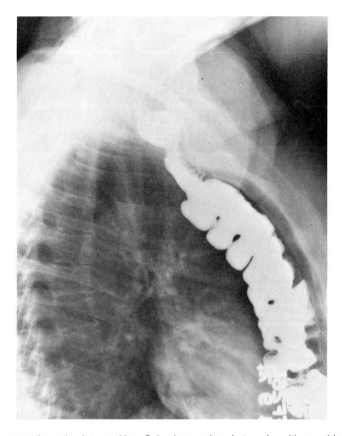

Fig. 8-31. Postoperative colon interposition. Colon is seen in substernal position on this lateral film.

time results in a deformity in the antral and pyloric regions. This may often be confused with severe scarring from previous ulcer disease. An alternate form of drainage procedure is the gastrojejunostomy, in which a loop of jejunum is anastomosed with the greater curvature of the stomach.

Patients who have had repeated episodes of severe peptic ulcer disease with or without perforation may require a subtotal gastrectomy, especially if they show signs of obstruction. Although several procedures have been designed, they are collectively referred to as Billroth I or Billroth II type subtotal gastrectomies. A Billroth I procedure (Fig. 8-32) is recognizable as a direct continuation of an amputated distal stomach with the duodenum. The base of the duodenal bulb is removed at the time of surgery. In a Billroth II procedure (Fig. 8-33) a subtotal gastrectomy is performed, with anastomosis of the gastric stump to a loop of jejunum. An afferent loop drains the pancreatobiliary system through the duodenum. The base of the duodenal bulb usually is removed in this procedure.

Anastomoses between the distal ileum and colon (ileocolostomy) are performed for inflammatory bowel disease or carcinoma. These are easily recognized by the filling of small bowel from a portion of colon other than the cecum.

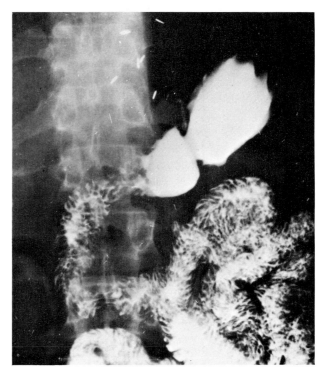

Fig. 8-32. Postoperative Billroth I subtotal gastrectomy and gastroenterostomy. Note absence of duodenal bulb. Note also vagotomy clips.

SUMMARY

The gastrointestinal tract is a tubular structure that allows recognition of patterns of disease that may be seen in any portion. In each area the appearance of these lesions will be quite similar. However, the incidence varies from location to location, depending on the disease. These abnormalities include polypoid lesions, mucosal tumors, ulcerations, diverticula, extrinsic compression, and benign stricture. A discussion of special procedures and their application to the gastrointestinal tract was also presented.

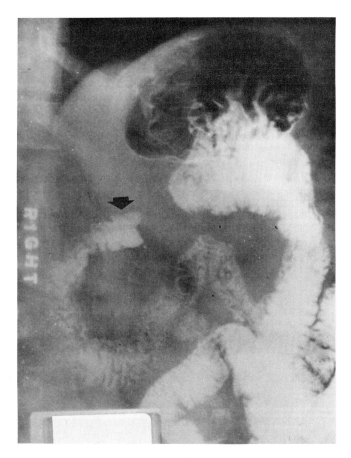

Fig. 8-33. Postoperative Billroth II subtotal gastrectomy and gastroenterostomy. Note blind ending of afferent loop (arrow).

Selected case studies

For your case studies, consider three different groups of patients who have similar findings.

Cases 8-1 to 8-3: DYSPHAGIA

The patients in this group all have a similar history of dysphagia. All three are middle-aged women who have a variety of aches and pains and who have visited your office many times.

Patient 1, in describing her dysphagia, states that she has been having difficulty swallowing for the past 3 months. At first she had difficulty only with solid foods. She changed to a liquid diet. Now she is having difficulty swallowing even water. Concomitant with her symptoms is a 40-pound weight loss over the past 3 months. Her esophagogram is shown in Case 8-1.

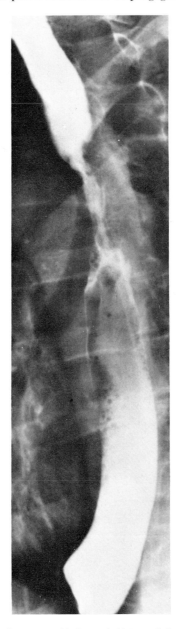

Case 8-1. Patient 1. Middle-aged woman with 3-month history of dysphagia. What does the esophagogram show?

Patient 2 gives a history of having a sensation of food catching in the midportion of the chest. She is frequently awakened by chest pains that are relieved by antacids. She has a long history of "heartburn." There is no appreciable weight loss. This patient is markedly obese. Her esophagogram is shown in Case 8-2, A.

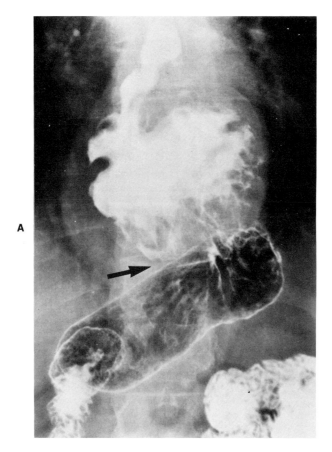

A

Case 8-2. Patient 2. **A,** Detail of gastroesophageal region in middle-aged woman with dysphagia. Arrow indicates level of diaphragm. What is the main abnormality?

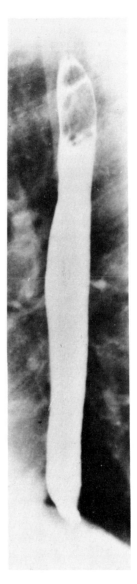

Case 8-3. Patient 3. Esophagogram in patient with "lump in the throat." Lucency within upper esophagus is air bubble.

Patient 3 complains of having a "lump stuck in her throat." Her review of systems is remarkable in that it is *totally positive*. Physical examination is entirely unremarkable. Her esophagogram is shown in Case 8-3.

What are the radiographic findings in each case? What is your diagnosis? Do you see the value of combining the radiographic examination with a careful history and physical examination?

ROENTGEN DIAGNOSIS

Patient 1. There is a normal swallowing mechanism at fluoroscopy. There is an 8 cm area of narrowing in the mid- to distal portion of the esophagus. There is an abrupt change in the mucosa at the beginning of the narrow area, with irregularity of the lesion as it encircles the esophagus. The findings are consistent with a diagnosis of carcinoma of the esophagus.

Patient 2. Radiographic and fluoroscopic examinations demonstrate a normal swallowing mechanism and normal esophageal motility. A moderate-sized sliding-type hiatal hernia is present in the distal esophagus. Gross gastroesophageal reflux was present at fluoroscopy.

Patient 3. Radiographic and fluoroscopic examinations show a normal swallowing mechanism, normal motility, and normal mucosal pattern. There is no reflux. This study is normal. The findings are consistent with a diagnosis of "globus hystericus."

DISCUSSION

These three patients report the same complaint. On close examination of their histories, significant weight loss accompanies the symptoms of patient 1. Benign conditions of the esophagus generally do not result in weight loss. The history given in this patient is quite characteristic of an obstructing lesion: difficulty swallowing solids progressing to the point where only liquids could be taken by mouth. The radiographic findings are typical of an infiltrating mucosal lesion with extension around the lumen of the viscus, as noted previously in the chapter.

Patient 2, who has a hiatal hernia, also complained of dysphagia. However, the history elicited was more of postprandial burning and "heartburn." Hiatal hernia by itself may not cause symptoms; however, gastroesophageal reflux can and often does cause significant symptoms. Patients with reflux may develop peptic ulcerations in the distal esophagus (Case 8-2, *B*) or in some instances may even develop aspiration pneumonitis, a condition frequently seen in patients with scleroderma.

Patient 3 complained of the classic "lump in the throat." Additional history suggests an overlying psychogenic disorder. However, you must be prepared to rule out an organic lesion in any patient before making a diagnosis of psychogenic disorder. Her examination was entirely normal.

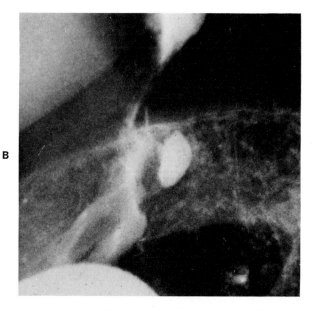

B

Case 8-2. B, Patient with peptic ulceration in distal esophagus caused by gastroesophageal reflux. Although this is unusual site for ulcer, features of typical benign ulcer are present.

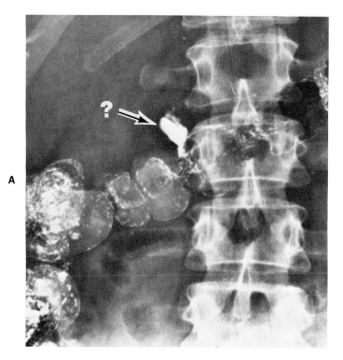

Case 8-4. Patient 4. **A,** Detail view of scout film taken as part of gallbladder series. Unabsorbed chole-cystographic contrast material is present in colon. What is the arrow pointing to?

Cases 8-4 to 8-6: EPIGASTRIC PAIN

The patients in this group all give similar histories of epigastric pain that is worse at night and is relieved by antacids.

Patient 4 is a 45-year-old man who also claims to have fatty food intolerance. A gallbladder series was ordered (Case 8-4, *A*).

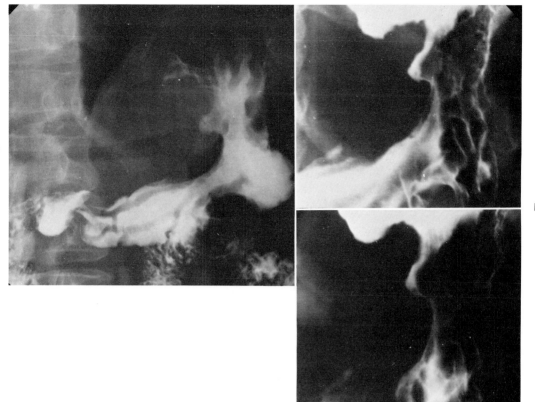

Case 8-5. Patient 5. **A,** Static radiograph of stomach of 50-year-old man with abdominal pain and occult blood in stool. **B,** Fluoroscopic spot films. Note that abnormality remains constant and does not change with fluoroscopy.

Patient 5 is a 50-year-old man who, in addition to the symptoms noted, has physical findings of occult blood on stool examination. He gives a history of weight loss over the past few months and decreasing appetite. His gallbladder examination was normal. Films from his upper GI series are shown in Case 8-5, *A* and *B*.

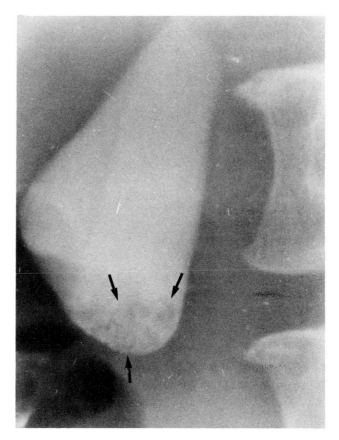

Case 8-6. Patient 6. Oral cholecystogram. What are the arrows pointing to?

Patient 6 gives a history identical to that of patient 4. His oral cholecystogram is shown in Case 8-6.

What are the radiographic findings in each case? Would you order any additional studies? What is your diagnosis?

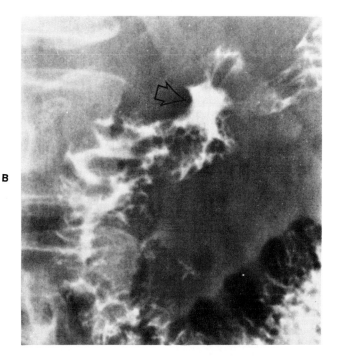

Case 8-4. Patient 4. **B,** Spot film of duodenal bulb from upper GI series. There is an irregular ulcer cra-ter in duodenal bulb (arrow). This area trapped cholecystographic contrast material seen in **A.**

ROENTGEN DIAGNOSIS

Patient 4. A plain film of the abdomen shows no contrast medium within the gallbladder. Contrast medium is seen within the colon in a flocculant pattern representing nonabsorbed cholecystographic material. There is, in addition, a concentrated collection of contrast medium just above this area, which suggests trapping of the contrast agent by a peptic ulcer. An upper GI series was performed and showed a normal stomach. However, there is an *ulcer crater* within the duodenal bulb (Case 8-4, *B*). Mucosal edema is present around the crater, suggest-ing an active ulcer.

A subsequent oral cholecystogram showed a normal gallbladder.

Patient 5. Detail films of the stomach in this patient show a mass along the lesser curva-ture of the stomach projecting into the lumen. Ulceration is present in this mass. The borders of the mass have an abrupt transition with the gastric mucosa. These are the findings of an ulcerating carcinoma. Endoscopic examination confirmed the presence of an ulcerating adeno-carcinoma of the stomach.

Patient 6. Oral cholecystogram showed multiple radiolucent gallstones. An upper GI series was also performed on this patient and was normal.

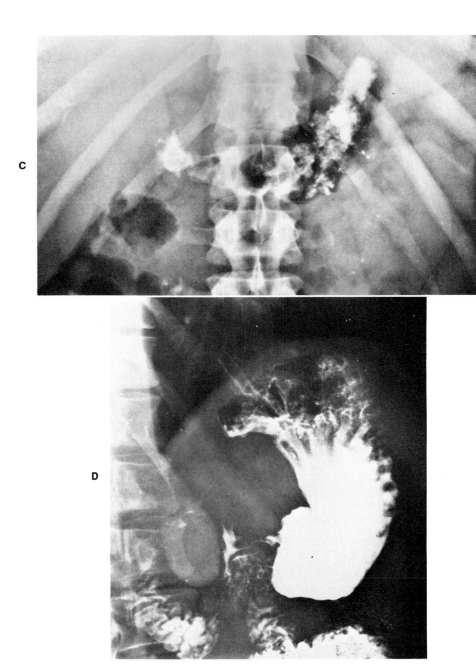

Case 8-4. Another patient. **C,** Gallbladder scout film. Oral cholecystographic contrast material taken previous night remains in stomach. **D,** Upper GI series shows near total gastric outlet obstruction. Normal gallbladder is seen as well. (Case 8-4, **A** to **D,** from Daffner, R. H.: New Physician **23:**45, 1974. Reproduced with permission of the publisher.)

DISCUSSION

Once again you have three patients with similar symptoms. They illustrate the need to combine oral cholecystography with an upper GI series. Quite often, symptoms of gallbladder disease simulate GI disease and vice versa.

The failure of a gallbladder to opacify following ingestion of oral contrast material does not necessarily mean there is intrinsic biliary disease. There are many nonbiliary causes of non-opacification. In Chapter 3 we discussed the physiology of cholecystographic material. By understanding this physiology, you can see that there are many conditions that might prevent opacification of the gallbladder. One of the most common causes of nonopacification is that the patient may not have taken the contrast agent the night before. Generally there is not 100% absorption of the material, and flecks of unabsorbed contrast medium, as shown in Case 8-4, *A*, may be seen within the GI tract. If the patient takes the tablets immediately before coming to the x-ray department, the material will be seen within the stomach. When the radiologist makes this observation, he must ask the patient when the material was ingested. If there is a lesion producing gastric outlet obstruction (Case 8-4, *C* and *D*), all the material taken the night before will remain in the stomach.

Vomiting is a common side effect after the ingestion of oral cholecystographic material. Thus a patient who took the tablets as directed may have vomited them back up, resulting in nonopacification.

Another cause of nonopacification is diarrhea, which may occasionally result from the contrast agent. This may also occur in patients with hypermotility syndromes. In these patients the contrast material would have passed through the duodenum and small intestine too rapidly for adequate absorption. Malabsorption may occur in patients with severe pancreatic disease.

Finally, one must always make sure that the patient has not had a cholecystectomy. The reader will be amazed at how many requests come to an x-ray department for an oral cholecystogram for patients who have had their gallbladders removed.

Patient 5 has symptoms suggesting peptic ulceration. However, the real culprit was a large carcinoma that had ulcerated. The findings illustrated in Case 8-5, *A* and *B*, are characteristic of an ulcerating malignancy. Contrast this with a benign gastric ulcer in which there is penetration of the ulcer crater beyond the lumen, radiation of folds toward the crater, and a gentle sloping edematous collar surrounding the lesion (Case 8-5, *C*). These are all signs of benign

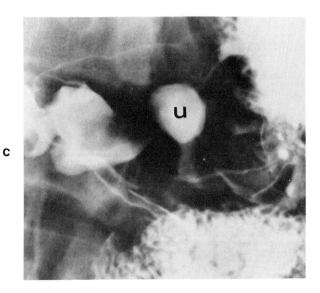

Case 8-5. C, Detail view of benign lesser curvature ulcer *(u)* in another patient. Note radiation of folds toward ulcer crater.

ulcer. Table 5, earlier in the chapter, compares benign gastric ulcers with ulcerating malignancies.

Patient 6 has gallstones. He has a normally functioning gallbladder. However, gallstones are indicative of biliary disease. The upper GI series was performed in this patient because, as mentioned before, the symptoms of biliary and GI disease may mimic each other.

Cases 8-7 to 8-9: ACUTE ABDOMEN

The patients in this group all came to the emergency room with the following history: acute onset of abdominal pain accompanied by nausea and vomiting. On physical examination there is distention of the abdomen and decreased bowel sounds and the abdomen is tympanic.

Patient 7 is a 79-year-old woman. Her plain film is shown in Case 8-7, A.

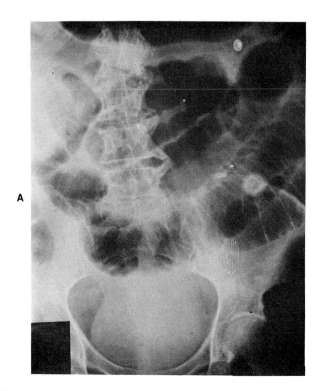

Case 8-7. Patient 7. **A,** Abdominal plain film of 79-year-old woman with "acute abdomen."

Patient 8 is an 82-year-old woman who has a history of chronic laxative use. She has a 4-day history of abdominal pain. Her plain film is shown in Case 8-8, *A* and *B*.

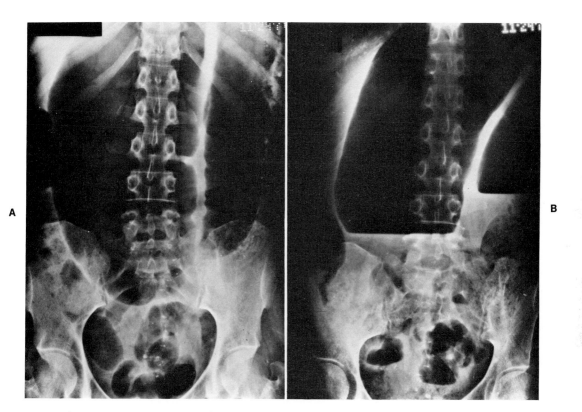

A

B

Case 8-8. Patient 8. **A** and **B**, Abdominal plain films in elderly woman with "acute abdomen."

Patient 9 is a 11-year-old boy with acute onset of epigastric abdominal pain radiating into the right groin. On physical examination there is a point tenderness over the right lower quadrant of the abdomen. His plain film is shown in Case 8-9.

What are the radiographic findings? Will you order any additional studies? What is your diagnosis?

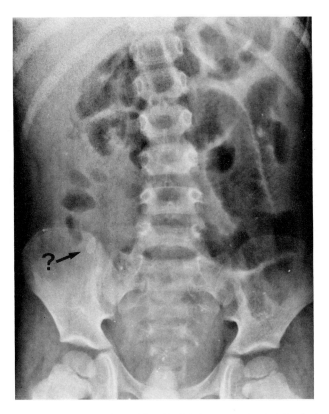

Case 8-9. Patient 9. Abdominal plain film in child with right lower quadrant abdominal pain. What is the arrow pointing to?

ROENTGEN DIAGNOSIS AND DISCUSSION

Patient 7. The plain film of the abdomen shows small bowel dilatation. The pelvis is relatively free of gas. A large calcific density is present in the left midabdomen. This calcific density represents a gallstone, the cause of this patient's gallstone ileus. Other abnormalities that may be seen in this entity but are not present on this film include gas within the biliary tree and air-fluid levels on horizontal beam films.

Gallstone ileus is really a misnomer. In truth, the disorder is a mechanical obstruction. It results from erosion of a large gallstone through the wall of a chronically inflamed gallbladder into the duodenum, which has become adherent secondary to the adjacent inflammatory process. The stone passes easily through the small bowel until it reaches the ileocecal valve. At this point the stone is usually too large to pass and impacts, resulting in a bowel obstruction. Occasionally the stone is lucent and is not seen on plain films. In these cases, it may be necessary to perform a barium enema to make the diagnosis. Occasionally a pseudodiverticulum representing the tract of the stone is seen on the antimesenteric side of the duodenum (Case 8-7, *B* and *C*).

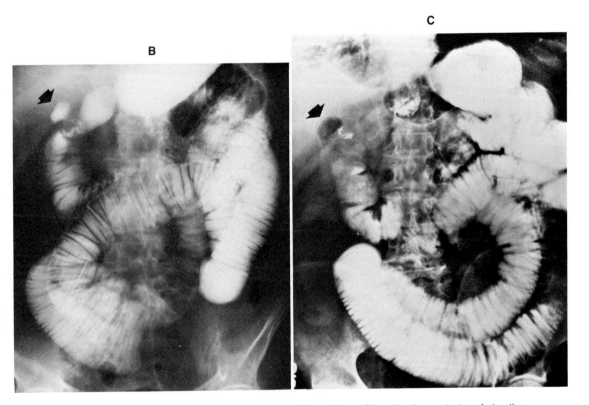

Case 8-7. B and **C,** Another patient with gallstone ileus. Upper GI series demonstrates obstructive changes in small bowel. Pseudodiverticulum is seen in both views on antimesenteric side of duodenum (arrows).

Patient 8. The plain film of the abdomen shows massive dilatation of the colon with air-fluid levels. A barium enema was performed on this patient and demonstrated total obstruction to the passage of barium in the sigmoid colon in a beaklike manner (Case 8-8, *C* and *D*) This finding is characteristic of a sigmoid volvulus.

Sigmoid volvulus occurs in older patients, often with a history of long-term laxative use. In these patients the sigmoid colon becomes redundant and floppy and is able to twist on itself.

Cecal volvulus may occur in patients who have a hypermobile cecum, that is, one not bound down by mesentery. Clincal findings are similar to those of sigmoid volvulus. However, there is more small bowel dilatation. There is not a great degree of colonic dilatation because the obstruction is proximal to the remainder of the colon. Both these entities are surgical emergencies. If undetected, ischemic necrosis or cecal rupture may occur.

Patient 9. The plain film of the abdomen shows scoliosis to the right. There is a localized ileus in the right lower quadrant. A small calcified density is present in this region. In view of the history, which also included fever and elevated white count, the most likely diagnosis is acute appendicitis with impacted fecalith in the appendix. A subsequent laparotomy confirmed this diagnosis.

The plain film and barium enema findings in acute appendicitis are listed in the following outline.

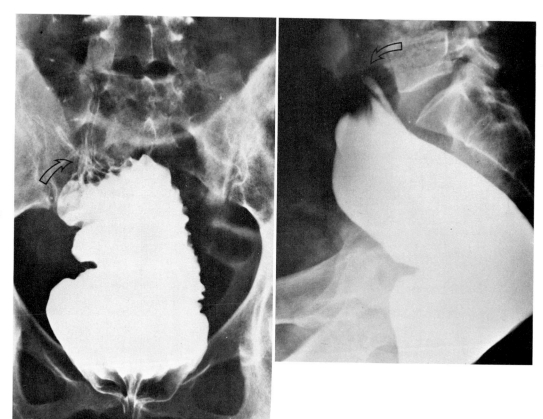

C

D

Case 8-8. Patient 8. Barium enema. **C,** Frontal and, **D,** lateral views of rectosigmoid colon demonstrate complete occlusion secondary to sigmoid volvulus. Twisted mucosa can be seen (arrows).

RADIOGRAPHIC FINDINGS OF ACUTE APPENDICITIS

I. Plain film
  A. Ileocecal changes: localized ileus
    1. Distention
    2. Thickened, edematous wall
    3. Fluid level
    4. Haziness in right lower quadrant from fluid accumulation
  B. Distal ileus
  C. Small bowel obstruction
  D. Gas in appendiceal lumen
  E. Free intraperitoneal air
  F. Fecalith of the appendix
  G. Scoliosis to the right
  H. Loss of psoas shadow on the right
  I. Obliteration of properitoneal fat line on right
II. Barium enema
  A. Changes in cecum
    1. Pressure (extrinsic) on cecum: single defect or "reverse three"
    2. Persistence of indentation when distended with air
  B. Absent filling of appendiceal lumen
  C. Patent appendiceal lumen: complete filling rules out appendicitis
  D. Segmental appendiceal obstruction: sharp cutoff

These findings have been discussed elsewhere and will not be repeated here. I would like to emphasize, however, that barium enema is a useful adjunct in the diagnosis of appendicitis, particularly when the clinical findings and plain film findings are equivocal. In general, if an appendix can be visualized on the barium enema, the patient does not have appendicitis. Furthermore, an inflammatory mass in the vicinity of the appendix and cecum may aid in making the diagnosis of appendicitis.

References

Balthazar, E. J., and Schechter, L. S.: Gallstone ileus: the importance of contrast examinations in the roentgenographic diagnosis, Am. J. Roentgenol. **125:**374, 1975.

Daffner, R. H., Gehweiler, J. A., and Carden, T. S., Jr.: Case studies in radiology, New York, 1975, Appleton-Century-Crofts.

Dodd, G. D.: Double contrast examination of the upper gastrointestinal tract. In American College of Radiology syllabus: categorical course on gastrointestinal radiology, Chicago, 1977, American College of Radiology.

Ferrucci, J. T., Jr.: Radiology of the pancreas 1976, Radiol. Clin. North Am. **14:**543, 1976.

Ferrucci, J. T., Jr., and Wittenberg, J.: Refinements in Chiba transhepatic cholangiography, Am. J. Roentgenol. **129:**11, 1977.

Fetouh, S. A., Daffner, R. H., Postlethwait, R. W., and Millar, R. C.: Radiologic aspects of Beck gastric tube in esophageal reconstruction, Am. J. Roentgenol. **129:**425, 1977.

Goldberg, H. I., and Sheft, D. J.: Abnormalities in small intestine contour and caliber. A working classification, Radiol. Clin. North Am. **14:**461, 1976.

Goldstein, H. M.: Double-contrast gastrography, Am. J. Dig. Dis. **21:**797, 1976.

Goldstein, L. I., Sample, W. F., Kadell, B. M., and Weiner, M.: Gray-scale ultrasonography and thin-needle cholangiography. Evaluation in the jaundiced patient, J.A.M.A. **238:**1041, 1977.

Haaga, J. R., Alfidi, R. J., Havrilla, T. R., Tubbs, R., Gonzolez, L., Meaney, T. F., and Corsi, M. A.: Definitive role of CT scanning of the pancreas, Radiology **124:**723, 1977.

Hatfield, P. M., and Wise, R. E.: Radiology of the gallbladder and bile ducts, Baltimore, 1976, Williams and Wilkins Co.

Havrilla, T. R., Haaga, J. R., Alfidi, R. J., and Reich, N. E.: Computed tomography and obstructive biliary disease, Am. J. Roentgenol. **128:**765, 1977.

Malini, S., and Sabel, J.: Ultrasonography in obstructive jaundice, Radiology **123:**429, 1977.

Margulis, A. R., and Burhenne, H. J., editors: Alimentary tract roentgenology, ed. 2, St. Louis, 1973, The C. V. Mosby Co.

Miller, R. E.: Detection of colon carcinoma and the barium enema, J.A.M.A. **230:**1195, 1974.

Miller, R. E., Chernish, S. M., Skukas, J., Rosenak, B. D., and Rodda, B. E.: Hypotonic colon examination with glucagon, Radiology **113:**555, 1974.

Nathan, M. H., Newman, A., Murray, D. J., and Camponovo, R.: Cholecystokinin cholecystography, Am. J. Roentgenol. **110:**240, 1970.

Nelson, S. W.: A crescent-shaped collection of residual cholecystographic contrast material: a new sign of benign gastric ulcer? Am. J. Roentgenol. **116:**293, 1972.

Nelson, S. W.: Abnormal small bowel fold patterns. In American College of Radiology syllabus: categorical course on gastrointestinal radiology, Chicago, 1977, American College of Radiology.

Sheedy, P. F. II, Stephens, D. H., Hattery, R. R., and MacCarty, R. L.: Computed tomography in the evaluation of patients with suspected carcinoma of the pancreas, Radiology **124:**731, 1977.

Sickles, E. A.: Cholecystographic diagnosis of duodenal ulcer: the incomplete ring sign, Radiology **124:** 27, 1977.

Stanley, R. J., Sagel, S. S., and Levitt, R. G.: Computed tomographic evaluation of the pancreas, Radiology **124:**715, 1977.

Stein, L. A., and Margulis, A. R.: The spheroid sign. A new sign for accurate differentiation of intramural from extramural masses, Am. J. Roentgenol. **123:**420, 1975.

Stephens, D. H., Gisvold, J. J., and Carlson, H. C.: Tomography of the gallbladder in oral cholecystography, Gastrointest. Radiol. **1:**93, 1976.

Stephens, D. H., Sheedy, P. F. II, Hattery, R. R., and MacCarty, R. L.: Computed tomography of the liver, Am. J. Roentgenol. **128:**579, 1977.

Varley, P. F., Rohrmann, C. A., Jr., Silvis, S. E., and Vennes, J. A.: The normal endoscopic pancreatogram, Radiology **118:**295, 1976.

9 Uroradiography

In evaluating the urinary tract radiographically, you must keep in mind that there are basically two types of abnormalities you may encounter: "physiologic" and morphologic. The so-called *physiologic abnormalities* include a wide variety of diseases referred to collectively as the "medical nephropathies." These include diseases of the glomeruli, tubules, and interstitial tissues. Also included are forms of tubular and cortical necrosis. In patients with these diseases, intravenous urography shows poor function or none at all; diagnosis is best made by biopsy. Furthermore, intravenous urography may be detrimental.

The *morphologic abnormalities* constitute the other large group in which urography is definitely of value. These will be discussed under pathologic considerations.

TECHNICAL CONSIDERATIONS

There are basically six types of studies commonly used to evaluate the urinary tract: the intravenous urogram; the retrograde pyelogram; the cystogram, which is often combined with a study of the urethra as a voiding cystourethrogram; the renal arteriogram; ultrasound; and CT scanning. Isotope studies are also used, but less frequently.

Since intravenous urography (IVP) is the most frequently performed of these examinations, the technique will be reiterated briefly. Before starting an IVP a scout film of the abdomen should be taken to determine the degree of bowel cleanliness. As with the colon examination, scrupulous preparation of the bowel is necessary to eliminate overlying gas and fecal shadows that could obscure the renal outlines. The cleansing regimen is the same as for colon examination.

Once you are assured that the patient's bowel has been satisfactorily prepared for the examination, you must question the patient regarding a history of allergy in general and allergy to iodinated radiopaque drugs specifically. It is very important to ask these patients if they have ever had their "kidneys x-rayed before." A history of allergy to seafood and fish is suggestive of an iodine allergy. If a history of a previous reaction to contrast material is elicited, a decision must be made by the radiologist, in consultation with the referring physician, whether the study requested is absolutely necessary. If it is deemed that the study is needed, the patient may be "prepared" by the referring physician with several days' dosing of steroids and a dose of antihis-

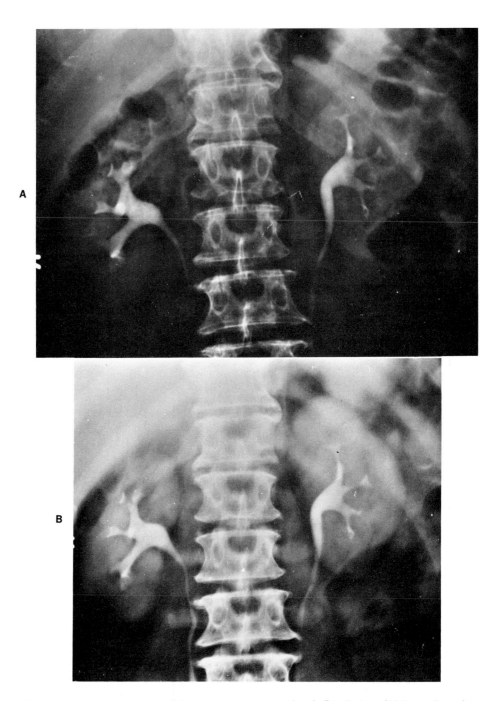

Fig. 9-1. Value of tomography during intravenous urography. **A,** Detail view of kidneys shows bowel gas obscuring renal borders. **B,** Tomography blurs overlying gas and bowel content, revealing smooth, normal-appearing renal borders.

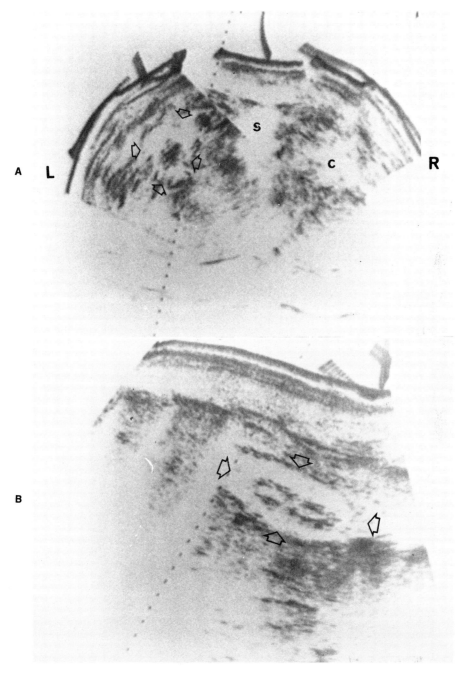

Fig. 9-2. Ultrasonic examination of kidney. **A,** Transverse scan made with patient in prone position. Normal left kidney shows as rounded echo-free area (arrows). Zone of echoes within it represents collecting system. There is cyst *(c)* in right kidney. Spine *(s)* is indicated. **B,** Longitudinal scan of normal left kidney shows typical renal shape (arrows). Internal echoes represent collecting system.

tamine before the study. The effectiveness of this regimen has been questioned, however. There is recent evidence to suggest that the majority of the reactions to contrast material may be psychologically induced.

During the typical urogram, tomography of the kidneys should be used routinely to show renal outlines that may otherwise be obscured by overlying gas or bowel content (Fig. 9-1). The filming sequence employs tomography during the nephrogram or earliest phase when contrast material is in the small vessels and nephrons. This method offers the best opportunity to evaluate the renal parenchyma as well as the renal size and shape. Two or more static films (without tomography) are obtained usually at 5-minute intervals to examine the collecting systems, the ureters, and the bladder. Additional views of the kidneys or of the bladder are taken as needed to delineate any areas still in question. Occasionally, oblique tomography will be performed in this regard. In this way the examination is "tailored" to each patient.

The urinary tract is easily studied by B-mode ultrasonography. Renal size may be evaluated as well as renal shape. Fig. 9-2 shows a transverse and longitudinal scan of the kidneys. Renal ultrasound is used primarily in assessing the nature of a renal mass by searching for internal echoes within the mass. Renal cysts that have only fluid within them have no internal echoes and are referred to as sonolucent (Fig. 9-3). Solid tumors, on the other hand, will frequently show internal echoes, indicating their solid nature (Fig. 9-4).

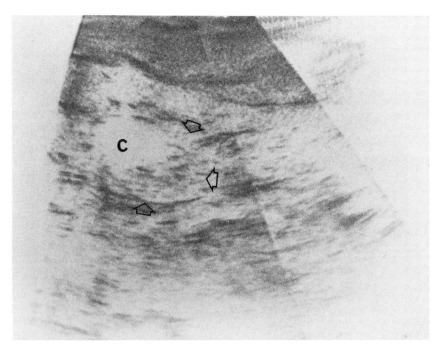

Fig. 9-3. Renal cyst. Longitudinal ultrasonic examination shows echo-free area *(c)* in upper pole of this patient's kidney. Arrows outline remainder of kidney.

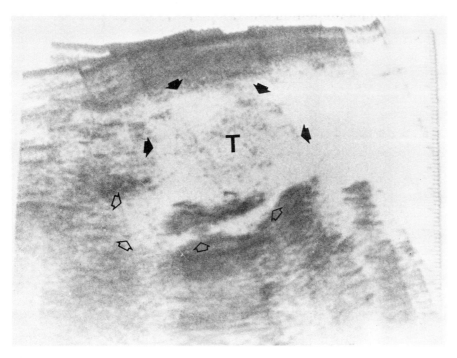

Fig. 9-4. Renal carcinoma. Longitudinal ultrasound examination shows mass (solid arrows) that contains many internal echoes *(T)* on upper pole of this kidney. Compare this appearance with that in Figs. 9-2 and 9-3. Remainder of kidney is outlined by open arrows.

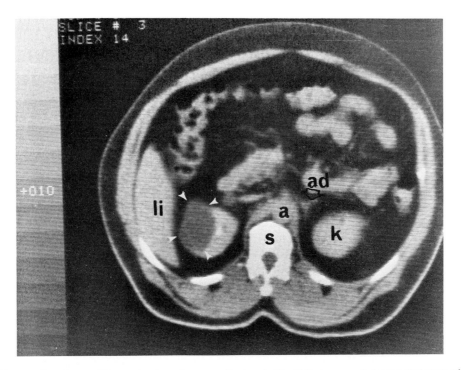

Fig. 9-5. Renal cyst. CT examination of same patient as in Fig. 9-3 shows well-demarcated zone of lucency in upper pole of right kidney (arrowheads). Other easily recognizable structures include aorta *(a)*, liver *(li)*, left kidney *(k)*, lumbar spine *(s)*, and left adrenal gland *(ad)* (open arrow).

Abdominal CT scanning has proved a useful tool for the evaluation of renal mass lesions. In addition, the CT scan may be used to determine the etiology of masses that are distorting or displacing normal urinary tract, such as enlarged abdominal

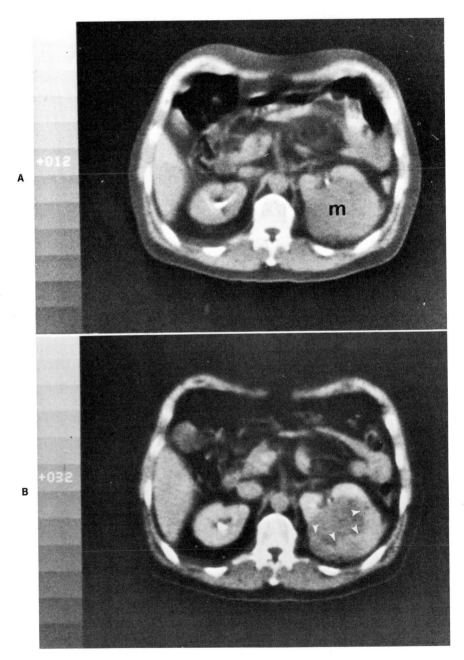

Fig. 9-6. Renal cell carcinoma. CT scan shows effect of enhancement on large tumor in left kidney of this patient. **A,** Unenhanced scan shows large mass *(m)* in left kidney. Contrast medium seen in both kidneys is residual from previous intravenous urogram. **B,** Contrast-enhanced study shows enhancement of edge of tumor (arrowheads) surrounding necrotic center.

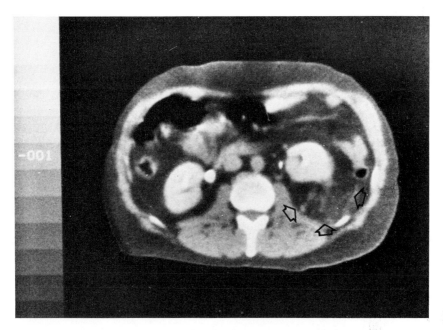

Fig. 9-7. Renal cell carcinoma. Same patient as in Fig. 9-6. There is extrarenal extension of tumor on left (arrows). Notice normal retrorenal area on right. Ability to detect extrarenal extension of tumor is one of advantages of CT scan in evaluation of renal mass lesions.

lymph nodes. CT characteristics of renal cysts show that they are of low density and of CT number 0 to 8, which corresponds to that of urine. On intravenous injection of contrast material there is no enhancement of the mass. Indeed the mass stands out as a prominent "lucency" against the contrast-containing parenchyma (Fig. 9-5). Renal cell carcinoma is, on the other hand, generally isodense (density same as renal tissue) on the unenhanced scan and with enhancement may show hypervascularity, manifest by increased density of the lesion (Fig. 9-6). Contrast enhancement often aids in demonstrating necrotic areas within the mass. It is often possible to determine the extent of extrarenal involvement by tumor (Fig. 9-7).

ANATOMIC CONSIDERATIONS

The kidneys in a normal adult measure 11 to 14 cm in length from pole to pole. They are invested in their own fascia, with their upper poles oriented slightly medially. There may be a normal difference in size between the right and left kidney; the left kidney is often 0.5 to 1.5 cm longer than the right.

The collecting system consists of three to five major calyces draining a minor calyx. The minor calyx forms a sharply defined "cup" around the papilla, which it drains (Fig. 9-8). These are easily discernible on the normal urogram. The calyces drain into the renal pelvis, which terminates in the ureter.

The ureters course down on either side of the spine, generally in a vertical pattern, until they reach the pelvis. On reaching the pelvis, they may make a slight lateral deviation before turning medially to enter the bladder at the trigone. The ureters are not bound down by fascia and are relatively free to move, a fact that is useful in the evaluation of retroperitoneal disease.

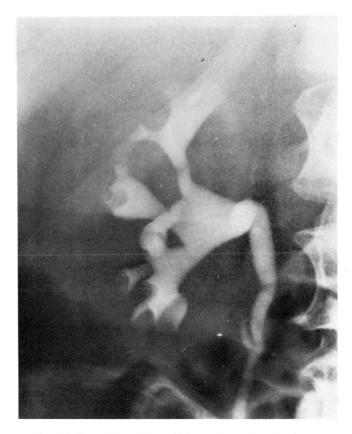

Fig. 9-8. Normal right kidney. Note gentle cupping of calyces.

The urinary bladder in the pelvis should be smooth and ovoid. There are normal variations in the shape of the bladder that occasionally result in a bizarre configuration.

The prostate lies immediately inferior to the bladder and when enlarged may indent and elevate the floor of the bladder (Fig. 9-9). The urethra courses through the prostate. The membranous portion of the urethra between the prostatic and bulbous urethra is fixed in the urogenital diaphragm. This area is subject to laceration from trauma to the pelvis.

The vascular supply to the kidney generally consists of a single pair of renal arteries. However, occasionally two or more arteries to each kidney are present. This is of significance when it is necessary to evaluate the kidney by arteriography or for renal surgery. A single renal vein drains each kidney. On the right the vein drains directly into the inferior vena cava without anastomosis with other veins. On the left there is communication of the renal vein with the left adrenal and gonadal veins. These two communications form a collateral pathway for blood to drain the kidney in the event of renal vein thrombosis. There are collateral channels in the arterial system as well, which may enlarge in stenotic lesions of the renal artery. The foremost of these is the ureteric artery.

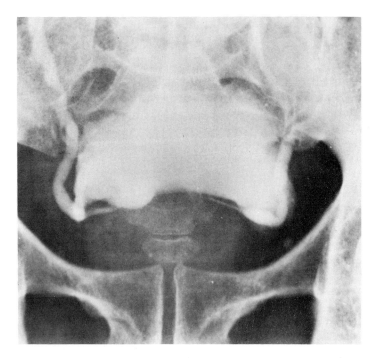

Fig. 9-9. Prostatic enlargement. Floor of bladder is elevated by enlarged prostate gland. Note "fish-hooking" of distal ureters as they enter bladder.

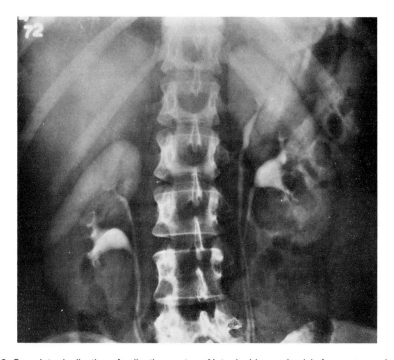

Fig. 9-10. Complete duplication of collecting system. Note double renal pelvis from upper pole of each kidney and duplicated ureter. This duplication extended to ureterovesical junction (not shown on this film).

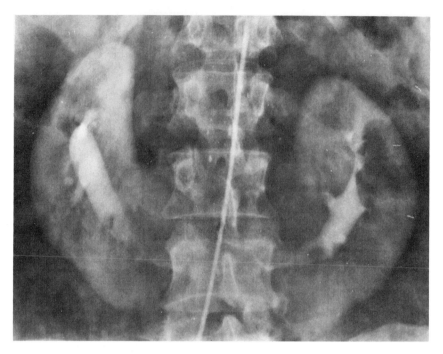

Fig. 9-11. Horseshoe kidney. Nephrogram phase from arteriogram shows abnormal axis of each kidney, with lower pole oriented medially. Functioning isthmus tissue is faintly visible coursing toward midline. A pair of kidneys oriented in this manner should suggest diagnosis of horsehoe kidney.

PATHOLOGIC CONSIDERATIONS

As previously mentioned, the so-called physiologic abnormalities will uniformly result in a decrease or absence of renal function. The only morphologic change that may be discerned is the decrease in the size of a kidney. This discussion will concentrate on diseases that produce recognizable morphologic abnormalities, including:

1. Congenital abnormalities
2. Obstructive lesions with or without calculi
3. Infections
4. Mass lesions: cysts and tumors
5. Vascular lesions
6. Traumatic lesions
7. Extrinsic compression

Renal transplants will also be discussed.

Congenital abnormalities

Congenital anomalies of the urinary tract are not uncommon. The complex development of the genitourinary tract in embryonic life provides opportunities for anomalous development to occur. Anomalies may be relatively benign, such as duplication of the collecting system (Fig. 9-10) or uncomplicated horseshoe kidney (Fig. 9-11), or severe, such as posterior urethral valves with secondary hydroureter and hydrone-

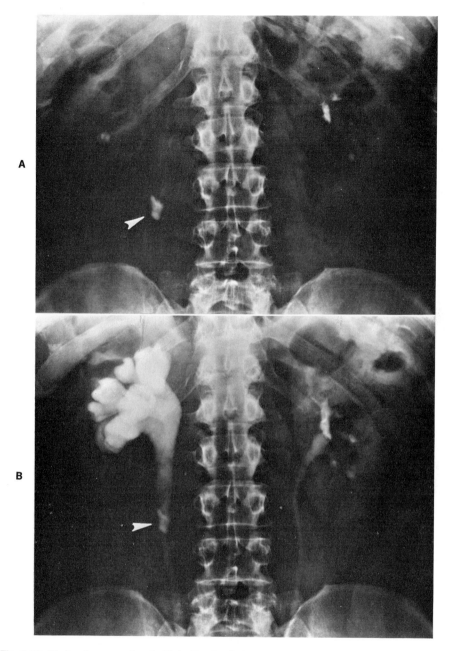

Fig. 9-12. Obstructive uropathy. **A,** Plain film detail shows multiple calculi overlying renal shadows. In particular, note large calculus adjacent to L3-4 interspace (arrowhead). **B,** Intravenous urogram demonstrates obstruction on right secondary to ureteral stone (arrowhead). Left kidney is not obstructed.

phrosis in a newborn male infant. Other anomalies include ectopic kidneys and ectopic ureteroceles. For an in-depth discussion of these, you are referred to the section on these abnormalities in *Emmett's Clinical Urography* (Witten, Hyers, and Utz, 1977).

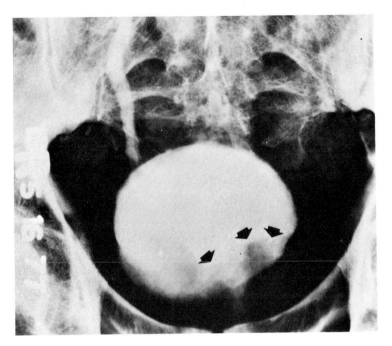

Fig. 9-13. Carcinoma of bladder (arrows), with obstruction of left ureter. Right ureter is clearly visible. On subsequent films, there was never visualization of left kidney.

Obstructive lesions with or without calculi

Obstruction of the urinary tract may be either congenital or acquired. The acquired variety is more common and is usually the result of urinary calculus (Fig. 9-12). Other causes are tumor (Fig. 9-13) and operative manipulation.

Whatever the etiology, obstruction produces a series of pathophysiologic changes that result in characteristic radiographic appearances. These changes, which are described in detail in *Urologic Radiology* (Sussman and Newman, 1976), will determine the radiographic appearance, depending on the degree of renal parenchymal destruction.

Radiographic changes of acute obstruction include initial nonvisualization, with subsequent delayed visualization on the abnormal side, or prompt visualization, with evidence of dilatation (calicectasis) of the collecting system (Fig. 9-12). Frank hydronephrosis usually indicates a long-standing obstruction. If the obstruction is caused by a stone, very frequently that stone may be demonstrated. It is occasionally necessary to obtain oblique films to be certain that a calcification seen on the abdominal film is indeed present within the urinary tract.

Ultrasonography and CT are useful techniques for diagnosing hydronephrosis. Ultrasound is also particularly useful in evaluating newborns and infants with palpable abdominal masses.

Urinary calculi are the most common causes of obstruction. They may be opaque or nonopaque. Populations of certain areas, such as North Carolina, have a high incidence of urinary stones. Interestingly the composition of stones varies with the

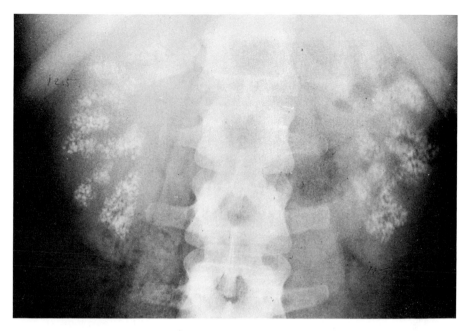

Fig. 9-14. Nephrocalcinosis. Note fine deposition of calcium within renal pyramids of both kidneys. This is a reversible condition.

locale. In the "stone belt" of North Carolina, 85% of the stones are formed of oxalate, whereas only 40% are of that composition in New York state.

Most stones contain a mineral deposit embedded in an inorganic matrix. This matrix has been found to be elevated in the urine of patients with hyperparathyroidism, renal infection, and patients undergoing steroid therapy in an amount that ranges from 3 to 15 times that of normal patients.

Urinary stones must be differentiated from nephrocalcinosis, a pathophysiologic condition in which calcium is deposited *within* renal tissue. It results from an underlying disease that elevates the serum calcium level. In most instances the calcification is limited to the distal convoluted tubules. These calcifications appear as fine stippled deposits that should be easily differentiated from stones by their appearance and location. There are many causes of this condition, but the most common ones include hyperparathyroidism, renal tubular acidosis, tuberculosis, and milk-alkali syndrome. Medullary sponge kidney, a disease that produces microlithiasis, is included in the gamut of nephrocalcinosis. The condition is fully reversible once the underlying disorder has been treated successfully. Nephrocalcinosis is illustrated in Fig. 9-14.

Infections

Infection is a common disease of the urinary tract. It is often seen as a complication of obstruction. Acute pyelonephritis may be difficult to recognize radiographically because of the subtle changes it produces on the collecting system. Occasionally, acute pyelonephritis may be detected on a radiograph if it produces a large swollen kidney. More commonly, however, the effects of chronic pyelonephritis are seen: marked cortical irregularity to the kidney; focal cortical scarring;

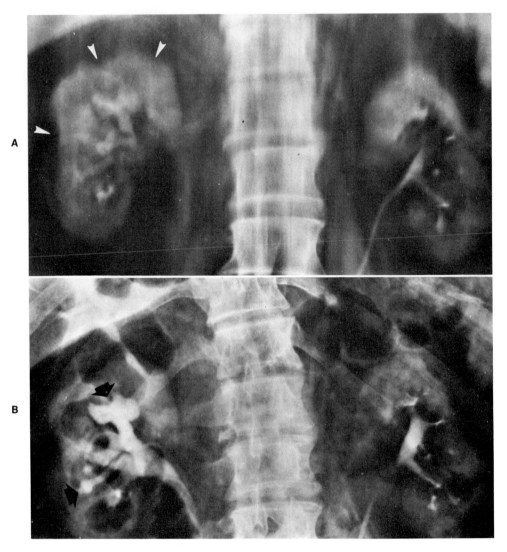

Fig. 9-15. Chronic pyelonephritis with scarring. **A,** Tomogram shows marked cortical irregularity, more severe on right than on left (arrowheads). **B,** Static film shows blunting and clubbing of calyces on right (arrows).

clubbed, irregular calyces; and loss of renal volume (Fig. 9-15). Other complications of infections in the collecting system include the development of a renal carbuncle or abscess (Fig. 9-16), pyonephrosis, and papillary necrosis. This last condition results from anoxia of the renal papilla, causing sloughing of that papilla. Characteristic findings include a filling defect in a calyx, a ring of contrast medium surrounding a filling defect, and an abnormal blunted calyx. Often there is poor excretion of contrast medium by the abnormal kidney (Fig. 9-17).

Tuberculosis of the kidney in its early stages may produce nonspecific changes such as papillary necrosis. With progression of the disease the more characteristic findings of stricture across a calyx, calyceal amputation, and cavitation may occur.

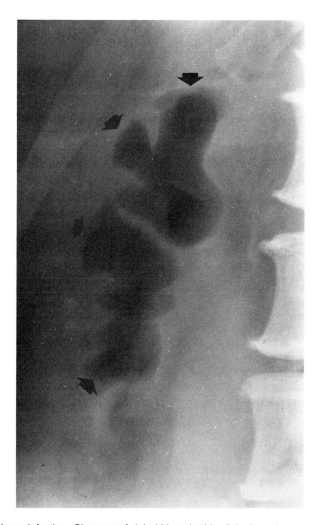

Fig. 9-16. Renal gas infection. Close-up of right kidney in this diabetic patient reveals gas outlining collecting system of upper pole (arrows).

Tuberculosis also causes ureteral strictures. The combination of renal and ureteral abnormalities such as strictures should suggest the diagnosis. The end stage of renal tuberculosis is a small, shrunken, nonfunctioning kidney that often contains calcific debris ("putty kidney") (Fig. 9-18).

Changes of chronic inflammation of the bladder include thickening and irregularity of the wall secondary to hypertrophy of the bladder trabeculae and spasticity.

Mass lesions: cysts and tumors

Mass lesions in the kidneys represent either cysts or tumors. Filling defects elsewhere in the urinary tract generally are tumors. Renal cysts are extremely common in older individuals and are found in a high percentage of these patients undergoing autopsy. They are frequently incidental findings on abdominal CT scans. In the kidney, renal cysts appear as bulges along the cortical margin (Fig. 9-19) or as absent

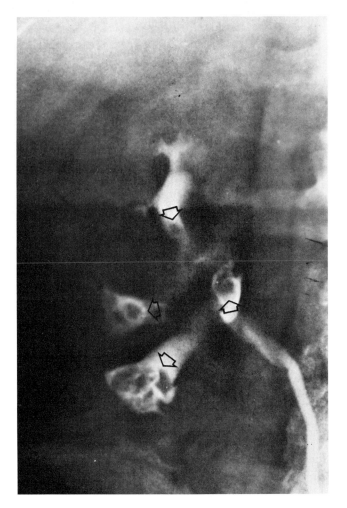

Fig. 9-17. Papillary necrosis. Multiple filling defects (arrows) are present within collecting system. These filling defects represent sloughed papillae.

portions of the kidney (Fig. 9-20). Quite frequently on the tomogram a thin, beaklike collection of contrast material representing compressed parenchyma may be seen along the margin (Fig. 9-19). A cyst may also displace the calyceal structures.

Prior to the early 1970s, when a cyst was suspected, the diagnosis was confirmed mainly by angiography. However, newer diagnostic techniques, including ultrasound, CT, and cyst puncture, have reduced the need for arteriography. Once a renal mass lesion is detected on an IVP, the next logical step should be an ultrasound examination to determine whether the mass is cystic or solid (Fig. 9-21). In many institutions, CT examination is also used. The CT appearance of a benign renal cyst includes a homogenous, smooth, rounded appearance of uniform radiographic density with a CT value of 0 to 8. There is no enhancement of the mass following the intravenous injection of contrast material (Fig. 9-22).

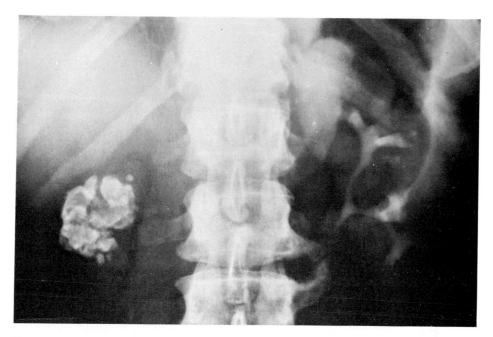

Fig. 9-18. Renal tuberculosis. Small, nonfunctioning right kidney containing calcific debris ("putty kidney") is present.

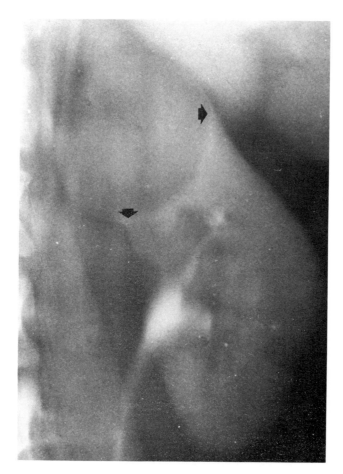

Fig. 9-19. Benign renal cyst. Cyst produces bulge along upper pole of this kidney. Note beaklike appearance along parenchymal margin of cyst (arrows).

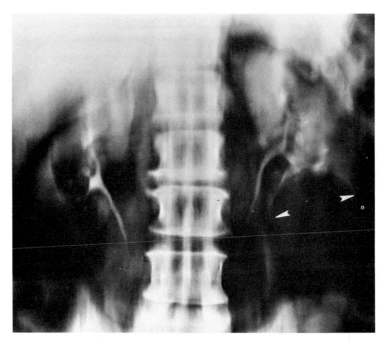

Fig. 9-20. Renal cyst. Tomogram shows large lesion with beak (arrowheads) in lower pole of left kidney.

Renal tumors, on the other hand, have a considerably different radiographic appearance. On the intravenous urogram, they may produce an abnormal contour to the renal outline and distortion or displacement of the calyceal system similar to those findings seen with renal cysts. However, the similarity ends here. In addition to the distortion of the calyceal system, calyces often appear amputated. Quite often on the tomogram the mass appears mottled and not lucent, as seen with a renal cyst (Fig. 9-23, *A*). On ultrasound examination the mass appears as a solid lesion with many internal echoes (Fig. 9-23, *B*). This is contrary to the echo-free picture seen in a simple renal cyst.

CT has contributed greatly to the differentiation between renal cyst and tumor. On an unenhanced study, distortion of the renal architecture may be plainly seen (Fig. 9-23, *C*). Furthermore, when the study is enhanced by the intravenous injection of contrast material, the lesion becomes more dense, indicating it is quite vascular. This is quite contrary to the appearance of a cyst (Fig. 9-22). Furthermore, on a CT examination, we may often see extrarenal extension of a large tumor (Fig. 9-24).

Angiographic examination of renal carcinoma demonstrates abnormal vessels that are of a nonuniform size and show aneurysmal dilatations, pooling, and early venous drainage (Fig. 9-23, *E*). Compare the angiographic findings of a renal cell carcinoma with those of a cyst, which demonstrates stretching of vessels and no neovascularity (Fig. 9-25).

Cyst puncture (Fig. 9-26) is a procedure performed with increasing frequency for

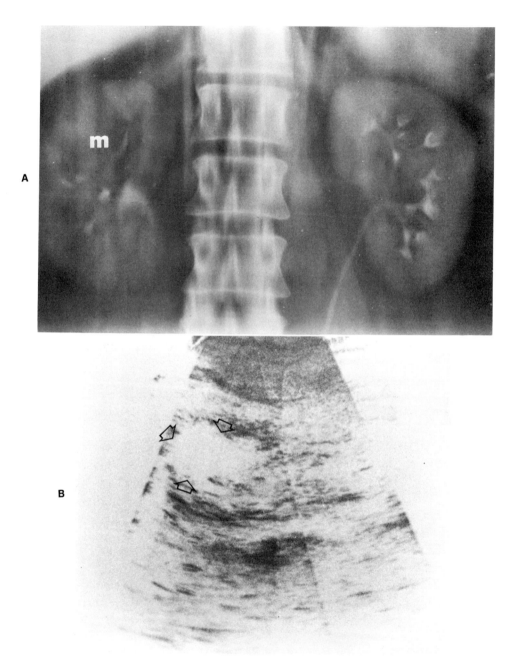

Fig. 9-21. Renal cyst. **A,** Tomogram shows mass *(m)* distorting upper pole collecting system on right. **B,** Gray scale ultrasound examination shows echo-free area in upper pole of kidney (arrows).

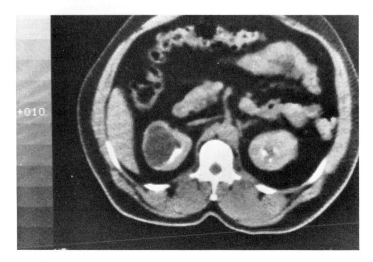

Fig. 9-22. Renal cyst. Same patient as in Fig. 9-21. Renal cyst is visible as area of low density in right kidney. It does not enhance with intravenous contrast material. Thin rim of normal cortex surrounds cyst on its lateral margin.

the evaluation of renal mass lesions. Frequently, these are performed under ultrasonic or CT guidance. Whatever the method, the purpose of cyst puncture is for aspiration of cyst contents, which are then sent for chemical and cytologic analysis. If the fluid is clear or straw colored, has a specific gravity of urine, is free of cellular debris containing malignant cells, and has a smooth outline on injection of positive contrast medium and/or air, you may be assured you are dealing with a benign cyst. A cystic malignancy, on the other hand, generally has a hemorrhagic aspirate that is positive for malignant cells, often contains debris, and has a high fat content. Furthermore, on injection a mass may be seen within the cyst.

Table 6 lists the differential features in the roentgenographic diagnosis of renal cysts versus renal tumors.

Vascular lesions

The most common renal vascular disease you will encounter is occlusive disease of the renal arteries. In most instances, this will be discovered in patients you are evaluating for hypertension. The most common cause of renal artery stenosis is the atherosclerotic plaque. This most often occurs near the origin of the vessel. There are, however, intrinsic diseases of the renal arteries that may result in renovascular hypertension, including fibromuscular dysplasia, a whole spectrum of stenosing diseases.

There are two types of screening imaging examinations that may be used in evaluating patients with hypertension: hypertensive urogram and isotope renogram or renal scan. The hypertensive urogram is performed by rapid injection of contrast medium followed immediately by filming at 1, 2, 3, 4, and 5 minutes. There are four radiographic criteria used in making the diagnosis of renovascular hypertension: (1) a difference in renal size greater than 1.5 cm, (2) delayed appearance of contrast medium in one kidney, (3) persistence of the pyelogram phase in the same kidney

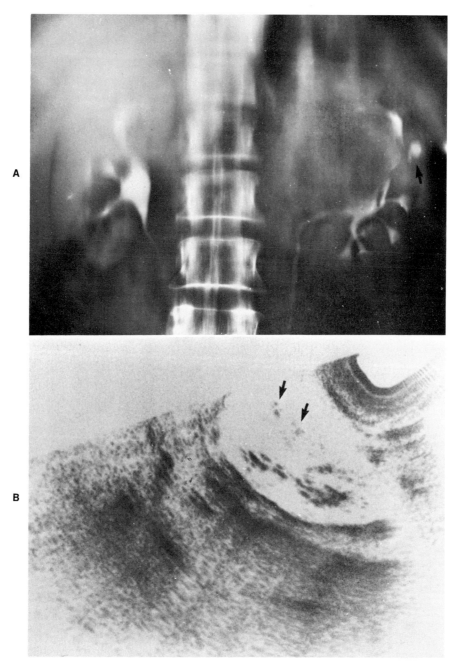

Continued.

Fig. 9-23. Renal cell carcinoma. **A,** Tomogram reveals mass distorting calyces in upper pole of left kidney. One calyx appears to be amputated (arrow). **B,** Ultrasound examination shows echoes within mass (arrows). **C,** CT scan shows mass *(m)* distorting calyceal system on left. **D,** With scanner in "interrogation mode," mass has density of 20 attenuation (CT) units (arrows), a number much higher than that of cyst. **E,** Angiogram demonstrates neovascularity and pooling of contrast material, features not seen in renal cyst.

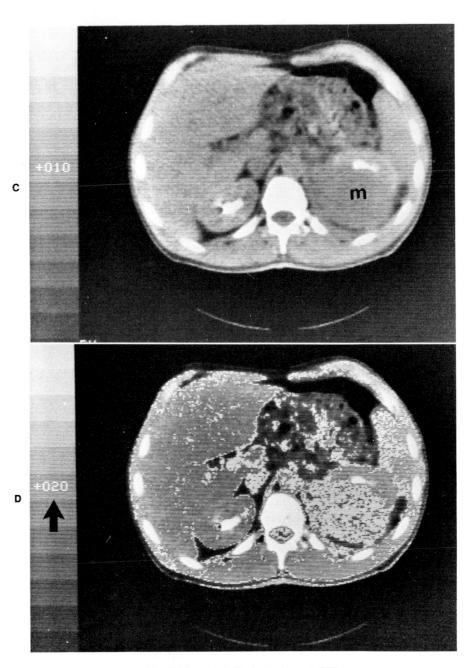

Fig. 9-23, cont'd. For legend see p. 275.

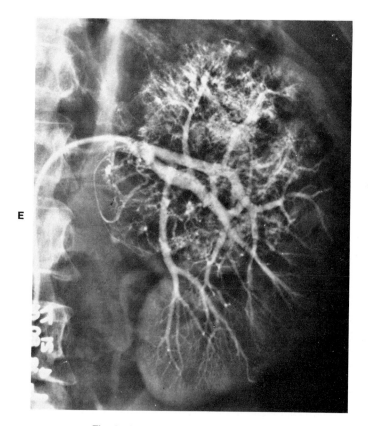

E

Fig. 9-23, cont'd. For legend see p. 275.

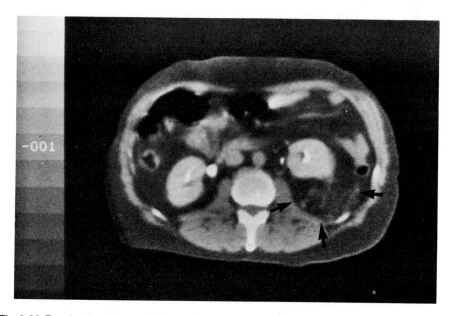

Fig. 9-24. Renal cell carcinoma. CT scan shows extrarenal extension into perirenal tissues (arrows).

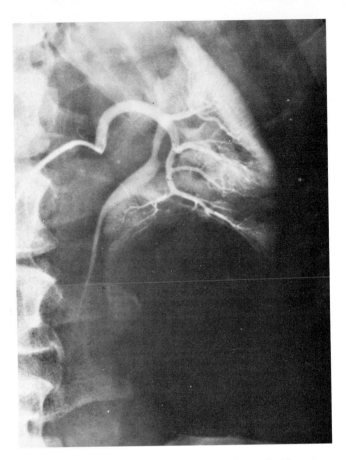

Fig. 9-25. Renal cyst. Angiogram shows stretching of intrarenal vessels. There is no neovascularity. Cyst is "avascular." Compare with Fig. 9-23, *E.*

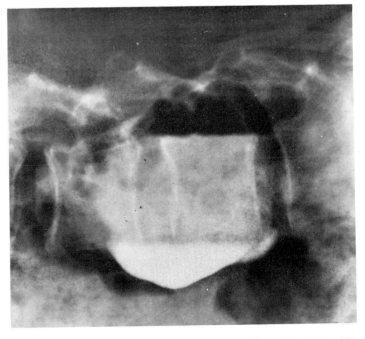

Fig. 9-26. Cyst puncture. Contrast material and air pool in this renal cyst (decubitus view).

Table 6. Imaging criteria in differentiating renal cyst and renal cell carcinoma

Examination	Renal cyst	Renal cell carcinoma
Nephrotomogram	Radiolucent mass Thin, smooth, well-defined wall Sharp margins "Claw sign" or "beak sign" at cyst/cortex junction	Mass same density as adjacent parenchyma Thick, irregular wall Poorly defined margins
Ultrasound	Interior sonolucent (no internal echoes) Well-defined border	Many internal echoes Less well-defined border
CT	Smooth, well-defined border Density low (CT No. 0 to 8) Avascular on contrast enhancement No invasion of perirenal tissues	Less well-defined border May be isodense (same as kidney) Usually enhances, may show areas of necrosis Invasion of perirenal tissues may be seen
Angiography	Avascular mass No neovascularity Vasoconstriction with epinephrine injection Vessels stretched and displaced	Usually vascular Neovascularity: irregular, nonuniform, serpentine; pooling of contrast medium; early venous filling; aneurysm-like dilatations No response to epinephrine injection
Cyst puncture and injection	Clear, straw-colored fluid No cellular debris, negative cytologic evidence Smooth inner border, no filling defects on injection	Cloudy or hemorrhagic fluid Cellular debris, positive cytologic evidence Irregular inner border with filling defects on injection

with delayed appearance (delayed washout), and (4) evidence of collateral circulation.

In general, one may accept a difference in renal size of up to 1.5 cm, especially if the left kidney is larger. In most instances where there is a significant stenotic lesion the difference in renal size will be considerably greater than that.

Delayed appearance and delayed washout of contrast material result from a stenotic lesion in the renal vascular tree. Consequently, less contrast material goes to the affected kidney, which results in a delayed nephrogram. The overall delay in function of the affected kidney results in a delayed "washout" on that side because of increased sodium and water reabsorption.

Collateral circulation to a kidney with a stenotic renal artery may be derived from the ureteral, renal capsular, or adrenal vessels. The most common manifestation seen on a positive hypertensive urogram exhibiting this is ureteral notching from hypertrophy of ureteral arteries. The positive findings in a hypertensive urogram are demonstrated in Fig. 9-27.

The radioisotope renogram is performed by the rapid intravenous injection of orthoiodohippuric acid, which has been labled with [131]I. Detectors are placed over each kidney, and a comparison is made between the appearance time and the washout time of the isotope in each kidney. There are three phases in the normal curve

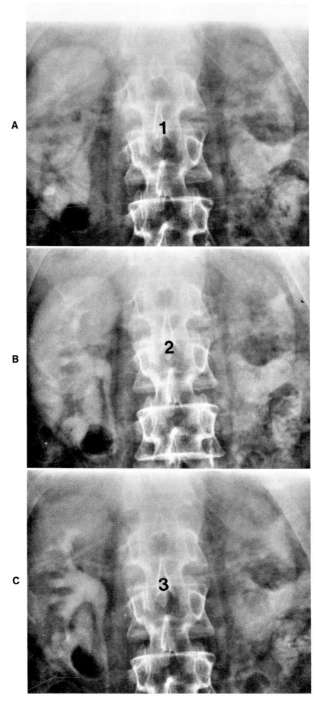

Fig. 9-27. Renovascular hypertension. Rapid-sequence intravenous urogram demonstrates findings in this patient with hypertension. Note difference in size of two kidneys and delayed appearance of contrast material in collecting system on abnormal left side. Subsequent films showed delayed washout of contrast material on left side as well. Films taken 1, 2, and 3 minutes after injection.

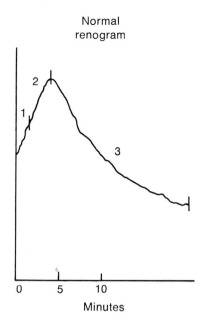

Normal
renogram

0   5   10

Minutes

Fig. 9-28. Normal radioisotope renogram. *1,* Vascular phase; *2,* secretory phase; *3,* excretory phase.

(Fig. 9-28): a vascular phase with a rapid slope; a secretory or functional phase, usually 2.5 to 4.5 minutes; and an excretory phase, during which time the labeled material is excreted. This generally plateaus in 20 minutes. A positive study in renovascular hypertension shows prolongation of this second phase (Fig. 9-29). Other criteria include delayed peaking of counts over a kidney, delayed drainage from a kidney, and differences in renal size. These are quite similar to the criteria used in urography.

Technetium-99m may be used in a chelated form for renal scanning. When a rapid-sequence injection is followed with the gamma camera, we may infer diminished blood flow by delayed appearance of the isotope in the affected kidney.

Traumatic lesions

Trauma to the urinary tract may result from a variety of causes. These include blunt trauma from a direct blow; penetrating injuries by a bone fragment (Fig. 9-30), a foreign object (bullet, knife), or instrumentation or a biopsy; or pathologic rupture or fracture of a diseased kidney.

Trauma to the urinary tract may be very slight, such as a renal contusion, or catastrophic, such as a shattered kidney (Fig. 9-31) or ruptured bladder (Fig. 9-30). You should be aware that these entities occur in major trauma to the abdomen and pelvis. A detailed discussion of urinary tract trauma is contained in *Urologic Radiology* (Sussman and Newman, 1976), to which you are referred.

Extrinsic diseases

Diseases in organs adjacent to the urinary tract often produce morphologic alterations on the urogram. These include displacement of a kidney by a suprarenal mass

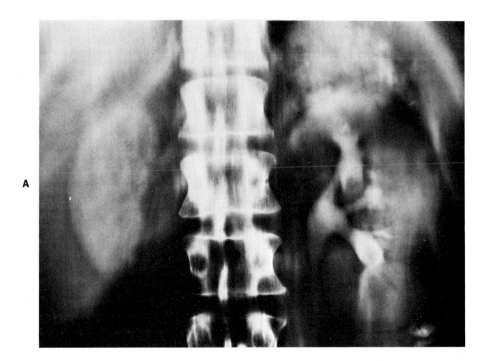

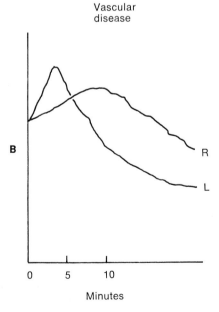

Fig. 9-29. Renovascular hypertension. **A,** Tomogram of intravenous urogram shows delayed function on right. Note difference in size between kidneys. **B,** Radioisotope renogram shows normal curve for left kidney. There is lengthening of vascular and secretory portions of curve on right side.

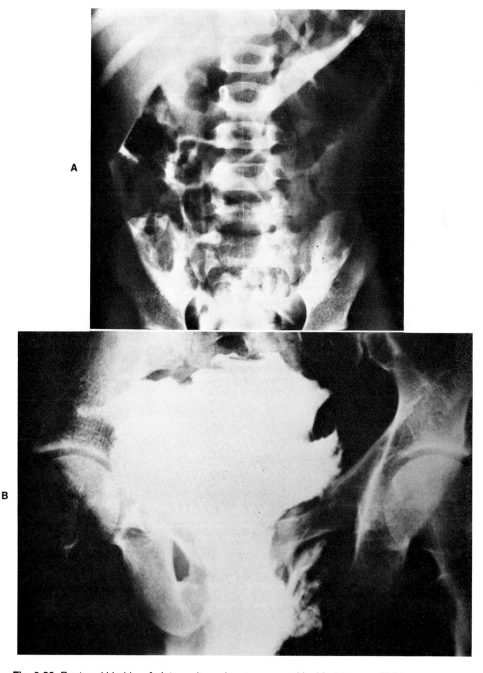

Fig. 9-30. Ruptured bladder. **A,** Intraperitoneal rupture caused by blunt trauma. Light areas represent contrast material extravasated into abdomen. **B,** Extraperitoneal rupture in patient with pelvic fractures.

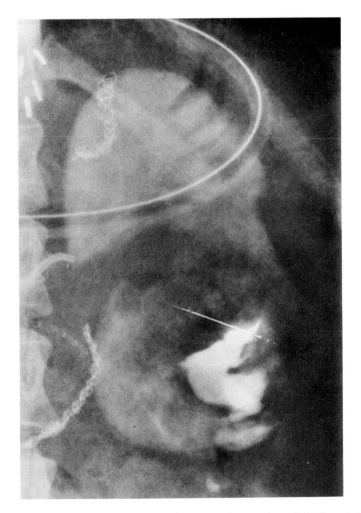

Fig. 9-31. Fractured kidney. Nephrogram phase of renal arteriogram shows left kidney to be bisected. There is no contrast material in collecting system of upper portion.

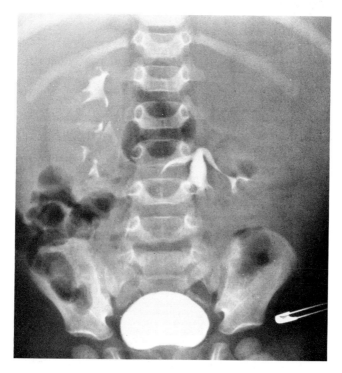

Fig. 9-32. Neuroblastoma. Note downward displacement of left kidney by large adrenal mass.

(Fig. 9-32), displacement of a ureter by enlarged lymph nodes (Fig. 9-33), compression of a ureter with obstructive uropathy secondary to abdominal or pelvic masses, compression of the bladder by pelvic masses, and elevation of the bladder floor by an enlarged prostate (Fig. 9-34). Abdominal CT scanning has made evaluation of these displacements somewhat easier. Furthermore, ultrasound has been used to determine whether a mass displacing portions of the urinary tract is cystic or solid.

Renal transplants

Renal transplantation is now common in most large medical centers. You will undoubtedly treat many of these patients at some time in your medical career. Imaging studies are used to evaluate transplants and to determine their function as well as whether or not rejection is taking place.

There are three critical areas that may affect the function of a transplanted kidney. The first of these is the rejection process itself. This will ultimately lead to a decrease in or absence of function in the transplanted kidney. Obstruction at the site of ureteric reanastomosis is a second cause of decreased function. Third, a vascular abnormality at the site of graft may adversely affect the function of a transplant. A normal renal transplant is shown in Fig. 9-35. The spectrum of diagnostic examinations performed on normal kidneys is performed on renal transplants.

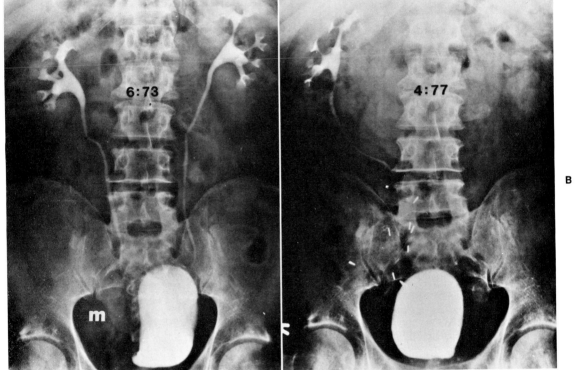

Fig. 9-33. Metastatic melanoma. **A,** June 1973. There is leftward compression of bladder by pelvic soft tissue mass *(m).* **B,** April 1977. Metal clips mark site of removal of enlarged lymph nodes on right. Note lateral deviation of right kidney and proximal ureter. This was secondary to enlarged para-aortic lymph nodes. Compare with **A.**

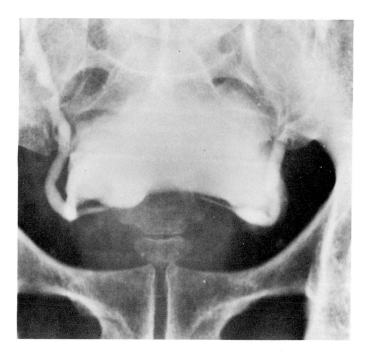

Fig. 9-34. Prostatic enlargement. There is elevation of floor of bladder and "fishhooking" of distal ureters by enlarged prostate gland.

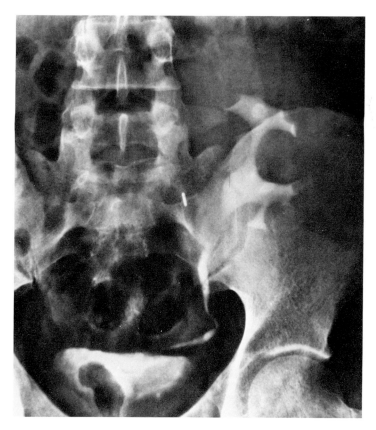

Fig. 9-35. Normal renal transplant. Transplanted kidney is placed in left iliac fossa.

SUMMARY

The urinary tract is one area of the body where a wide variety of imaging procedures is used. The diagnostic accuracy of these studies when used in combination is exceedingly high. The various types of pathologic abnormalities you will encounter in a daily practice have been discussed. The case studies that follow are designed to illustrate the application of the material presented.

Selected case studies

Cases 9-1 to 9-3: BACK PAIN AND HEMATURIA

Three patients are seen in the emergency department following separate automobile accidents. All are complaining of back pain. On routine urinalysis, patients 1 and 2 reveal gross hematuria, and patient 3 shows microscopic hematuria.

Patient 1 is a 54-year-old man who passed out at the wheel of his automobile. He is in no acute distress but does complain of back pain. On physical examination, he is noted to be pale. His hematocrit is 22%.

Patient 2 is a 40-year-old man who was struck in the left side by an automobile while crossing the street. He complains of severe left-sided abdominal and back pain. On examination a large ecchymosis is noted over the left lower rib cage posteriorly and over his left flank. His laboratory studies, aside from the urinalysis, are normal.

Patient 3 is a 60-year-old man who was a passenger in an automobile that was involved in an accident. He complains of pain over the upper lumbar region. Physical examination reveals an enlarged liver and tenderness over the L2 region. He is found to be slightly anemic.

What radiographic studies would you order for each of these patients? Lumbar spine films were ordered for all three patients. In addition, pelvic films were made of patients 1 and 2. An intravenous urogram was performed on all three patients. The lumbar spine and pelvic films were normal in patients 1 and 2.

Case 9-1 is a detailed view of the bladder in patient 1. Case 9-2, *A* and *B*, shows the left kidney in patient 2. Case 9-3, *A*, is the lumbar spine in patient 3. Case 9-3, *B*, is the scout film from his urogram; Case 9-3, *C*, is the tomogram of his kidneys. *What are the radiographic findings in each case? What additional studies would you order? What is your diagnosis?*

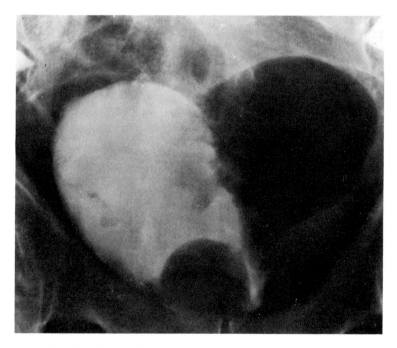

Case 9-1. Detail of bladder from intravenous urogram of patient 1.

Case 9-2. Detail views of left kidney in patient 2. **A,** Conventional radiograph. **B,** Tomogram. What are the arrows pointing to?

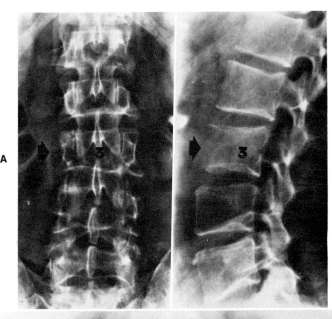

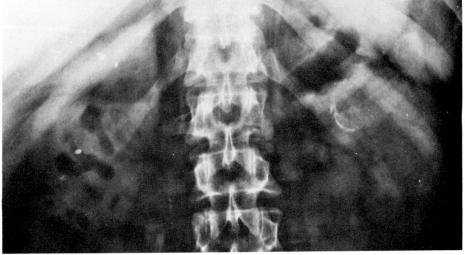

Case 9-3 A, Lumbar spine film of patient 3. What is the arrow at L3 pointing to? **B,** Detail of scout film of urogram of patient 3.

Continued.

C

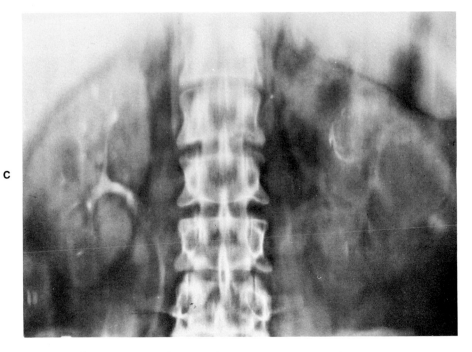

Case 9-3, cont'd. C, Detail of tomogram at urography of patient 3.

ROENTGEN DIAGNOSIS AND DISCUSSION

Patient 1. A detailed view of the bladder (Case 9-1) reveals a filling defect along the floor of the bladder on the left. The appearance is that of a mucosal lesion. There is an obstruction of the left ureter, which resulted in a left-sided hydronephrosis (not shown). The clinical history coupled with the findings of anemia in a middle-aged man suggest a lesion that has been present for some time. In view of the findings the most likely diagnosis is that of a bladder tumor. The patient underwent cystoscopy, where a large transitional cell carcinoma of the bladder was encountered. At subsequent surgery the tumor was found to have completely obstructed the left ureter.

Carcinoma of the bladder is relatively rare, occurring at a rate of approximately 17:100,000 population. Men are much more frequently affected than women. It occurs more commonly in the older age groups.

Hematuria is the most frequent sign. Other symptoms include frequency and pain. Occasionally the patient may first come to medical attention because of complications of blood loss, as in this case. Although the definitive diagnosis rests with cystoscopy, urography will usually demonstrate the lesion.

The majority of these lesions are papillary transitional cell carcinomas. The prognosis depends on the histology and the stage of disease. It is likely that CT scanning will play an important role in the staging and follow-up of patients with these lesions.

Patient 2. The urogram (Case 9-2, *A* and *B*) revealed diminished function in the left kidney. There is a streaky collection of contrast medium in the midportion of the kidney adjacent to an upper pole calyx. On delayed films (not shown), this collection became more prominent. In view of the history and radiographic findings, a diagnosis of renal laceration was made. A CT scan (not shown) demonstrated an intact renal capsule. Arteriography was not performed. Because the patient's vital signs were stable, conservative management was elected. A subsequent urogram 6 months later (Case 9-2, *C*) demonstrated a cortical scar in an otherwise normally functioning kidney. The patient did not become hypertensive.

Trauma to the kidney results most often from a blunt injury sustained in automobile accidents, athletics, and falls. Other less common injuries result from penetrating trauma or iatrogenic causes such as instrumentation or renal biopsy.

Four types of injury may be sustained by the kidney: parenchymal injury, vascular pedicle injury, rupture of the renal pelvis, or a combination of these (Case 9-2, *D*). By far parenchymal injury is the most common. This may be manifest as renal contusion, renal laceration, or renal fracture.

Renal contusion is a relatively benign injury that may be intrarenal or subcapsular; the former is more common. Urography shows distortion of the collecting system ("mass effect") or a bulge in the renal outline. If arteriography is performed, deviation of the intrarenal or capsular vessels would be seen.

Renal laceration is a more serious injury. The most common type is a tear through the renal capsule, resulting in intra- and perirenal hematoma. Less common is a laceration through the collecting system, in which intrarenal and peripelvic extravasation occurs (Case 9-2, *A* and *B*). In these patients, partial nephrectomy may be necessary if the bleeding is severe.

Fracture or shattering of the kidney is a serious injury that, fortunately, is uncommon. Urographic and angiographic findings are similar to those seen in the less severe injuries but with more extensive extravasation. Usually, nephrectomy is required for treatment.

Vascular pedicle injuries are uncommon. They occur either as thrombosis of an artery or vein or as an avulsion from the renal pelvis. Arteriography is usually required to make the diagnosis.

Rupture of the renal pelvis is a very unusual injury and occurs most often in patients with an obstruction at the ureteropelvic junction and hydronephrosis. This injury is seen more commonly in children who have this type of preexisting urologic abnormality.

There are other nonspecific signs that may be seen on urography in patients who have sustained renal trauma. These include a fracture of the twelfth rib and/or transverse process of a lumbar vertebra, obliteration of all or part of the psoas line, and scoliosis and elevated hemidiaphragm on the affected side. If the injury is severe or if the patient is in shock, a deeply staining nephrogram that persists may be the only urographic finding.

Traditionally, intravenous urography, meticulously performed, and angiography have formed the diagnostic mainstay in managing patients with renal trauma. However, CT scanning has been shown to provide diagnostic information about the damaged kidney in a new perspective. Actual laceration, hematoma, etc. may now be demonstrated with little discomfort to the patient.

The follow-up examination in patients who have sustained a renal injury often demonstrates a return of full function to the damaged kidney. There may be scarring (Case 9-2, *D*) or a decrease in size of the affected kidney. These patients must be carefully watched for the possibility of developing renovascular hypertension (Page kidney). Another late complication is urinoma, a peripelvic collection of urine resulting from a tear in the collecting system or ureter.

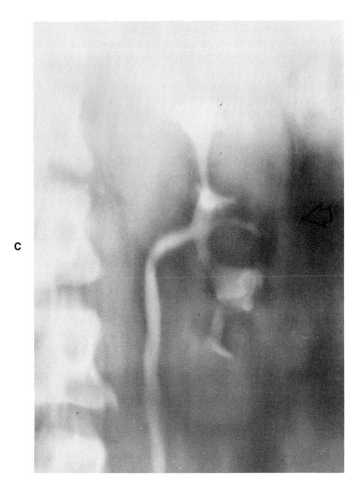

C

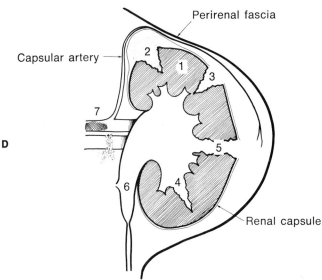

Perirenal fascia

Capsular artery

Renal capsule

D

Case 9-2. Patient 2. **C,** Detail of tomogram at urography of same patient 6 months later. Deep parenchymal scar is present at site of laceration (arrow). **D,** Drawing of various forms of renal trauma. *1,* Renal contusion; *2,* laceration with intracepsular hematoma—note stretching of capsular artery; *3,* laceration extending across renal capsule; *4,* internal laceration communicating with collecting system; *5,* renal fracture ("shattered kidney")—injuries *3* and *5* would result in enlargement of "renal" shadow with extensive hemorrhage into perirenal space; *6,* pelvic rupture, usually in patient with ureteropelvic obstructing lesion; *7,* vascular pedicle injury.

Patient 3. Films of the lumbar spine (Case 9-3, A) show a destructive lesion of the body of the L3 vertebra. A scout film of the abdomen shows an enlarged left renal outline with a rounded, rimlike calcific density over the upper pole (Case 9-3, B). An intravenous urogram (Case 9-3, C) shows a mass in the left kidney distorting the collecting system. Ultrasonography (not shown) demonstrated that the mass was solid. A CT scan showed a large mass within the kidney, extending outside the confines of the kidney and invading the perirenal tissue (Case 9-3, D). Furthermore, destruction of the L3 vertebra was shown. The mass was enhanced with intravenous contrast medium, indicating its vascular nature. Multiple scan cuts were made through the liver and lungs and demonstrated multiple metastatic lesions from this renal cell carcinoma. Angiography was not performed in this patient, who was subsequently treated by nephrectomy and chemotherapy.

Renal cell carcinoma (hypernephroma) is the most common malignant tumor of the kidney. It occurs in older patients, with a predominance in men. Patients with these lesions may be detected in a variety of ways, including incidental discovery of metastases on a "routine" chest film, renal mass found as part of a workup for hypertension, or following renal trauma, often minor. The classic triad of hematuria, flank mass, and pain are absent in the majority of patients.

The radiographic findings on the various diagnostic imaging studies were discussed earlier in the chapter and will not be repeated here.

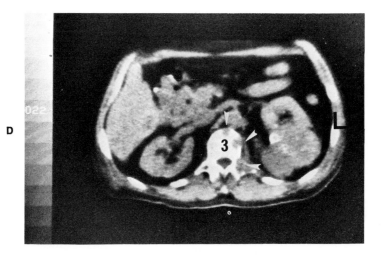

Case 9-3. Patient 3. **D,** Abdominal CT scan. There is large mass containing calcium in left kidney posteriorly. Note multiple metastatic lesions of L3 vertebra (arrowheads). Findings are compatible with large renal cell carcinoma.

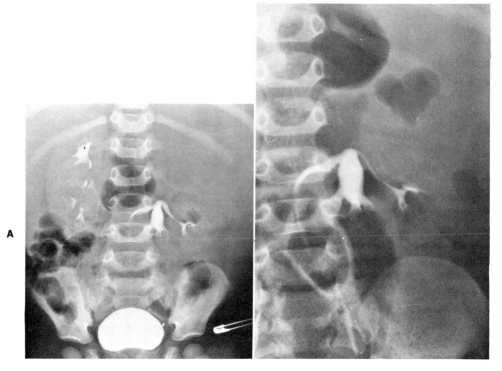

Case 9-4. Intravenous urogram in patient 4. How do the findings compare with those in Case 9-5?

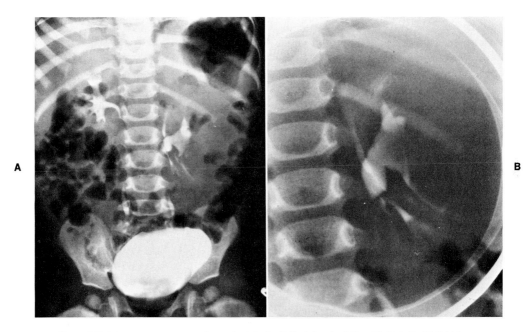

Case 9-5. Intravenous urogram in patient 5. **A,** Full abdominal film. **B,** Detail of left kidney.

Cases 9-4 to 9-6: ABDOMINAL MASSES IN INFANTS

Patients 4 through 6 are all infants. Patients 4 and 5 are 6 months of age and were brought to the clinic for a "well-baby" checkup. They have been gaining weight and developing appropriately for their age. An abdominal mass is palpated on the left side in each of them. Patient 6 is a newborn infant, the product of a normal pregnancy. During his examination prior to discharge an abdominal mass is palpated on the right side. *What are the diagnostic considerations regarding the etiology of the masses in each of these patients? What diagnostic imaging studies would you order?*

An intravenous urogram was performed on each patient. Case 9-4 is of patient 4, Case 9-5 is of patient 5, and Case 9-6 is of patient 6. *What are the radiographic findings? What is your diagnosis? Would you order any additional imaging studies?*

ROENTGEN DIAGNOSIS

Patient 4. A preliminary film of the abdomen (not shown) revealed a mass without calcification on the left. Following the intravenous injection of contrast material, the left kidney was demonstrated to be displaced downward by a large mass (Case 9-4). The intrarenal architecture was normal. An ultrasound study (not shown) was then performed and showed a large solid mass anterior and above the left kidney. The findings are most consistent with neuroblastoma. This diagnosis was confirmed at surgery.

Patient 5. The intravenous urogram (Case 9-5) revealed enlargement of the left kidney. The collecting system was distorted and splayed by a large intrarenal mass. The opposite kidney was normal. Ultrasonic examination confirmed an enlarged kidney containing a solid mass. The findings are most suggestive of Wilms tumor, a diagnosis that was confirmed at surgery.

Patient 6. A preliminary film of the abdomen (Case 9-6, A) shows gaseous distention of the bowel, a normal finding in a newborn. Following intravenous injection of contrast material a

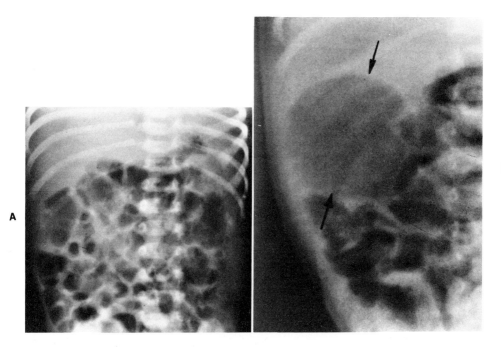

Case 9-6. A, Abdominal scout film prior to intravenous injection of contrast material in patient 6. **B,** Detail film of right upper quadrant during "total bodygram" phase of intravenous urogram. What are the arrows outlining? How does this film differ from that of **A?**

film reveals a relative lucency in the right upper quadrant during the "total bodygram" phase of the examination (Case 9-6, *B*). The effect is striking when you compare this area with the same area of the plain film. Ultrasonography demonstrated a multiloculated cystic mass consistent with a diagnosis of multicystic kidney. This was confirmed at subsequent surgery.

DISCUSSION

The evaluation of abdominal masses in children requires a variety of diagnostic imaging modalities to determine whether or not the mass is of neoplastic origin. The most common mass in newborns is multicystic kidney and in older children, hydronephrosis. The majority of malignant masses in infants and young children are of renal or adrenal origin. Hence the diagnostic studies will be directed at defining the structures of the urinary tract. The majority of these studies are noninvasive. Grossman (1975, 1976) has written extensively on the subject, and his approach to these lesions will be summarized here. For an in-depth discussion of the topic, you are referred to his articles, which are listed in the references.

The abdominal plain film is the first diagnostic study in the evaluation of patients with palpable abdominal masses. Usually, this is the scout film of the intravenous urogram. The plain film can provide information regarding the location of the mass, the relationships of the mass to the kidney, the distortion or displacement of normal anatomic contours, and the presence of calcium. Calcification, whenever present, is highly suggestive of neuroblastoma or neonatal adrenal hemorrhage. In the latter condition the calcification develops after several days. As the hematoma resolves, the calcific mass is seen to contract and shrink.

The intravenous urogram makes use of the techniques of "total body opacification" and nephrotomography. The total body opacification effect occurs within the first minute following injection of a bolus of contrast medium and results from the high concentration of the contrast medium within the capillary beds of the abdominal viscera. This is usually sufficient to outline the mass or to show it as a "negative" shadow against the remainder of the opacified abdomen

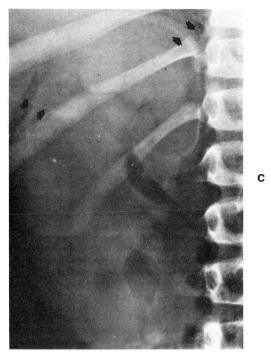

C

Case 9-6. Patient 6. **C,** Detail of kidney in patient with hydronephrosis. Arrows outline rim of parenchyma surrounding hydronephrotic calyces.

(Case 9-6, *B*). Nephrotomography likewise is a useful procedure for showing the renal outlines, particularly in patients with a large amount of abdominal gas. It is particularly helpful in demonstrating the "rim sign" of hydronephrosis—a rim of contrast-filled parenchyma around a hydronephrotic calyx (Case 9-6, *C*).

Ultrasonography is usually the next study performed to determine whether a mass is cystic (sonolucent, anechoic), mixed, or solid (echoic). Anechoic renal masses usually represent hydronephrosis or multicystic kidney in a neonate. A mass with mixed echoes may be an infantile polycystic kidney. A solid renal mass in a child suggests Wilms tumor. A solid

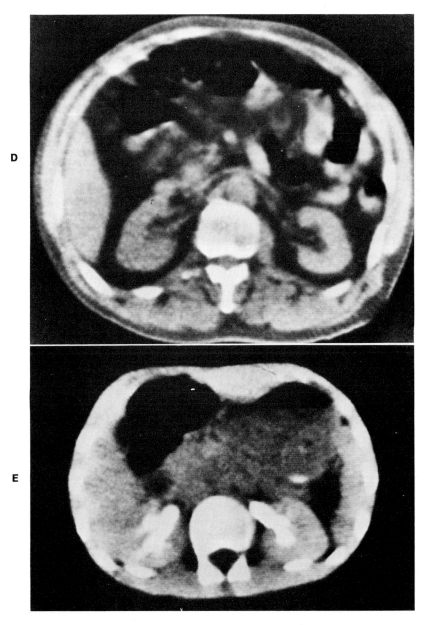

Case 9-6. Abdominal CT scans on an adult and a child. **D,** In adult, adequate amount of body fat clearly delineates kidneys and renal vessels from surrounding tissues. **E,** In child, paucity of soft tissue fat makes parenchymal differentiation considerably more difficult.

suprarenal mass generally represents a neuroblastoma. Rarely, however, will the homogenous nature of a neuroblastoma give a sonolucent picture.

Arteriography was used in the past for the evaluation of patients with suspected pheochromocytoma in an attempt to locate multiple tumors. It was also used to evaluate patients with hepatic masses. However, arteriography provides little additional useful information for the medical or surgical management of Wilms tumor or neuroblastoma and has been superseded by CT.

CT is now used frequently in evaluating children with abdominal masses. The greatest benefit may be in determining the extent of disease and in evaluating the liver for hepatic metastases. It is also used for evaluating the size of the mass or of enlarged lymph nodes in serial fashion for those tumors not totally removed at surgery. However, the paucity of body fat in most children has been a limiting factor in the ability of the scan to delineate body planes (Case 9-6, *D* and *E*). In these instances, ultrasound may be a better diagnostic modality.

References

Bosniak, M. A.: Nephrotomography: a relatively unappreciated but extremely valuable diagnostic tool, Radiology 113:313, 1974.

Daffner, R. H., Gehweiler, J. A., and Carden, T. S., Jr.: Case studies in radiology, New York, 1975, Appleton-Century-Crofts.

Davidson, A. J.: Radiologic diagnosis of renal parenchymal disease, Philadelphia, 1977, W. B. Saunders Co.

Doust, V. L., Doust, B. D., and Redman, H. C.: Evaluation of ultrasonic B-mode scanning in the diagnosis of renal masses, Am. J. Roentgenol. 117:112, 1973.

Freimanis, A. K., and Asher, W. M.: Ultrasonic diagnosis in and about the kidney, J.A.M.A. 234:1263, 1975.

Grossman, H.: The evaluation of abdominal masses in children with emphasis on noninvasive methods. A roentgenographic approach, Cancer 35:884, 1975.

Grossman, H.: Evaluating common intra-abdominal masses in children—a systematic roentgenographic approach, CA 26:219, 1976.

Hare, W. S. C., and Poynter, J. D.: The radiology of renal papillary necrosis as seen in analgesic nephropathy, Clin. Radiol. 25:423, 1974.

Harris, J. H., Jr., Loh, C. K., Perlman, H. C., and Rotz, C. T., Jr.: The roentgen diagnosis of pelvic extraperitoneal effusion, Radiology 125:343, 1977.

Hessel, S. J., and Smith, E. H.: Renal trauma: a comprehensive review and radiologic assessment, CRC Crit. Rev. Clin. Radiol. Nucl. Med. 5:251, 1974.

Kollins, S. A., Hartman, G. W., Carr, D. T., Segura, J. W., and Hattery, R. R.: Roentgenographic findings in urinary tract tuberculosis. A 10 year review, Am. J. Roentgenol. 121:487, 1974.

Korsower, J. M., and Reeder, M. M.: Filling defect in the urinary bladder, J.A.M.A. 231:408, 1975.

Korsower, J. M., and Reeder, M. M.: Nonvisualization or nonfunctioning of one kidney on intravenous pyelogram, J.A.M.A. 232:746, 1975.

Leopold, G. R., and Asher, W. M.: Fundamentals of abdominal and pelvic ultrasonography, Philadelphia, 1975, W. B. Saunders Co.

Maklad, N. F., Chuang, V. P., Doust, B. D., Cho, K. J., and Curran, J. E.: Ultrasonic characterization of solid renal lesions: echographic, angiographic and pathologic correlation, Radiology 123:733, 1977.

McDonald, E. J., Korobkin, M., Jacobs, R. P., and Minagi, H.: The role of emergency excretory urography in evaluation of blunt, abdominal trauma, Am. J. Roentgenol. 126:739, 1976.

Pollack, H. M., Goldberg, B. B., Morales, J. O., and Bogash, M.: A systematized approach to the differential diagnosis of renal masses, Radiology 113:653, 1974.

Richter, M. W., Lytton, B., Myerson, D., and Grnja, V.: Radiology of genitourinary trauma, Radiol. Clin. North Am. 11:593, 1973.

Roylance, J., Penry, J. B., Davies, E. R., and Roberts, M.: The radiology of tuberculosis of the urinary tract, Clin. Radiol. 21:163, 1970.

Sagel, S. S., Stanley, R. J., Levitt, R. G., and Geisse, G.: Computed tomography of the kidney, Radiology 124:359, 1977.

Sussman, M. L., and Newman, A.: Urologic radiology, ed. 2, Baltimore, 1976, The Williams & Wilkins Co.

Witten, D. M., Hyers, G. H., Jr., and Utz, D. C.: Emmett's clinical urography. An atlas and textbook of roentgenologic diagnosis, ed. 4, Philadelphia, 1977, W. B. Saunders Co.

10 Skeletal radiology

One of the most common x-ray examinations you will encounter is that of the skeletal system. Indeed, skeletal radiographs constitute the second largest group of films seen in a busy radiology practice. (Chest is first.) Analysis of the skeleton can provide considerable information regarding your patients. In addition to obvious abnormalities of the skeleton itself, bone radiography may provide clues to the presence of occult inflammatory, metabolic, and neoplastic diseases.

This chapter will outline an approach useful in the interpretation of skeletal radiographs. You should keep in mind that, as in the gastrointestinal tract, lesions in the skeleton appear similar to one another no matter where their location. The incidence may vary with the location, but the basic appearance is the same.

TECHNICAL CONSIDERATIONS

Conventional radiography is not the only means of investigating the skeletal system. Radiology of the skeleton encompasses the entire spectrum of diagnostic examinations, with the exception of ultrasound. In conventional radiography there are two basic techniques: screen and "cardboard." These were mentioned briefly in Chapter 2 and will be reiterated here. Screen technique uses intensifying screens that fluoresce when bombarded by x-rays; the visible light given off by the screen makes the exposure. This technique has the advantage of requiring smaller amounts of x-ray and shorter periods of time for a given exposure. "Cardboard," or nonscreen, technique refers to exposure of the x-ray film directly by the x-ray beam. The film is held in a lighttight cardboard container. This technique requires a longer exposure time but produces films of much better detail, which is desirable in examining the hands and feet. A comparison of screen versus cardboard technique is given in Fig. 10-1.

Xerography is a useful procedure for evaluating bone lesions and associated soft tissue abnormalities. Although xerography is used mainly for examination of the breast, there are applications for the skeletal system. Fig. 10-2 shows conventional radiographs and xerographs of a metastatic bone lesion. Note the better detail seen on the xerograph. Xerography is not used more extensively, however, because the exposure time necessary to obtain a quality xerograph is several times longer than that required for conventional radiographs.

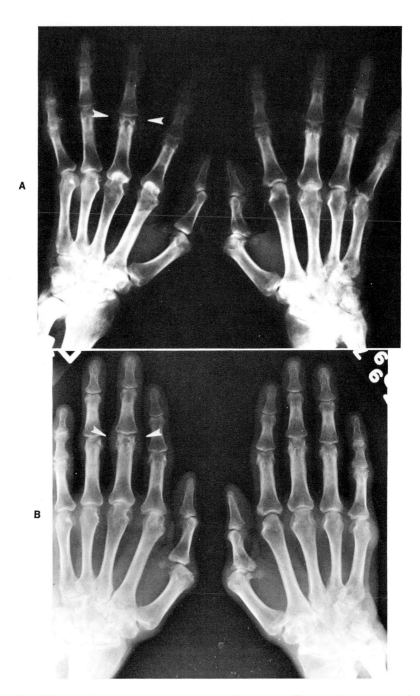

Fig. 10-1. Differences between screen and cardboard techniques. These radiographs are of same patient with rheumatoid arthritis. **A,** Film of hands made using screen technique. Note loss of soft tissue detail. Compare proximal interphalangeal joint of third digit on left (arrowheads) with its appearance in **B. B,** Radiograph of hands made using cardboard technique. Note improved detail. In addition to demonstration of soft tissues (arrows), note how well demonstrated bony trabeculae are.

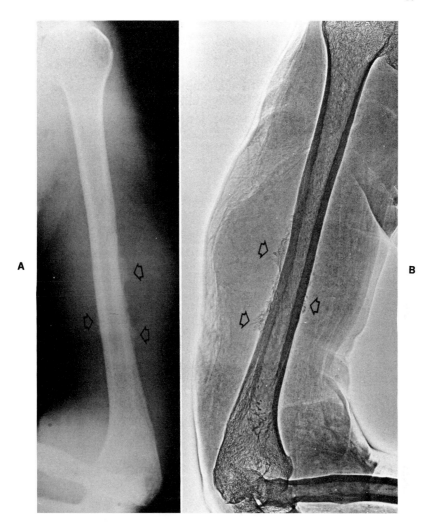

Fig. 10-2. Value of xerography. **A,** Conventional radiograph of humerus in man with metastatic carcinoma to shaft of humerus. There is irregular periosteal reaction along midshaft (arrows). **B,** Xerograph of same limb. Note improved detail in area of periosteal reaction (arrows). In addition, note marked improvement in bony as well as soft tissue detail on this examination. (Image is reverse of radiographic image because of nature of xerographic process.)

Tomographic examination provides additional detail that may be obscured by overlying soft tissues or other portions of bony structures (Fig. 10-3).

CT scanning is being used with increasing frequency in the evaluation of skeletal lesions. This examination can provide diagnostic information of bones and soft tissues in another dimension (Fig. 10-4). CT has also shown promise in evaluating the spinal canal in patients with suspected spinal stenosis (Fig. 10-5) and in providing further information in the evaluation of clubbed feet and congenital hip dislocations.

Invasive studies of the skeletal system include the radioisotope bone scan, arthrography, and angiography. The *bone scan* is a valuable and useful tool for detecting areas of abnormal metabolic activity within bone. With the introduction of tech-

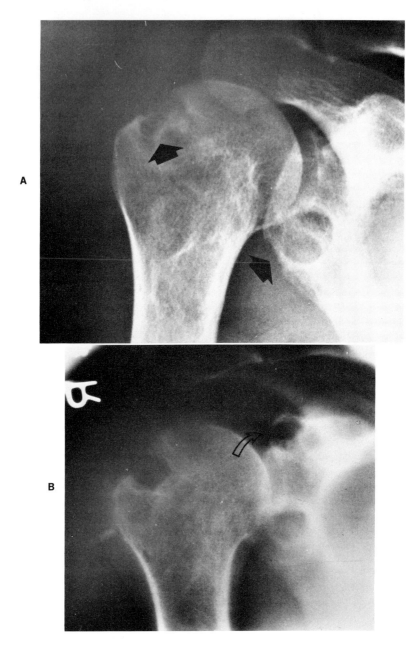

Fig. 10-3. Use of tomography. **A,** Patient with tuberculosis of shoulder. There are cystic lesions in humeral head and glenoid cavity (arrows). **B,** Tomogram of shoulder demonstrates additional areas of cystic tuberculosis in glenoid cavity (arrow).

netium-99m–labeled phosphorus compounds a new dimension of safety and accuracy was accomplished. The phosphorus contained within the isotope is exchanged in areas of rapid bone turnover: destructive lesions such as osteomyelitis and tumors, arthritis, and areas of growing bone. Although the scan itself is not specific for a particular disease, it indicates an area of bony abnormality to which radiography may be

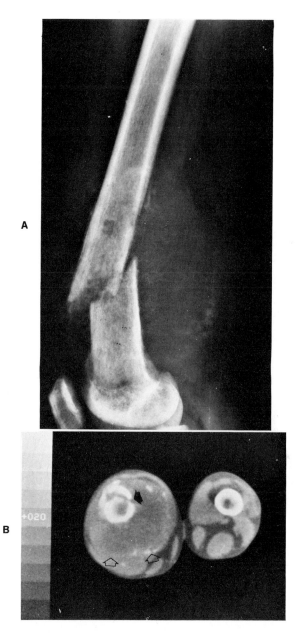

Fig. 10-4. Use of CT scan in skeletal radiology. **A,** Pathologic fracture through osteogenic sarcoma of distal femur. **B,** CT scan shows pathologic fracture in femur (solid arrow). In addition, note extent of soft tissue mass invading and replacing normal tissues (open arrows).

directed. The bone scan is positive before the conventional radiograph shows any abnormality in a particular bone. It should be used as the primary screening examination for the detection of metastases (Fig. 10-6).

Arthrography is the study of joints utilizing positive contrast medium, with or without air, which is injected into the joint space. It is most often used to evaluate the

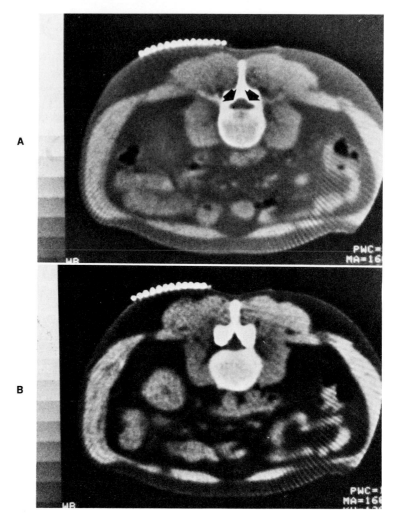

Fig. 10-5. Value of CT scan in patient with spinal stenosis. **A,** There is narrowing of the vertebral canal of lumbar spine (arrows). **B,** Compare this with normal segment 2 cm craniad. White dots on patient's back are catheters used for localization, which are responsible for streaks on study.

knee for meniscal and ligamentous tears (Fig. 10-7). Arthrography is also used in the shoulder to detect tears of the rotator cuff (Fig. 10-8) and in the hip in evaluating patients with painful total hip prostheses (Fig. 10-9).

Angiography is used to evaluate patients with suspected bone tumors. The proponents of this procedure are quite enthusiastic regarding its value in the preoperative evaluation of these lesions. Arteriography is also used to evaluate blood vessels in severe skeletal trauma where vascular injury is suspected.

ANATOMIC CONSIDERATIONS

The specific anatomy of each of the 206 bones in the skeleton will not be reviewed. For that purpose, consult a good textbook of anatomy. However, you should

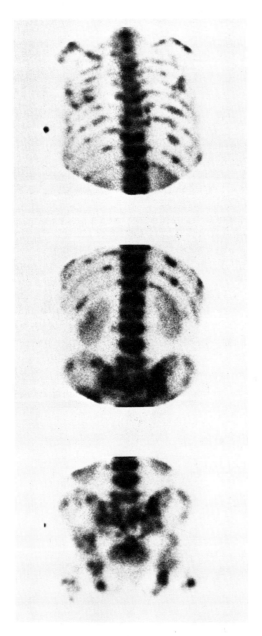

Fig. 10-6. Bone scan in patient with multiple metastases of carcinoma of breast. Metastatic lesions are represented by increased concentration of isotope.

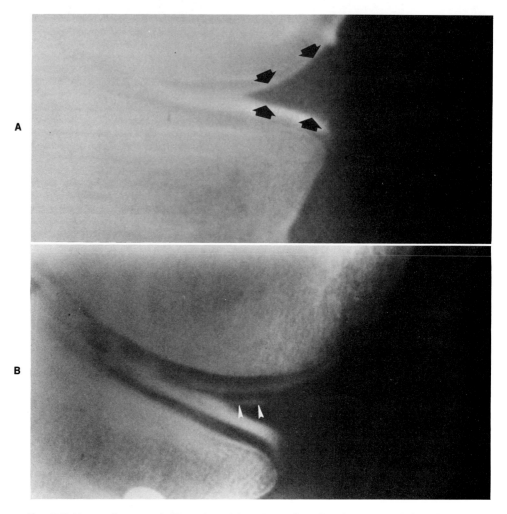

Fig. 10-7. Knee arthrogram. **A,** Normal medial meniscus. Spot film shows normal triangular shape of meniscus (arrows). **B,** Linear tear of medial meniscus. Tear is represented by streak of contrast material within meniscal "triangle" (arrowheads).

remember that because you are dealing with three-dimensional structures in the skeleton, many bony projections may overlap and produce "strange" shadows with which you are not familiar. The best way to avoid this confusion is to have a thorough knowledge of the anatomy of the bone being studied.

There are five types of bone, based on their shapes:
1. Long bones, which have two ends and a shaft (femur, humerus, and, interestingly, phalanges, which are miniature long bones)
2. Short bones, which are six sided, as a rule (carpal and tarsal bones)
3. Flat bones (calvaria, ribs, and sternum)
4. Irregular bones, which have many sides (vertebrae)
5. Sesamoid bones, which lack periosteum (largest is the patella)

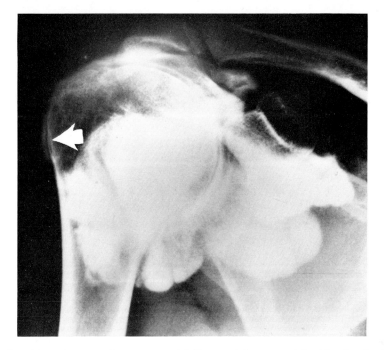

Fig. 10-8. Shoulder arthrogram. Contrast material fills synovial spaces of shoulder. Small collection of contrast material just lateral to humeral head (arrow) represents extravasation secondary to tear of rotator cuff.

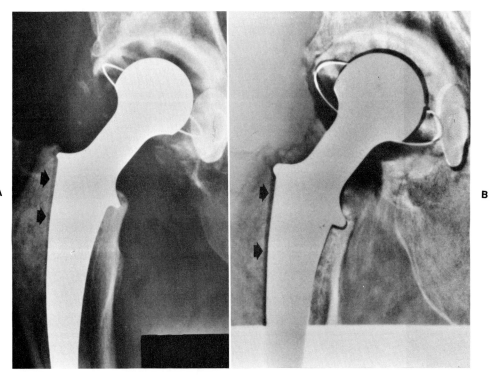

A

B

Fig. 10-9. Hip arthrogram in patient with loose total hip prosthesis. **A,** Preliminary film shows lucent zone between bone and stem of prosthesis (arrows). **B,** Subtraction technique arthrogram shows contrast material to fill this area (arrows). In subtraction mode, all images are reverse of normal black and white. Prosthesis appears gray because of subtraction.

Furthermore, bone may be of two architectural types: compact (dense) bone or cancellous (spongy) bone. The distribution of these types of bones depends on the stress to which each bone is subjected.

There are three locations within a bone: the epiphysis, or growth center; the metaphysis, an area that lies just beneath the epiphyseal plate; and the diaphysis, or shaft. As you will see later, these locations are of considerable importance in predicting the nature of some bone lesions.

PATHOLOGIC CONSIDERATIONS

Analysis of bone and joint lesions can be as simple as the ABCS. Forrester and Nesson (1973) in their monograph on arthritis developed a concept of using the mnemonic of ABC and S that applies to bone diseases as well as to arthritis:

A Anatomic appearance and alignment
B Bony mineralization and texture
C Cartilage (joint) space
S Soft tissues

These will be elaborated on as they apply to the analysis of bone lesions later in the discussion. Using this approach, however, you will find how adept you will be at recognizing and diagnosing many bone lesions.

There are six basic pathologic categories of skeletal disease: *congenital, inflammatory, metabolic, neoplastic, traumatic,* and *vascular.* A seventh category, *miscellaneous* or *other,* might be added to encompass those diseases that do not fall strictly into one of the first six.

The logical approach to skeletal radiology begins by defining the distribution of a lesion and by applying a number of factors that can further narrow the diagnostic choices. These factors have been termed "predictor variables" and have been used in making computer diagnoses of bone lesions.

Distribution

The distribution of a bone or joint lesion provides important clues to the etiology of that lesion. Lesions may be monostotic or monoarticular, that is, confined to one bone or joint; polyostotic or polyarticular, that is, located in many bones or joints; or diffuse, that is, involving virtually every bone or joint. Applying this distribution pattern to the six pathologic categories produces a scheme shown in Table 7. You can see by studying Table 7 that there are only two disease categories that may occur diffusely: neoplastic and metabolic. Metabolic disease by definition is a diffuse disease; however, occasionally monostotic or polyostotic forms occur. Examples of these lesions are shown in Table 8.

Predictor variables

There are 11 predictor variables that may be applied to any joint or bone lesion to aid in making the correct diagnosis. These are listed in the following outline.

FACTORS AFFECTING CORRECT ROENTGEN DIAGNOSIS OF BONE LESIONS

I. Behavior of the lesion
  A. Osteolytic
  B. Osteoblastic
  C. Mixed
II. Bone involved
III. Locus within bone
  A. Epiphysis
  B. Metaphysis
  C. Diaphysis
IV. Age, sex, and race of patient
V. Margin of lesion
  A. Sharply defined
  B. Poorly defined
VI. Shape of lesion
VII. Joint space crossed (?)

VIII. Bony reaction
  A. Periosteal
    1. Solid
    2. Laminated
    3. Spiculated, sunburst, "hair-on-end"
    4. Codman triangle
  B. Sclerosis
  C. Buttressing
IX. Matrix production
  A. Osteoid
  B. Chondroid
  C. Mixed
X. Soft tissue changes
XI. History of trauma

It will become apparent from the discussion that some of these variables apply to the diagnosis of bone tumors. You should keep in mind that primary bone tumors, exclusive of myeloma, are rare lesions. You should also remember that in many instances you may not be able to make a specific diagnosis even after applying all these factors. Radiologists should be satisfied that they have done their best when they have been able to categorize a difficult lesion as either aggressive or nonaggressive. In these instances, they will essentially have decided that the lesion is malignant or benign.

Table 7. Distribution of bone disease by pathologic category

Category	Distribution		
	Monostotic	**Polyostotic**	**Diffuse**
Congenital	X	X	
Inflammatory	X	X	
Neoplastic	X	X	X
Metabolic	(X)	(X)	X
Traumatic	X	X	
Vascular	X	X	

Table 8. Examples of distribution: pathologic relationships

Category	Monostotic	Polyostotic	Diffuse
Congenital	Cervical rib	Cleidocranial dysostosis	—
Inflammatory	Osteomyelitis	Congenital lues	—
Neoplastic	Any primary bone tumor	Myeloma	Metastasis
Metabolic	(Paget disease)	(Paget disease, fibrous dysplasia)	Osteopetrosis, hyperparathyroidism
Traumatic	Single fracture	Multiple fracture, battered child	Usually incompatible with life
Vascular	Perthes disease	Perthes disease	—

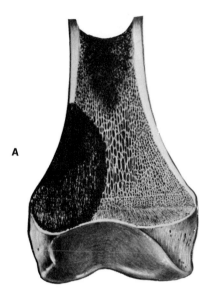

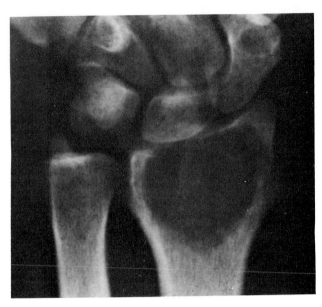

A

B

Fig. 10-10. Geographic destruction. **A,** Schematic drawing demonstrates large zone of bony destruction. (After Lodwick [1966].) **B,** Giant cell tumor of distal radius exhibits geographic destruction. Note large zone of bony destruction.

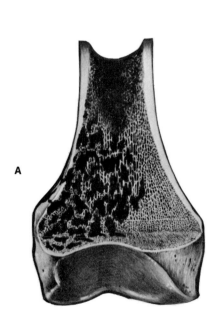

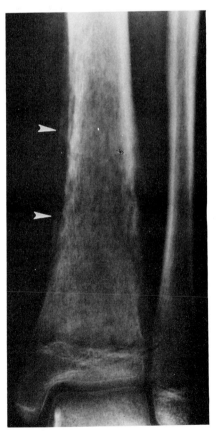

A

B

Fig. 10-11. Moth-eaten destructive pattern. **A,** Schematic drawing demonstrates multiple holes within bone. These are smaller than holes seen with geographic destruction. They are still visible to unaided eye on radiograph. (After Lodwick [1966].) **B,** Osteomyelitis of distal tibia. Note multiple holes within bone. Zone of periosteal reaction is seen on medial aspect of tibia (arrowheads).

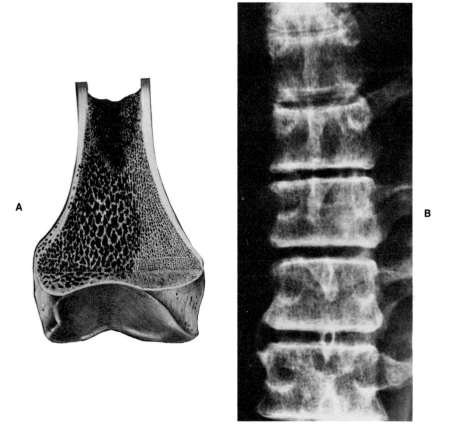

Fig. 10-12. Permeative destruction. **A,** Diagrammatic representation. Destruction is represented by multiple small holes within bone. (After Lodwick [1966].) **B,** Multiple myeloma. Permeative pattern is apparent within spine. This is not osteoporosis. There is actual bony destruction.

Behavior of the lesion

Bone lesions may be primarily osteolytic (bone destroying), osteoblastic (bone forming, reactive, or reparative), or, occasionally, a mixture of the two. There are three forms of osteolytic bone destruction: geographic (Fig. 10-10), moth-eaten (Fig. 10-11), and permeative (Fig. 10-12). *Geographic* destruction implies that large areas of bone have been destroyed and are easily visible with the unaided eye (Fig. 10-10). A *moth-eaten* appearance is one in which there are many discrete small holes throughout the bone, similar to a piece of clothing ruined by moth larvae. A moth-eaten appearance suggests a more aggressive lesion (Fig. 10-11). A *permeative* pattern is one in which there is fine bony destruction. Pathologically, this represents a lesion diffusely infiltrating bone through the haversian system. In many instances a magnifying lens is required to see the bone destruction. Permeative destruction implies a very aggressive process such as the round cell tumors of bone (Ewing tumor, myeloma, reticulum cell sarcoma) (Fig. 10-12).

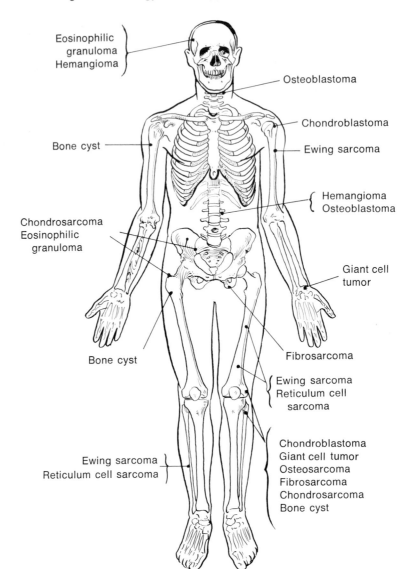

Eosinophilic
granuloma
Hemangioma

Osteoblastoma

Chondroblastoma

Bone cyst

Ewing sarcoma

Hemangioma
Osteoblastoma

Chondrosarcoma
Eosinophilic
granuloma

Giant cell
tumor

Bone cyst

Fibrosarcoma

Ewing sarcoma
Reticulum cell
sarcoma

Chondroblastoma
Giant cell tumor
Osteosarcoma
Fibrosarcoma
Chondrosarcoma
Bone cyst

Ewing sarcoma
Reticulum cell sarcoma

Fig. 10-13. Preferred location of common bone tumors.

Bone involved

Some diseases have a predilection for certain bones. Fig. 10-13 illustrates the preferred location of many common bone tumors. This information is quite useful in diagnosing many bone lesions. For example, chondrosarcomas (Figs. 10-14) favor the pelvis, whereas enchondromas (Fig. 10-15) favor the phalanges and metacarpals; Paget disease commonly affects the pelvis, skull, and spine, while sparing the fibula (Fig. 10-16); gout favors the bones of the feet (Fig. 10-17); rheumatoid arthritis affects the hands and feet (Fig. 10-18); and hyperparathyroidism commonly affects the skull, distal clavicles, and bones of the hands and feet (Fig. 10-19).

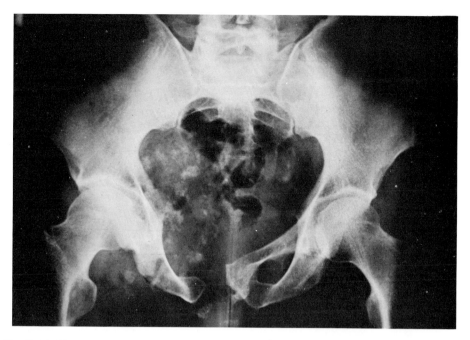

Fig. 10-14. Chondrosarcoma of pelvis. This is common location for this type of malignant tumor. Note massive bony destruction on right. Punctate calcific densities within pelvic cavity represent chondroid matrix.

Locus within bone

The location of a lesion within a bone can provide an important clue to the etiology. Many lesions have a predilection for the epiphysis, metaphysis, or diaphysis. The common locations of bone tumors are shown in Fig. 10-20. Certain benign lesions also have predilection for favored areas of bone; for example, osteoarthritis prefers the weight-bearing surfaces of the large joints (Fig. 10-21) whereas rheumatoid arthritis affects the entire surface of the same joint (Fig. 10-22).

Age, sex, and race of patient

The distribution of bone disease depends on the patient's age. A child with a permeative lesion of the shaft of the humerus is likely to have Ewing tumor (Fig. 10-23). A lesion of similar appearance in a much older patient should suggest reticulum cell sarcoma or malignant lymphoma of bone. Edeiken and Hodes believe they can predict the type of a malignant bone tumor on the basis of the patient's age. For example, under age 1 year, neuroblastoma is the most common type of tumor; in the first decade, Ewing tumor of tubular bone; ages 10 to 30 years, osteosarcoma and Ewing tumor of flat bones; between ages 30 and 40 years, most of the malignant sarcomas; and over age 40 years, metastatic carcinoma, along with multiple myeloma and chondrosarcoma.

Certain benign lesions also occur more commonly in different age groups. For example, Paget disease is almost never seen in patients under age 40 years. Infantile cortical hyperostosis (Caffey disease) is not seen in patients over age 1 year.

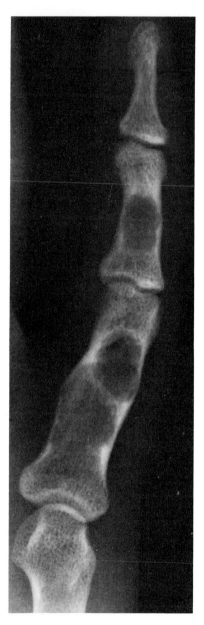

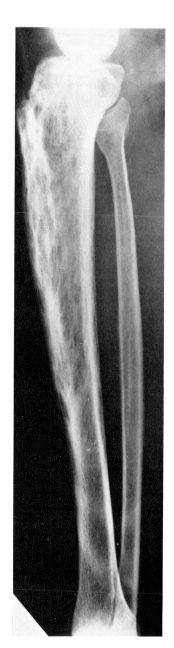

Fig. 10-15   **Fig. 10-16**

Fig. 10-15. Enchondromas of phalanges. Multiple lucent defects are seen within first and second phalanges of this fifth digit. There is expansion of cortex of proximal phalanx. This is common location for these benign tumors.

Fig. 10-16. Paget disease of tibia. Fibula is uninvolved.

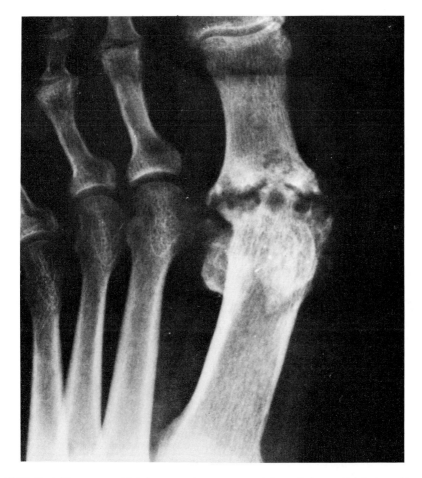

Fig. 10-17. Gout. There are multiple bony erosions across metatarsophalangeal joint of great toe. This is "classic" location for gout.

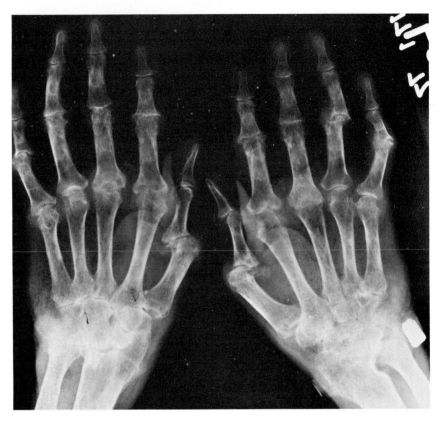

Fig. 10-18. Rheumatoid arthritis of hands and wrists. Rheumatoid arthritis has predilection for small bones of hands and wrists. In addition to bony destruction, subluxation is present at proximal inter-phalangeal joint of fourth digit on left.

Many lesions have a sex distribution. Paget disease is seen more commonly in males, for example.

In addition to sexual predominance, there is a racial predominance in some diseases, particularly sickle cell disease and thalassemia.

Margin of lesion

In general a sharp transition zone appearing as a dense zone of sclerosis between a lesion and normal bone or as a thin, well-defined line between normal bone and a lesion (Fig. 10-24) indicates a benign lesion. On the other hand a broad or wide, poorly defined zone between normal and abnormal bone indicates a more aggressive lesion (Fig. 10-25). The differences in the growth rate of these lesions accounts for the difference in the appearance. A slow-growing, benign lesion such as a fibroxanthoma of bone or a focus of tuberculosis progresses at a rate slow enough to allow the bone to react in an attempt to wall off the lesion. An aggressive lesion such as a malignant tumor or osteomyelitis progresses at a rapid rate, so that the bone is unable to respond adequately.

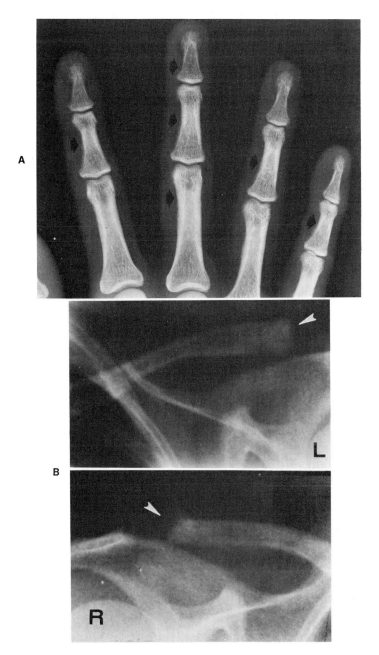

Fig. 10-19. Hyperparathyroidism. **A,** Preferred locations of bony resorption along radial aspects of phalanges (arrows). There has been some resorption of tufts of distal phalanges. **B,** Resorption of distal clavicle is also favorite site (arrowheads).

Locus within bone

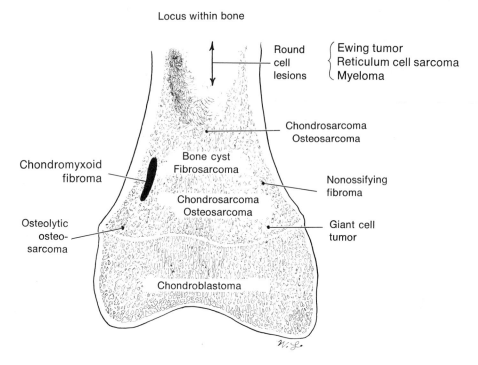

Fig. 10-20. Common location of bone tumors within particular bone.

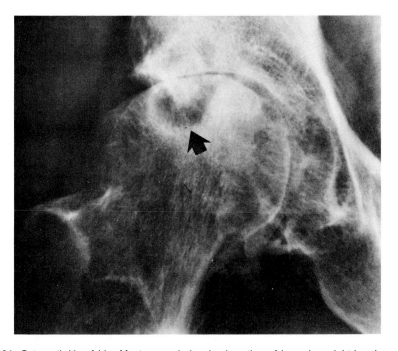

Fig. 10-21. Osteoarthritis of hip. Most severely involved portion of bone is weight-bearing surface. Aseptic necrosis, as manifest by lucency, is present within this area (arrow). Bony spurs are present inferiorly.

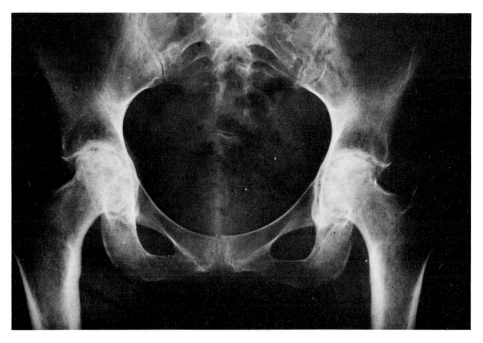

Fig. 10-22. Rheumatoid arthritis of hips. Hips are affected in bilateral symmetric manner. Entire joint space is affected rather than just weight-bearing surface, common in osteoarthritis.

Shape of lesion

The shape of a lesion helps in the same way that the margin does. A lesion that is longer than it is wide, that is, oriented with the shaft of the bone, is likely to be a benign process. In this situation the lesion is growing with bone and not faster than bone. On the other hand, a lesion that is wider than the bone, has broken out of the bone, and has extended into the soft tissues is a more aggressive type of lesion (Fig. 10-26).

Joint space crossed(?)

If a lesion has crossed the joint space, it is most likely a benign inflammatory process. This is generally the case no matter how aggressive or malignant a process may appear (Fig. 10-27). Infectious processes will extend across a joint space, but tumors will not. Tumors that have a predilection for the ends of bones, such as chondroblastoma and giant cell tumor (Fig. 10-28), will extend to the joint but will not cross it. Furthermore, even the most malignant bone tumors respect the cartilage of the growth plate area (Figs. 10-26 and 10-29).

Bony reaction

Bony response to insult includes periosteal reaction, sclerosis, and buttressing. Periosteal reaction is of four varieties: solid, laminated or onionskin, spiculated (sunburst or "hair-on-end"), or Codman triangle. *Solid* periosteal reaction (greater than 2 mm) indicates a benign process. It is most often seen in osteomyelitis and fracture

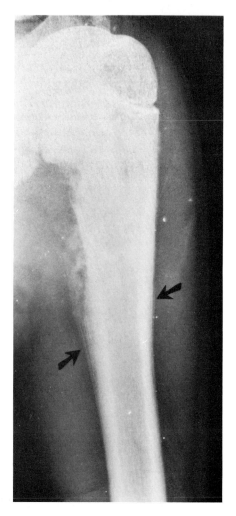

Fig. 10-23. Ewing tumor of proximal humerus. There is destructive lesion in diametaphysis of this bone in child. Open growth plate helps establish age. Note laminated periosteal reaction (arrows).

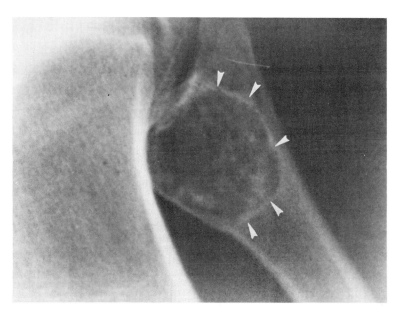

Fig. 10-24. Enchondroma of proximal fibula. Sharp sclerotic border defines normal from abnormal bone (arrowheads).

healing (Fig. 10-30). A *laminated or onionskin* type of periosteal reaction indicates repetitive injury to bone. Previously this was thought to be pathognomonic of Ewing tumor or reticulum cell sarcoma of bone. However, this type of reaction also occurs in any type of repetitive injury to bone such as in the "battered child" (Fig. 10-31). Once again the nature of the laminated periosteal reaction may be determined by its thickness. In a Ewing tumor the periosteum is quite thin (Fig. 10-32), whereas in a benign process such as osteomyelitis or battered child, the reaction is considerably thicker. A *spiculated*, sunburst, or "hair-on-end" appearance is almost always associated with a malignant bone lesion (Fig. 10-33), most often an osteogenic sarcoma. Occasionally this occurs in metastatic disease (Fig. 10-34). The *Codman triangle* represents triangular ossification of a piece of periosteum. In the past this was thought to be pathognomonic of tumor. However, it is seen in many benign conditions, including subperiosteal hemorrhage in scurvy and battered child.

Sclerosis is an attempt by the bone to wall off a diseased area. It generally indicates a benign process (Fig. 10-35). Buttressing is an attempt by the bone to reestablish architectural integrity. The term is derived from the flying buttresses of Gothic architecture. The most common example of this is the osteophyte of degenerative arthritis (Fig. 10-36).

Matrix production

Matrix is a substance produced by certain bone tumors. It may be chondroid (cartilaginous), osteoid (bony), or mixed. Chondroid matrix appears as fine stippled calcification or multiple popcornlike calcifications. Quite often it occurs in bulky masses of tumor within the soft tissues (Fig. 10-37). Osteoid matrix, on the other

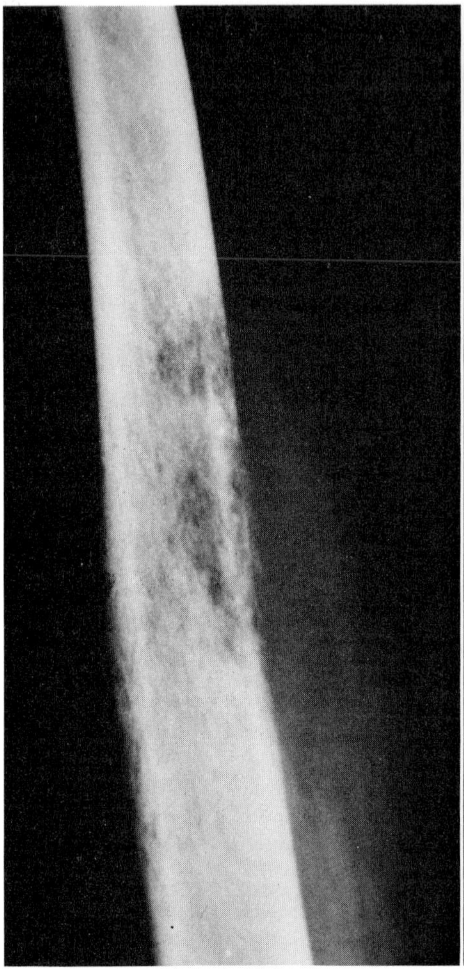

Fig. 10-25 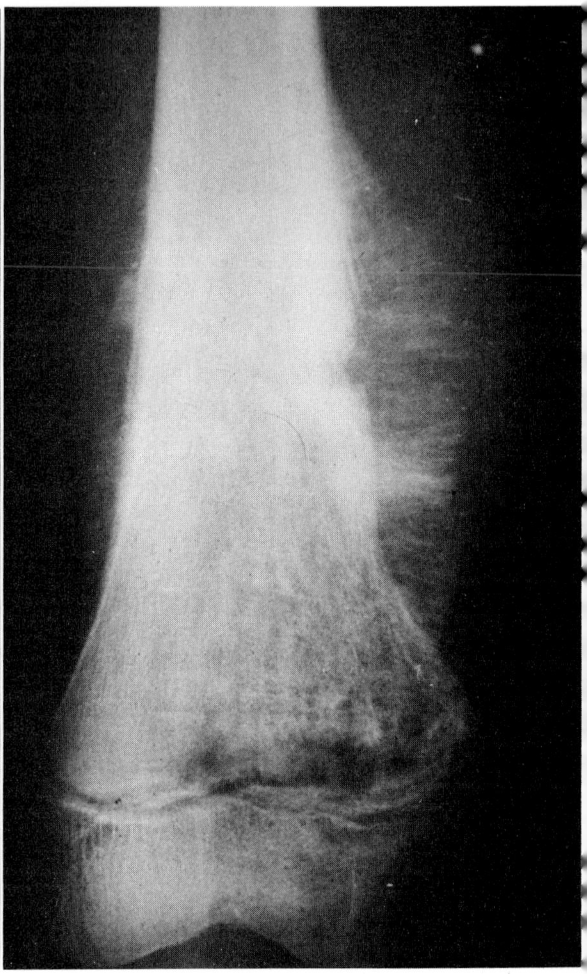   **Fig. 10-26**

Fig. 10-25. Metastatic carcinoma to humerus. Moth-eaten to permeative pattern is present. Lesion has no border. One is unable to differentiate transition between normal and abnormal bone.

Fig. 10-26. Osteogenic sarcoma of distal femur. Tumor has extended outward into soft tissues from bone. This is most apparent on one side where "hair-on-end" periosteal reaction is present. Note that tumor has not crossed growth plate.

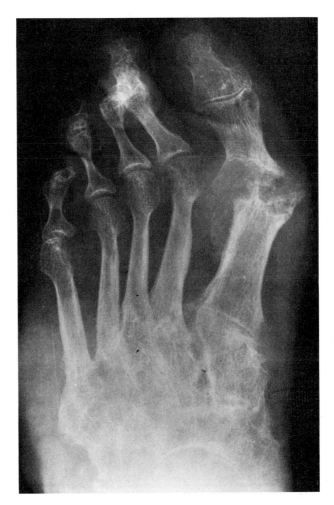

Fig. 10-27. Gout. There is aggressive lesion at metatarsophalangeal joint of great toe. However, the fact that process is present on both sides of joint space indicates that this is an inflammatory rather than a neoplastic lesion. Changes of gout are present in other joints. In addition, long history of gouty arthritis could be elicited.

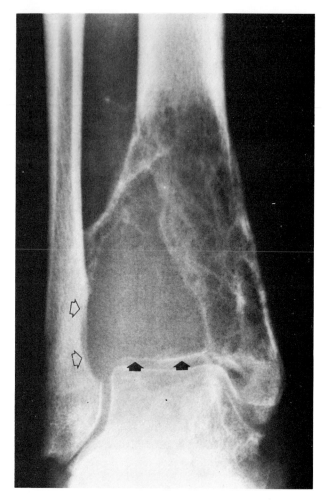

Fig. 10-28. Giant cell tumor of distal tibia. This aggressive-appearing lesion is poorly defined on its proximal end. It is extending into soft tissues and causing pressure changes on adjacent fibula (open arrows). Note, however, that subarticular bone is preserved (solid arrows). Infection would easily cross joint space.

hand, is dense and usually of the same radiographic density as bone. It occurs most often in osteogenic sarcoma (Fig. 10-38) but also may be seen in the benign ossifying condition myositis ossificans.

Soft tissue changes

By analyzing the soft tissues, you may obtain important clues regarding an underlying disease process or a specific bone disease. For example, diffuse muscle wasting suggests a patient with paralysis, primary muscle disease, or severe inanition caused by disseminated carcinomatosis. The presence of soft tissue swelling may be indicative of a mass lesion (Fig. 10-39), hemorrhage, inflammation, or edema. The loss or displacement of fat lines normally seen in the soft tissues is another indication of adjacent abnormality. For example, displacement or obliteration of the pronator

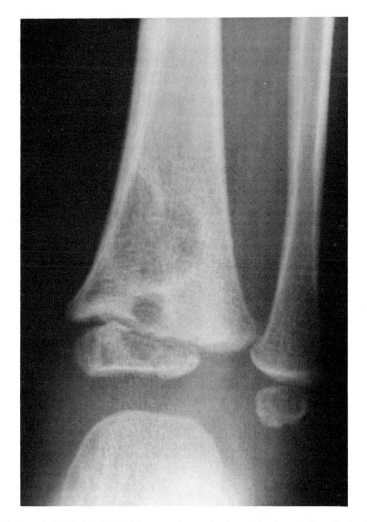

Fig. 10-29. Tuberculosis of distal tibia. There are lucencies in epiphysis and diametaphysis. The fact that this lesion has crossed growth plate indicates it is an inflammatory lesion. Compare with Fig. 10-26.

quadratus fat line in the wrist (Fig. 10-40) usually indicates a fracture of the wrist. Prominence of the fat pads of the elbow indicate fluid within the joint space, usually the result of trauma but sometimes seen in an inflammatory condition such as rheumatoid arthritis (Fig. 10-41). The presence of a fat-fluid level on a horizontal radiograph of the knee is indicative of a fracture communicating with the knee (Fig. 10-42).

Calcifications within the soft tissues may result from old trauma or connective tissue disorders. Occasionally, old parasitic disease will be manifest by soft tissue calcifications.

Gas in the tissues may indicate trauma or gas gangrene. Other soft tissue findings include the presence of foreign bodies or renal calculi in a patient being evaluated for back pain.

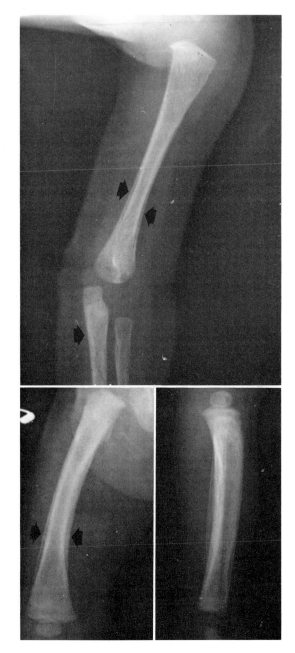

Fig. 10-30. Solid periosteal reaction (arrows) in patient with congenital syphilis.

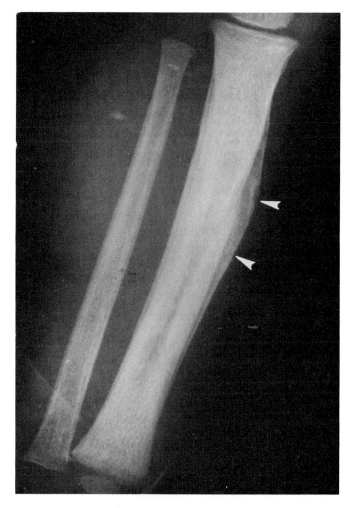

Fig. 10-31. Battered child. There is solid periosteal reaction across fracture of midshaft of this patient's tibia (arrowheads). Thick laminated periosteal reaction is present on opposite side of tibia.

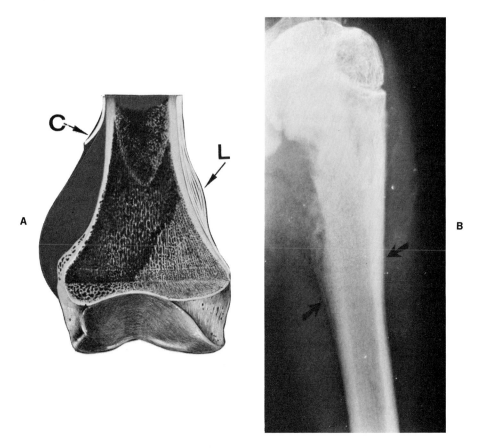

Fig. 10-32. Periosteal reaction. **A,** Drawing illustrating laminated reaction *(L)* and Codman triangle *(C).* (After Lodwick [1966].) **B,** Ewing tumor of proximal humerus. Note thin laminated periosteal reaction (arrows).

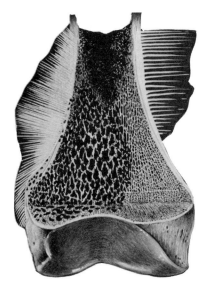

Fig. 10-33. Types of "hair-on-end" periosteal reaction. (After Lodwick [1966].)

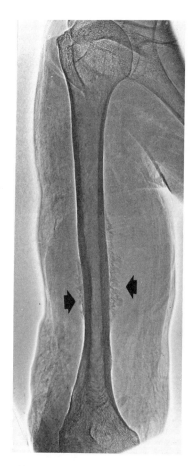

Fig. 10-34. Xerogram of patient with metastatic carcinoma of humerus. There is "hair-on-end" periosteal reaction along midshaft (arrows). See also Fig. 10-26.

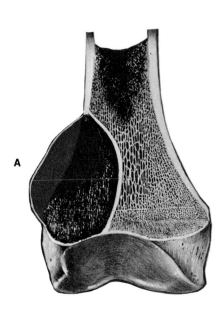
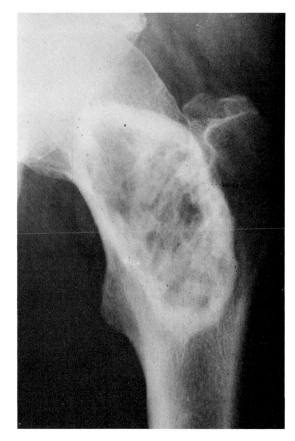

Fig. 10-35. Sclerosis around bony lesion. **A,** Schematic drawing. (After Lodwick [1966].) **B,** Fibrous dysplasia of proximal femur. Dense zone of sclerosis surrounds lesion.

History of trauma

Since trauma constitutes the most common bone "disease" you will see, it is very important to elicit a history of trauma whenever possible. A stress fracture may be misdiagnosed as a malignant bone tumor unless a specific history of "trauma" (pain with an unusual activity, condition worsening with that activity, and relief achieved by rest) is obtained. Occasionally, however, a history of trauma will be deliberately withheld as in the case of the battered child or of a child who, prior to injury, was doing something that was prohibited.

Additional observations
Bony anatomy and alignment

Deformities in a bone generally indicate congenital abnormality (Fig. 10-43). However, they may also be seen as a sequel of poorly treated trauma (Fig. 10-44). There are two types of malalignment that may occur in joints: subluxations and dislocations. *Subluxation* is a partial loss of continuity between articulating surfaces;

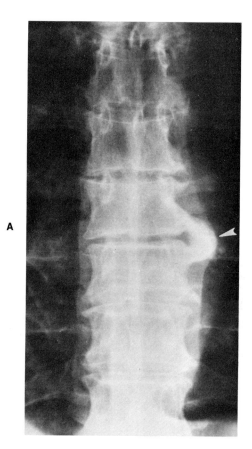

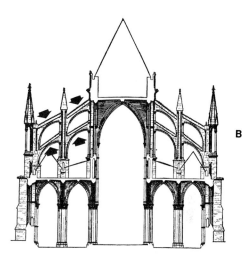

A

B

Fig. 10-36. Buttressing. **A,** Osteophytes of thoracic spine. This is most marked at level indicated by arrowhead. **B,** Schematic drawing of Gothic cathedral. Flying buttresses are indicated by arrows.

dislocation is the complete loss of continuity at that joint space. These are illustrated in Fig. 10-45.

Bony mineralization

The degree of mineralization of a bone is directly related to the patient's age, the physiologic state, and the amount of activity or stress being placed on that bone. Osteoporosis commonly occurs in the elderly and in postmenopausal women. However, an acute form of osteoporosis may occur following immobilization of a limb. Diminished mineralization is also a common manifestation of certain diseases such as scurvy and rheumatoid arthritis (Fig. 10-46). For an excellent in-depth discussion of bone mineral deposition, consult *Orthopedic Diseases* (Aegerter and Kirkpatrick, 1975).

Joint space changes

The width of the joint space and the appearance of the distal ends of articulating bones are important in the diagnosis of arthritis. The distribution, location, and

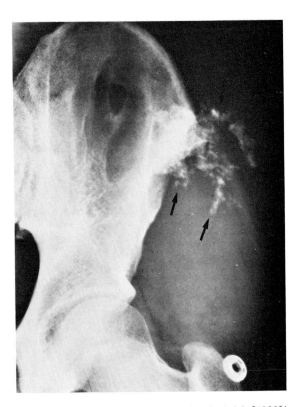

Fig. 10-37. Matrix production. **A,** Drawing showing chondroid-type matrix. (After Lodwick [1966].) **B,** Chondrosarcoma of iliac crest. Note matrix within soft tissue extension of tumor (arrows).

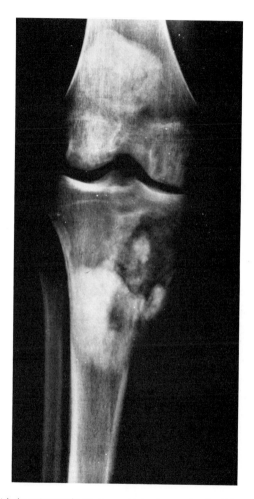

Fig. 10-38. Osteoid matrix in osteogenic sarcoma. Note dense cloud within zone of bony destruction.

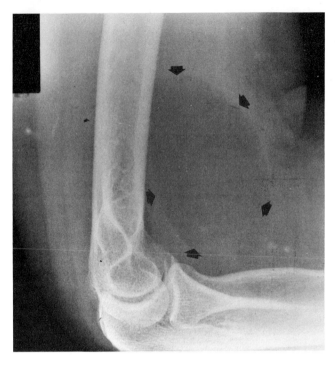

Fig. 10-39. Lipoma of antecubital fossa. Lucent soft tissue mass is present (arrows).

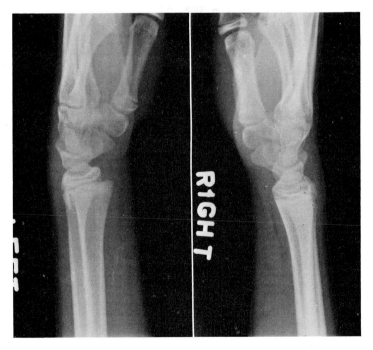

Fig. 10-40. Pronator quadratus fat pad sign. Pronator quadratus fat stripe is seen as lucent line anterior to radius in normal right wrist in this patient (arrowhead). It is absent in abnormal wrist on left, which has sustained fracture through distal radial epiphysis. Note also soft tissue swelling on left.

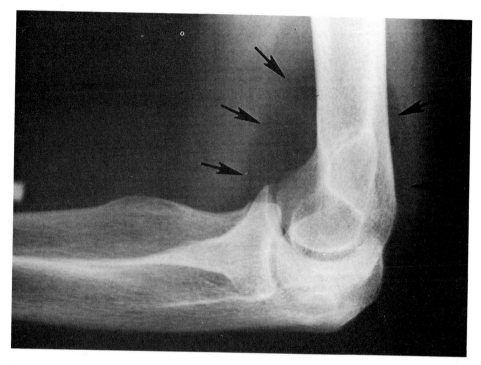

Fig. 10-41. Elbow fat pad sign. Anterior and posterior fat pads (arrows) are visible in this patient with rheumatoid arthritis. Positive fat pad indicates fluid in joint. Most often this is secondary to trauma. (From Daffner, R. H.: New Physician **24**:52, 1975. Reproduced with permission of the publisher.)

erosive patterns produced by the various arthritides allow considerable accuracy in radiologic diagnosis, particularly when correlated with clinical and laboratory findings. You should familiarize yourself with the changes in the three most common types of arthritis you will encounter: rheumatoid, degenerative, and gouty. The salient features of these diseases are summarized here.

Rheumatoid arthritis. The radiographic findings depend on the stage of the disease. Early findings include fusiform pericapsular swelling, joint effusion, and subtle demineralization of the subarticular bone. As the disease progresses, marginal erosions occur, usually associated with narrowing of the joint space (Fig. 10-47). The degree of osteoporosis has progressed. In the late form of the disease, considerable destruction has taken place about the joints, and subluxations occur. In the end stage, ankylosis occurs (Fig. 10-48).

Degenerative arthritis (osteoarthritis). There are three salient features of degenerative arthritis: narrowed joint spaces, subarticular reactive sclerosis, and spur formation (Fig. 10-49).

Gouty arthritis. In the early stages of gouty arthritis, soft tissue swelling is the only radiographic finding. Indeed the disease must be present for 5 to 7 years before erosive changes, large punched-out lesions, are seen. These erosions may be articular or para-articular and result from tophus formation. Often the erosions have overhanging edges (Fig. 10-50). The degree of mineralization is usually normal except in an acute attack.

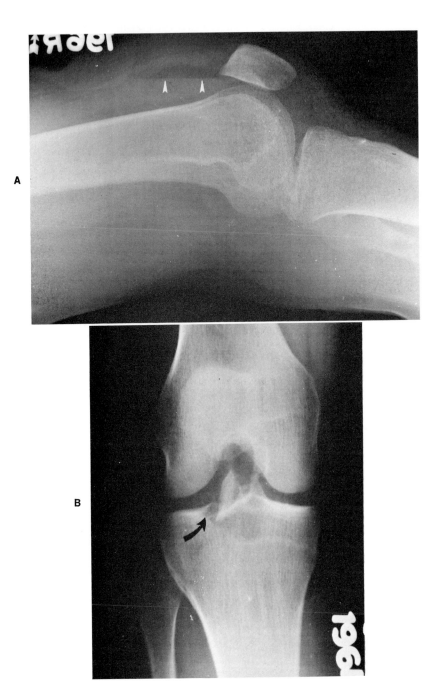

Fig. 10-42. Fat-fluid level of knee in patient with fracture of tibial plateau. **A,** Horizontal beam lateral view shows fat-fluid level (arrowheads). Fracture does not show in this view. **B,** Fracture near intercondylar spines is clearly seen (arrow).

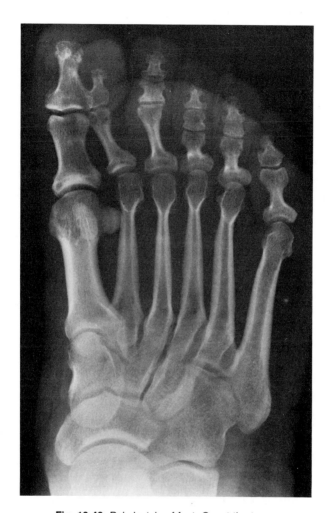

Fig. 10-43. Polydactyly of foot. Count the toes.

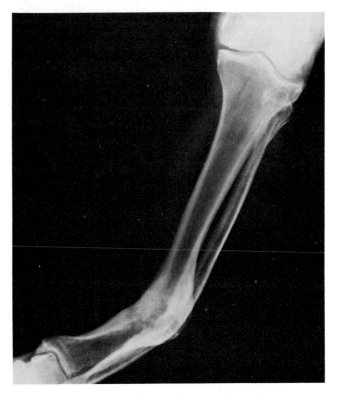

Fig. 10-44. Bad result of trauma resulting from poorly treated injury. There is too much angulation at site of healed fracture of tibia and fibula.

Trauma

As previously mentioned, skeletal trauma is the most common bone disorder. *A fracture is really a soft tissue injury in which a bone is broken.* In most instances the bone, if left by itself, would heal. However, in dealing with fractures, you must be concerned with associated soft tissue injury. For example, a fracture of the skull itself may be insignificant. However, if there is damage to the underlying meningeal vessels or brain, the injury is significant. Similarly, fractures of the spine are often associated with neurologic deficit from damage to the spinal cord. Therefore in evaluating a patient who has sustained skeletal trauma, it is important to assess the status of the adjacent soft tissue structures.

In trauma patients, views other than the routine ones may be necessary to demonstrate a suspected fracture. Furthermore, *comparison views* with the opposite uninjured limb may be necessary, particularly in evaluating possible epiphyseal injuries (Fig. 10-51). Occasionally, stress views to test ligamentous stability and arteriography to investigate the possibility of vascular injury may be necessary.

The descriptive terminology of fractures is important; the referring clinician, orthopedic surgeon, and radiologist must all speak the same language. Fractures are described by location within the bone, type (spiral, comminuted, oblique, greenstick) and position of the fragments (degrees of angulation, displacement, over-

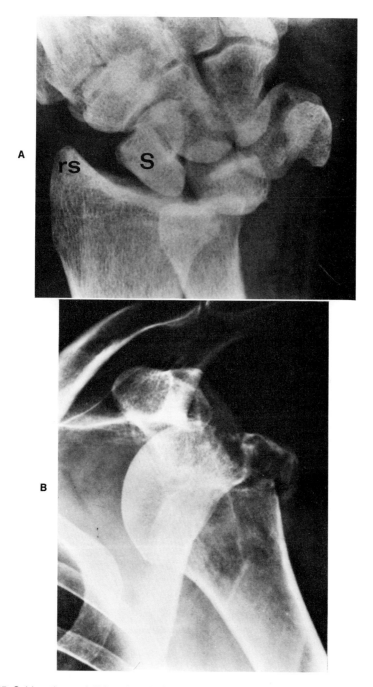

Fig. 10-45. Subluxation and dislocation. **A,** Subluxation of carpal bones in patient with systemic lupus erythematosus. Scaphoid bone *(S)* should be adjacent to radial styloid process *(rs)*. **B,** Dislocation of shoulder. Humeral head is dislocated anteriorly. Note complete loss of continuity between articular surfaces. Fracture of greater tubercle of humerus is also present.

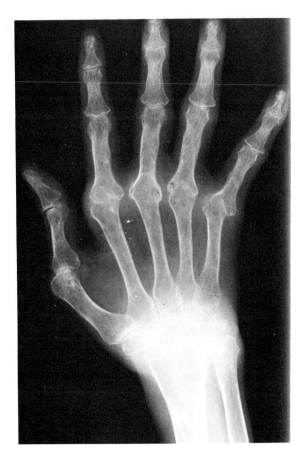

Fig. 10-46. Rheumatoid arthritis. There is marked osteoporosis in this patient with advanced rheumatoid arthritis. Note washed-out appearance of bones.

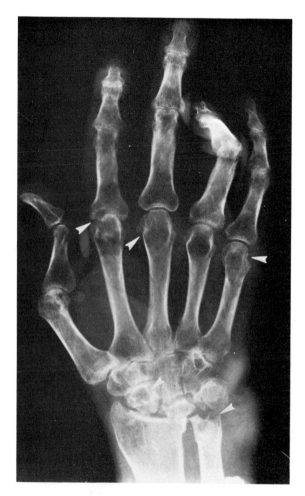

Fig. 10-47. Rheumatoid arthritis, moderately advanced. There are erosive changes in multiple sites (arrowheads). Note narrowing of joint spaces within wrist. There is subluxation of fourth digit at proximal interphalangeal joint.

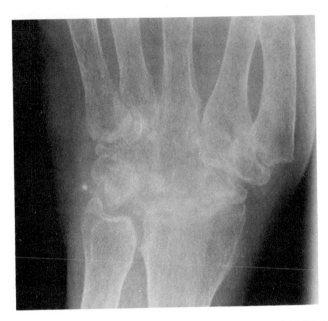

Fig. 10-48. Rheumatoid arthritis, late stage. There is ankylosis across wrist joint. Normal anatomic landmarks cannot be discerned. Note severe osteoporosis.

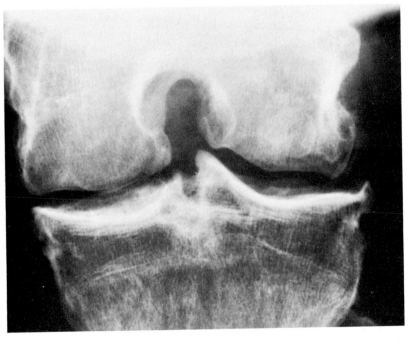

Fig. 10-49. Degenerative arthritis of knee. Salient features of joint space narrowing, subarticular sclerosis, and spur formation are present.

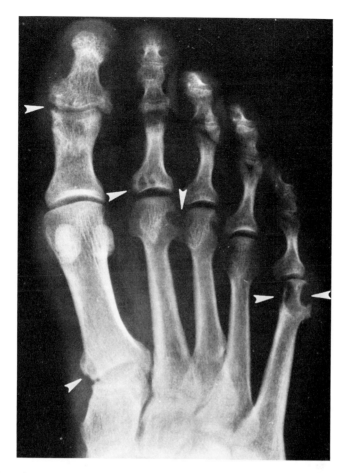

Fig. 10-50. Gout. Characteristic articular and para-articular lesions are present (arrowheads). Although foot is most common site of gout, similar changes may be seen in other joints.

riding, distraction). Fig. 10-52 shows several common types of fractures and their descriptive terminology. For a further discussion of terminology, refer to *The Language of Fractures* (Schultz, 1972).

Although an in-depth description of fractures is beyond the scope of this book, you should follow some of the principles listed here when evaluating patients with skeletal trauma. (1) Assume a fracture is present if there is pain, swelling, and discoloration over a bony surface in a child. It is best to treat patients for fracture and bring them back in 7 to 10 days for follow-up radiographs rather than to let them depart from your emergency department with an untreated fracture. (2) Comparison views should be made whenever you are uncertain about the presence or absence of a fracture (particularly in small children whose epiphyseal lines could be confused for a fracture). (3) Tomography is often useful in determining whether or not a fracture is present, particularly in the cervical spine, where a lucent line crossing the base of the dens and producing a Mach band could be misinterpreted as a fracture (Fig. 10-53).

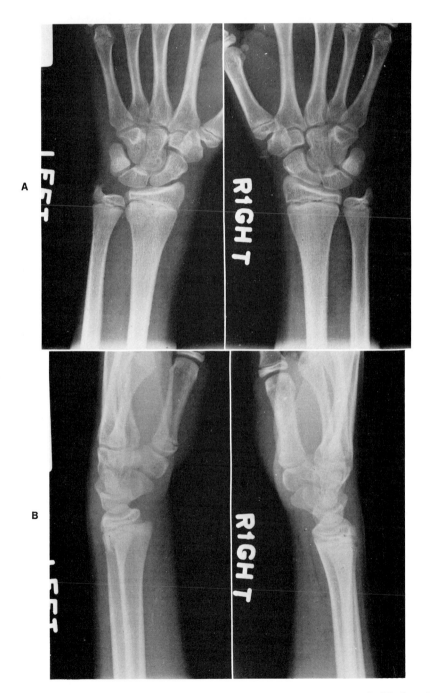

Fig. 10-51. This child fell and injured his left wrist. Epiphyseal fracture is present. **A,** PA view of both wrists. Note soft tissue swelling on left. There is narrowing of growth plate on left when compared to right. **B,** Lateral views demonstrate posterior displacement of distal radial epiphysis. In addition, there is positive pronator quadratus fat pad sign. Soft tissue swelling is present on left as well. Compare these findings with normal right side.

Postoperative changes

A large number of prostheses and appliances are used in orthopedics today. You should familiarize yourself with the more common of these and their appearance in bone (Fig. 10-54). Furthermore, the sites of previous screw holes, osteotomy, or prostheses may present a variety of bony defects that are easily recognizable if you are familiar with the types of procedures used in orthopedic surgery (Fig. 10-55).

SUMMARY

Most bone lesions fall into one of six basic pathologic categories: congenital, inflammatory, metabolic, neoplastic, traumatic, and vascular. By recognizing patterns of destruction and the use of a series of predictor variables, it is possible to reduce the complexities of skeletal radiology to a workable format. The application of the mnemonic ABCS was introduced to stress the analysis of bony Anatomy and alignment, *B*ony mineralization, *C*artilage (joint-space) changes, and *S*oft tissue changes. The principles of fracture diagnosis have been discussed.

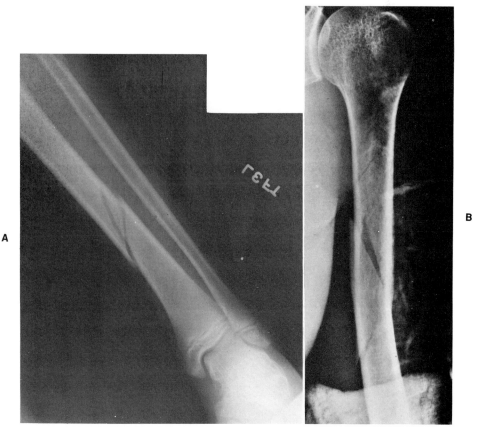

Continued.

Fig. 10-52. Types of fractures. **A,** Spiral fracture of tibia. **B,** Comminuted fracture of shaft of humerus. Patient is wearing hanging arm cast. **C,** Greenstick fracture of rib. Vertical line is artifact. **D,** Pathologic avulsion fracture of lesser trochanter (arrow). **E,** Pathologic oblique fracture in patient with osteogenic sarcoma.

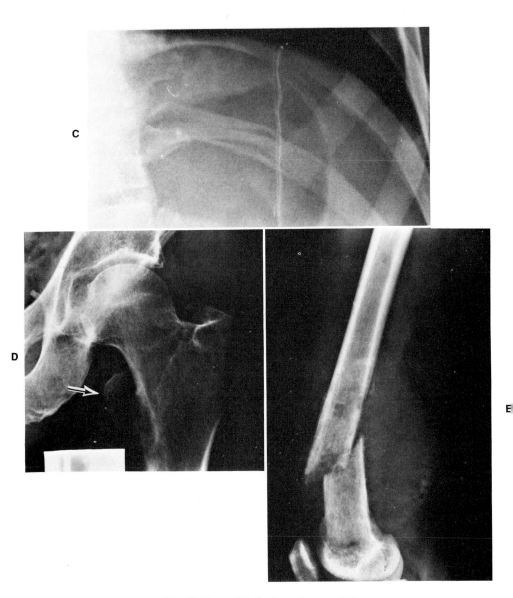

Fig. 10-52, cont'd. For legend see p. 347.

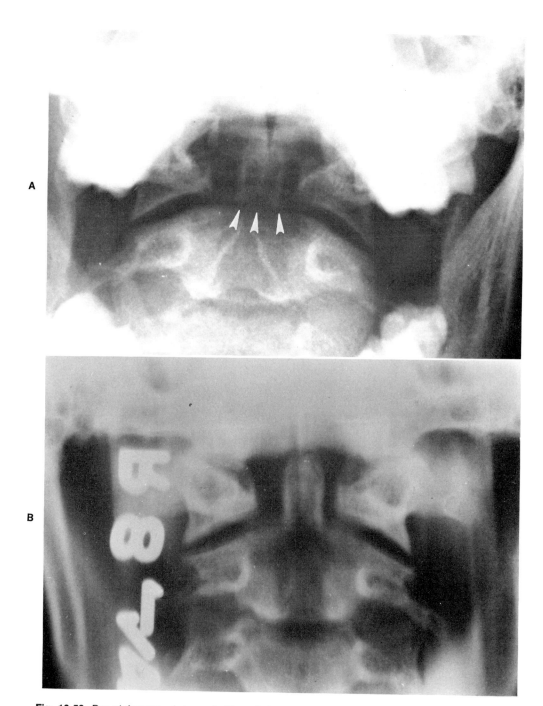

Fig. 10-53. Pseudofracture of dens. **A,** There is lucent line across base of dens (arrowheads). **B,** Tomogram of same area reveals no fracture of dens. This is common location for this pseudofracture. (From Daffner, R. H.: Am. J. Roentgenol. **128:**607, 1977. Reproduced with permission of the publisher.)

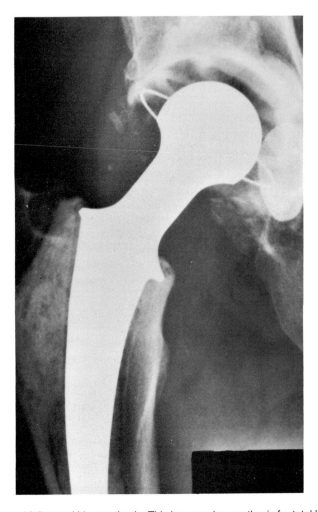

Fig. 10-54. Charnley-Müller total hip prosthesis. This is a popular prosthesis for total hip replacement.

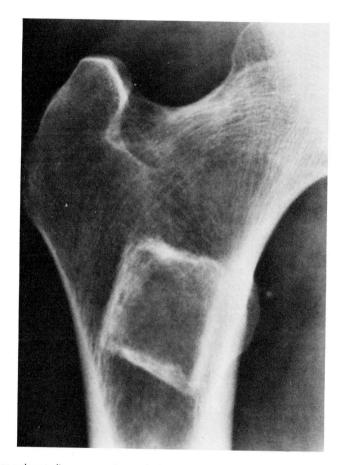

Fig. 10-55. Bone donor site seen postoperatively. Rectangular-shaped defect in intertrochanteric region of this femur is clue that this is an iatrogenic defect.

Selected case studies

The case studies of the skeletal system will have a slightly different format. The radiographs of 10 patients are given to you to examine. In each instance, study the radiographs, and describe the abnormalities present. You will be given the distribution of the disease in the history. Try next to determine the pathologic category to which the lesion belongs. If you can make a specific diagnosis, please do so. In some instances, you may only be able to determine whether the patient has a benign- or a malignant-appearing process.

Patient 1 is a 45-year-old man with a 2-month history of wrist pain (Case 10-1, *A*). No other bony abnormalities are detected on a bone scan (not shown). *What are the radiographic findings? What additional studies would you order?*

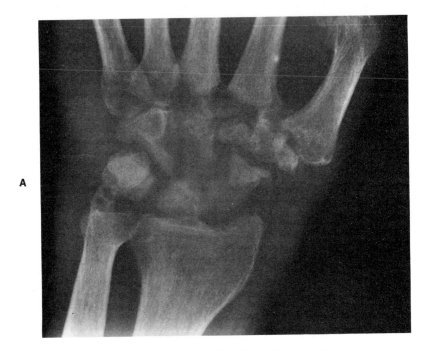

A

Case 10-1. Patient 1. **A,** PA radiograph of left wrist.

Patient 2 is a 1-month-old infant who was being evaluated for "failure to thrive." The skeletal survey (Case 10-2, *A* and *B*) was obtained because of an abnormal finding seen on a chest radiograph. *What are the radiographic findings?*

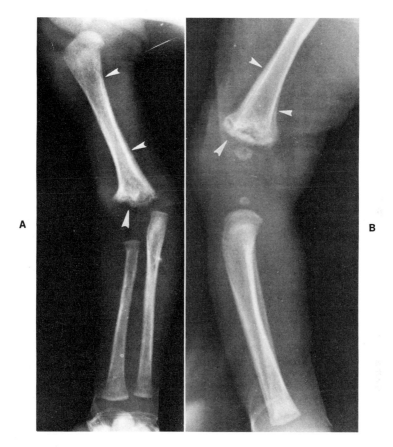

Case 10-2. Patient 2. Portions of skeletal survey in patient with failure to thrive. **A,** Radiograph of arm. **B,** Lateral radiograph of leg. What are arrowheads pointing to?

Patient 3 is a 21-year-old man who was examined because of recent onset of persistent pain in the foot (Case 10-3). The patient noted the onset of pain shortly after beginning a new job as a mailman. The pain is worse with walking and is relieved by rest. *What is the main radiographic finding? What is the differential diagnosis?*

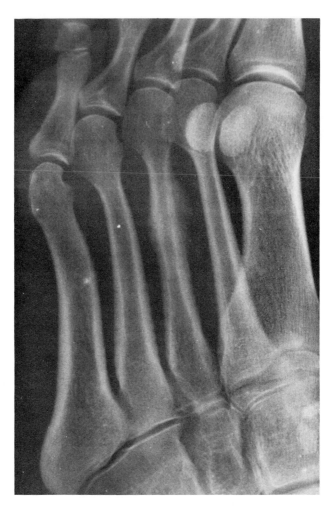

Case 10-3. Patient 3. Mailman with foot pain.

Patient 4 was seen in the emergency room because of pain in the wrist immediately following a fall on an outstretched hand (Case 10-4). *What is the main radiographic finding?*

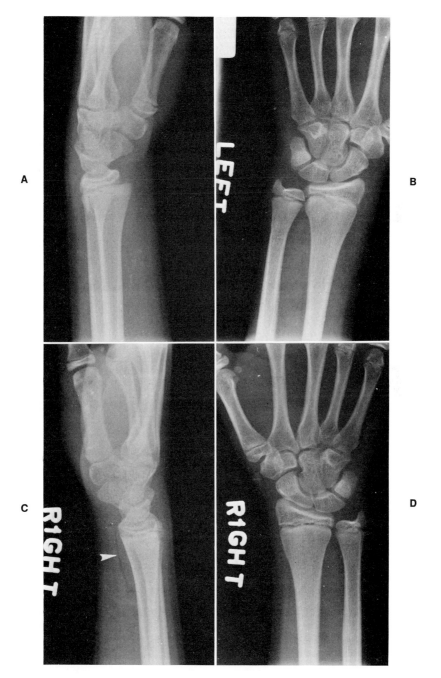

Case 10-4. A, Lateral and, **B,** PA views of left wrist of child after fall. **C,** Lateral and, **D,** PA views of opposite wrist in this same child. Arrowhead identifies pronator quadratus fat pad.

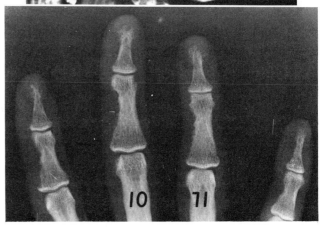

Case 10-5. A, Coned-down clavicular views from chest radiograph in patient 5. **B,** Lateral skull. **C,** Detail view of hands.

Patient 5 is a 35-year-old woman who is being evaluated for recurrent peptic ulcer disease and generalized malaise. An abnormality on her chest radiograph prompted the radiologist to suggest a skeletal survey (Case 10-5). *What are the radiographic findings? Can you correlate the clinical symptoms and the radiologic findings? What other studies would be useful in diagnosing this patient's disease?*

Patient 6 is a 54-year-old man with a long history of pain in multiple joints. Case 10-6, *A*, shows his foot; Case 10-6, *B*, shows his hand. *What are the main findings? What is your diagnosis?*

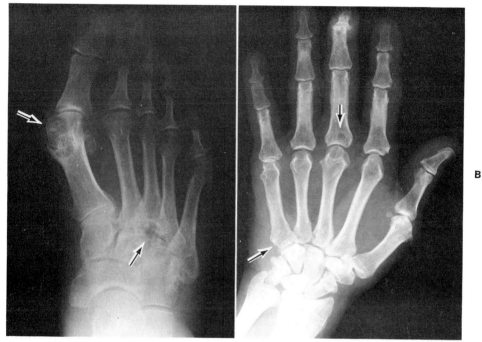

Case 10-6. Representative films of, **A,** foot and, **B,** hand in man with recurrent diffuse joint pain. Arrows point to main abnormalities.

Patient 7 is a 10-year-old child with pain in his arm following a fall. The remainder of the skeleton is normal (Case 10-7). *What is the main radiographic finding? Is there an underlying disease process?*

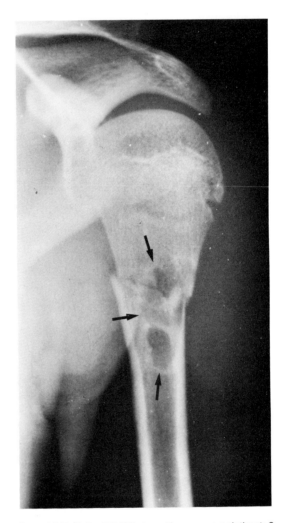

Case 10-7. Patient 7. What are the arrows pointing to?

Patient 8 is a 45-year-old man with a history of pain in his right arm for 2 months. Additional history is deliberately withheld in this case (Case 10-8, A). *What are the main radiographic findings? What additional imaging studies would you perform? What is your differential diagnosis?*

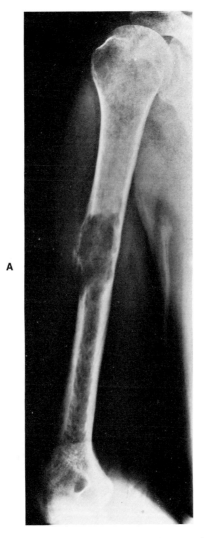

A

Case 10-8. Patient 8. **A,** AP radiograph of humerus in man with right arm pain.

Patient 9 has symptoms of a respiratory tract infection. A routine chest radiograph is obtained (Case 10-9). *What is the main radiographic finding?*

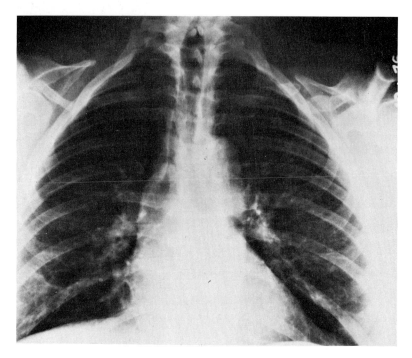

Case 10-9. Routine chest radiograph in patient with "cold."

Patient 10 is a 7-month-old infant who was seen in the emergency room because of a "cold." The pediatrician noted that the patient was reluctant to use his right arm. The film of the arm (Case 10-10, *A*) was ordered. On the basis of this film a skeletal survey (Case 10-10, *B* to *D*) was ordered. *What are the radiographic findings? What is your diagnosis?*

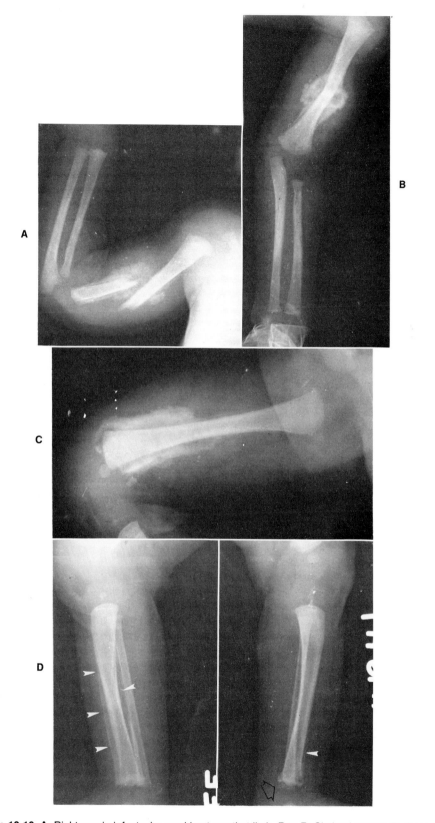

Case 10-10. A, Right arm in infant who would not use that limb. **B** to **D,** Skeletal survey. **B,** Opposite arm. **C,** Right femur. **D,** Legs. There are multiple fractures in various stages of healing. Note periosteal reaction in legs (arrowheads). These findings are hallmark of "battered child." More subtle finding is metaphyseal irregularity seen best in distal right ankle (open arrow). (**B** from Daffner, R. H., Gehweiler, J. A., and Carden, T. S., Jr.: Case studies in radiology, New York, 1975, Appleton-Century-Crofts. Reproduced with permission of the publisher.)

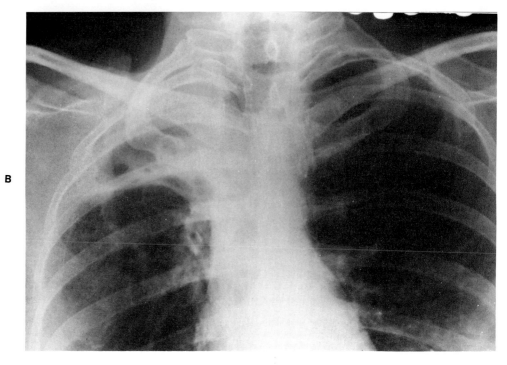

Case 10-1. Patient 1. **B,** Detail of chest radiograph. There is cavitary lesion in right upper lobe. Right hilum is retracted somewhat upward, suggesting volume loss. Combined findings of pulmonary cavitary lesion and bony lesion such as **A** make diagnosis of tuberculosis highly likely.

ROENTGEN DIAGNOSIS AND DISCUSSION

Patient 1. The wrist film (Case 10-1, *A*) demonstrates multiple destructive areas involving all the carpal bones, portions of the distal radius and ulna, and the bases of several metacarpals. The lesions are poorly defined. In addition, there is considerable bony debris and soft tissue swelling. When questioned closely, this patient admits to symptoms over a period of several months. A chest radiograph (Case 10-1, *B*) shows a cavitary lesion in the right upper lobe, suggesting cavitary tuberculosis. A skin test for tuberculosis was positive. Fungal skin testing was negative; the serum uric acid level was normal, as was his rheumatoid factor.

The radiographic appearance of this lesion should suggest an inflammatory process, since multiple joints are involved. Furthermore, the large amount of soft tissue swelling supports this diagnosis. Once you have decided that you are dealing with an inflammatory process, you must then decide whether you are dealing with one of the destructive arthritides or with a bacterial infection. The clinical history is important in helping you make this differentiation. None of the destructive arthritides (rheumatoid arthritis, gout, psoriasis, villonodular synovitis) produce a picture of widespread destruction in a short time period. Gout may be ruled out because the history of the complaint is not long enough in this patient. Destructive changes in gouty arthritis take 5 to 7 years to develop. Furthermore, the serum uric acid level of this patient was normal. Similarly, pigmented villonodular synovitis may be ruled out on the basis of history as well as radiographic appearance. The wrist is an uncommon location for this interesting disease, which primarily affects the large weight-bearing joints of young adults. The lesions are characteristically punched out and well defined. Unilateral joint involvement is unusual in rheumatoid and psoriatic arthritis, especially in the absence of clinical or laboratory findings of these diseases.

Bacterial arthritis can produce considerable bony destruction within a relatively short

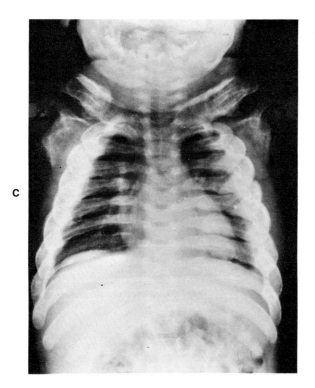

C

Case 10-2. C, Infantile cortical hyperostosis (Caffey disease). Generalized periosteal reaction. Thickening of bone is present in bony thorax, clavicles, and mandible. This is characteristic location for this unusual disease.

period of time. It is important to distinguish between pyogenic and tuberculous arthritis. In the majority of instances, pyogenic arthritis will be diagnosed and treated before significant bony destruction has occurred. The extensive proliferative reaction early in the disease causes considerable joint pain because of distention of the joint capsule, prompting the patient to seek early treatment. Tuberculous arthritis, on the other hand, has a slow course. Considerable infectious debris is produced by this disease, since hyaluronidase, which aids in removal of the debris, is not produced by the tubercle bacillus. An interesting finding, and one considered pathognomonic, is extensive bony destruction far out of proportion to the degree and severity of the patient's symptoms. In almost every case of osseous tuberculosis seen in the United States there is an accompanying focus in the lung.

Patient 2. The main radiographic findings in Case 10-2, *A* and *B*, are those of generalized periosteal reaction (small arrowheads). In addition, there is rarefaction in the metaphyseal areas (large arrowheads). Clinically the patient and his mother were known to have positive serology for syphilis. Furthermore, the patient had the stigmata of congenital lues: hepatosplenomegaly, bloody purulent nasal discharge (snuffles), and a maculopapular rash.

Congenital syphilis is one of the lesions that should come to mind when you are confronted with an infant with generalized periosteal reaction. Other conditions in this age group include the "battered child," infantile cortical hyperostosis (Caffey disease), and occasionally rubella. Of these conditions the most difficult one to radiographically differentiate from lues is Caffey disease. This condition, which was often confused with syphilis, is mainly manifest by periosteal reaction, particularly in the mandible and clavicles (Case 10-2, *C*). The serology is normal. The "battered child" (to be discussed later) generally has the characteristic radiographic picture of multiple healing fractures in various stages in a child who often has had multiple hospital visits. Rubella may be diagnosed serologically.

Table 9. Stress fractures: location and activities

Location	Activities
Metatarsals	Marching, running, prolonged standing, ballet dancing
Calcaneus	Prolonged standing, jumping, parachuting
Navicular bone of foot	Stomping on ground, marching
Distal fibula	Long-distance running
Tibia	Long-distance running, ballet
Proximal fibula	Parachuting or jumping
Patella	Hurdling
Femoral shaft	Marching, stomping on ground
Femoral neck	Ballet
Ribs	Coughing, carrying heavy pack, golfing
Coracoid process	Trap shooting
Humerus	Throwing a ball
Ulna	Pitchforking
Lumbar vertebra	Ballet, heavy lifting
Lower cervical/upper thoracic spinous process	Clay shoveling

Patient 3. The main radiographic finding in patient 3 is an area of increased density along the shaft of the third metatarsal (Case 10-3). The history is suggestive of a stress fracture, a common entity at this location. Stress fractures result from abnormal muscle action placed on a bone when the patient engages in an activity for which he is not physically prepared. The classic stress fracture occurs in the feet of new army recruits ("march fracture"). However, it is now recognized that stress fractures occur in many bones, including nonweight-bearing bones such as the fibula, and with a variety of physical activities.

Stress fractures are most often confused with malignant tumors such as osteogenic sarcoma. For this reason, it is important to learn the common locations of stress fractures and to include them in the differential diagnosis of any sclerotic bone lesion. Your best aid in differential diagnosis is time. Unless a patient is in a toxic condition, you can afford to wait several weeks to re-examine the abnormal bone for a change in appearance. In general, a bone tumor (benign or malignant) will not have changed within that short period of time. A stress fracture, on the other hand, will show progression to the healing stages.

Common locations for stress fractures are listed in Table 9. For an in-depth discussion of them, consult the article by Daffner (1978).

Patient 4. The salient feature in Case 10-4, *A* and *B*, is the positive pronator quadratus fat sign in the wrist. Under normal circumstances, this fat line (Case 10-4, *C*) appears as a thin lucent line on the volar surface of the wrist. Bleeding in and about the wrist or exudation of synovial fluid into the volar compartment of the wrist may result in obliteration or displacement of this line, as shown. The most common condition producing this finding is a fracture in and about the wrist joint. Many times the fat line sign may be the only evidence of trauma. Patients with this finding should be treated as if they have a fracture, even though one cannot be demonstrated on the initial examination, and then should be reexamined in 7 to 10 days. Careful examination of the frontal views in this patient demonstrate a fracture that is easily visible when compared with the opposite side.

Patient 5. The main radiographic finding in patient 5 is diffuse osteoporosis. In addition, there are erosions of the distal clavicles, a spotty form of osteoporosis in the skull referred to as "salt and pepper" pattern, and subperiosteal bone erosions along the radial aspect of the middle phalanges (Case 10-5, *A* to *C*). These findings are characteristic of hyperparathyroidism. Laboratory examination of this patient demonstrated an elevated serum calcium level and a diminished serum phosphorus level. Because there was no evidence of renal

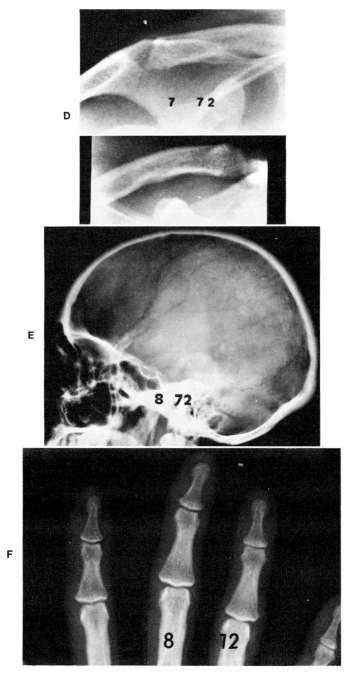

Case 10-5. Patient 5 after removal of parathyroid adenoma. **D,** Distal clavicles have remineralized. **E,** Skull is now normal. **F,** There has been remineralization of subperiosteal erosions in phalanges. Compare these findings with preoperative films, **A** to **C.**

disease, the patient was thought to have a primary parathyroid adenoma. An angiographic study was performed, during which time samples of venous blood from the neck and mediastinum were removed and analyzed for parathormone content. Elevated levels were found on the right side. At surgery a parathyroid adenoma was removed. This resulted in complete resolution of the patient's symptoms. A follow-up examination several months after surgery revealed the skeleton to be normal (Case 10-5, *D* to *F*). Note the difference between the pre- and posttreatment studies.

Patient 6. Patient 6 has classic gouty arthritis (Case 10-6). The findings are of well-defined punched-out lesions in the articular and para-articular spaces. Note that the lesions are not confined to the foot alone but are also seen in the hand and wrist. There is no osteoporosis, which helps to differentiate this condition from rheumatoid arthritis. Once again, the multiplicity of the lesions and the fact that the lesions cross the joint space tell us that we are dealing with an inflammatory disease.

Patient 7. The main radiographic finding in (Case 10-7) is a fracture in the proximal shaft of the humerus. Close examination of this fracture shows that it extends through a well-defined lucent lytic area that is oriented with the shaft and does not appear to have broken out into the periphery (arrows). There is a sharp zone of transition. The most likely diagnosis is a pathologic

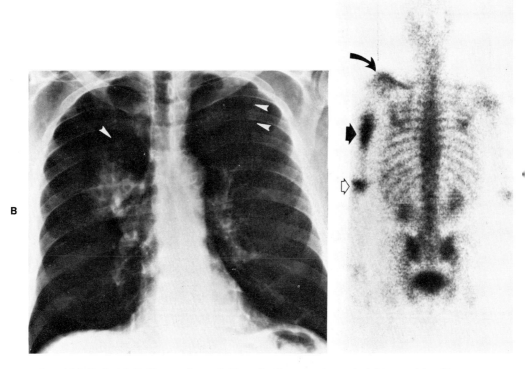

B

Case 10-8. Patient 8. **B,** Chest radiograph. There is a large carcinoma in right upper lobe. Closer examination of this radiograph revealed metastatic nodules in right upper and left upper lobes (arrowheads). **C,** Bone scan. Metastatic lesion in right humerus is apparent (short solid arrow). In addition, there is area of increased tracer concentration in right shoulder (curved arrow). Other areas of tracer concentration are normal. Site of injection was in right antecubital fossa (open arrow).

fracture in a benign bone cyst. This lesion was curetted; pathologic examination confirmed the diagnosis of a bone cyst. Recovery was uneventful.

It is not unusual for patients with benign bone cysts to have a pathologic fracture. These lesions are often discovered by accident when the patient is studied for another reason. Indeed, this patient had been studied several months prior to the fracture because of aspiration of a peanut. The lesion was noted at that time, but the family refused treatment then.

Patient 8. If you were given the clinical history of weight loss and cough in this patient, you would undoubtedly have made a diagnosis of metastatic lung carcinoma to the proximal humerus. The lesion depicted in Case 10-8, *A* has all the findings of an aggressive (malignant) lesion; it is poorly defined, is moth-eaten to permeative, and has sustained a pathologic fracture. Furthermore, there is a broad zone of transition. A chest radiograph (Case 10-8, *B*) reveals a large carcinoma in the right upper lobe. A radioisotope bone scan was performed (Case 10-8, *C*), revealing an additional metastatic lesion in the right shoulder. These lesions were confirmed on plain film examination. This case demonstrates the use of the isotope bone scan in the detection of metastatic lesions. The scan directs our attention to abnormal areas. This method is preferable to ordering blind skeletal surveys, particularly in a patient without skeletal symptoms.

Patient 9. The main radiographic findings in patient 9 are those of hypoplastic clavicles (Case 10-9). This patient worked as a "rubber man" for the circus. He and several members of his family suffered from cleidocranial dysostosis, a skeletal dysplasia that is often familial. The most striking abnormality seen in this disease is hypoplasia or absence of the clavicles.

Patient 10. Case 10-10 shows a fracture of the midshaft of the humerus in this patient. A skeletal survey revealed evidence of additional skeletal trauma manifest as periosteal reaction of the long bones and evidence of corner fractures in the metaphyses of the legs. A skull radiograph revealed a linear fracture in the parietal bone. The child is a victim of the "battered child" syndrome.

Child abuse has been known for centuries. However, it has only been in modern times and, in particular, within the past quarter century that a medical syndrome has been recognized and described. The medical, legal, and sociologic aspects of this interesting and tragic syndrome are quite extensive. It is now recognized that the skeletal manifestations of child abuse are only a small percentage of the radiographic findings that may be seen. Soft tissue findings include evidence of ruptured liver or spleen, duodenal hematoma, pancreatic injury, and urinary trauma. Skeletal manifestations previously mentioned include evidence of multiple skeletal trauma, usually over varying time periods. For further elucidation of this condition, the reader is referred to the articles by Caffey (1972) and Silverman (1972).

References

Aegerter, E., and Kirkpatrick, J. A.: Orthopedic diseases. Physiology. Pathology. Radiology, ed. 4, Philadelphia, 1975, W. B. Saunders Co.

American College of Radiology syllabus: categorical course on the skeletal system, Baltimore, 1976, American College of Radiology.

Caffey, J.: The parent-infant traumatic stress syndrome (Caffey-Kempe syndrome) (battered babe syndrome), Am. J. Roentgenol. **114**:217, 1972.

Corcoran, R. J., Thrall, J. H., Kyle, R. W., Kaminski, R. J., and Johnson, M. C.: Solitary abnormalities in bone scans of patients with extra-osseous malignancies, Radiology **121**:663, 1976.

Daffner, R. H.: Pseudofracture of the dens: Mach bands, Am. J. Roentgenol. **128**:607, 1977.

Daffner, R. H.: Stress fractures: current concepts, Skel. Radiol. **2**:221, 1978.

Daffner, R. H., Gehweiler, J. A., and Carden, T. S., Jr.: Case studies in radiology, New York, 1975, Appleton-Century-Crofts.

Edeiken, J., and Hodes, P. J.: Roentgen diagnosis of diseases of bone, ed. 2, Baltimore, 1973, The Williams & Wilkins Co.

Forrester, D. M., and Nesson, J. W.: The radiology of joint disease, Philadelphia, 1973, W. B. Saunders Co.

Kaye, J. J., and Freiberger, R. H.: Arthrography of the knee, Clin. Orthop. **107**:73, 1975.

Lodwick, G. S.: Solitary malignant tumors of bone, the application of predictor variables in diagnosis, Semin. Roentgenol. **1**:293, 1966.

Meszaros, W. T.: The many facets of multiple myeloma, Semin. Roentgenol. **9:**219, 1974.

Murphy, W. A., and Siegel, M. J.: Elbow fat pads with new signs and extended differential diagnosis, Radiology **124:**659, 1977.

Nelson, S.: Some important diagnostic and technical fundamentals in the radiology of trauma, with emphasis on skeletal trauma, Radiol. Clin. North Am. **4:**241, 1966.

Norman, A.: The use of tomography in the diagnosis of skeletal disorders, Clin. Orthop. **107:**139, 1975.

Osborne, R. L.: The differential radiologic diagnosis of bone tumors, CA **24:**194, 1974.

Osmond, J. D. III, Pendergrass, H. P., and Potsaid, M. S.: Accuracy of 99m Tc-diphosphonate bone scans and roentgenograms in the detection of prostate, breast and lung carcinoma metastases, Am. J. Roentgenol. **125:**972, 1975.

Schultz, R. J.: The language of fractures, Baltimore, 1972, The Williams & Wilkins Co.

Silverman, F. N.: Unrecognized trauma in infants, the battered child syndrome and the syndrome of Ambroise Tardieu, Radiology **104:**377, 1972.

Terry, D. W., and Ramin, J. E.: The navicular fat stripe. A useful roentgen feature for evaluating wrist trauma, Am. J. Roentgenol. **124:**24, 1975.

Wilkinson, R. H.: Pediatric skeletal trauma. In American College of Radiology syllabus: categorical course on trauma, Chicago 1977, American College of Radiology.

11 Neuroradiology

Neuroradiology is the subspecialty area concerned with radiologic investigation of the brain and spinal cord. Although abnormalities in other areas of the body may be grossly evident, the changes present on cerebral angiograms or pneumoencephalograms are often subtle. The student or house officer who is confronted with a neuroradiologic study is often frustrated and feels insecure. Remember, however, that neuroradiology is founded on the same principles of anatomy, physiology, and pathology as any other diagnostic area.

Previous chapters in this book have emphasized the spectrum of diagnostic examinations you would encounter in your daily practice. To do the same for neuroradiology and to do the subject justice is beyond the scope of this book, however. Consequently, the discussion will stress the one area with which you will have the most contact: the plain skull film examination.

TECHNICAL CONSIDERATIONS

There are a number of imaging examinations performed for evaluation of the nervous system and adjacent structures. The frequency with which these studies are used is variable in view of the impact that cranial computed tomography (CT) has made on the field of neuroradiology.

Conventional skull radiography concerns the bony vault as well as examinations of the facial bones, sinuses, mastoids, middle ears, and orbits. Tomography is used in a variety of clinical situations to study the sella turcica, the facial bones for fractures, and the middle and inner ear.

CT of the skull provides safe, rapid, accurate, and reliable diagnostic information for a wide variety of intracranial conditions: vascular lesions such as subdural and epidural hematomas, brain tumors, and infarcts. Cranial CT has revolutionized neuroradiology. One of the main effects of cranial CT has been a considerable reduction in the number of invasive studies performed on the brain, that is, cerebral arteriography and pneumoencephalography.

Arteriography may be performed by direct puncture of the carotid arteries or by catheterization of the vessels of the aortic arch. Catheter study is preferable and less traumatic to the patient because all four cerebral vessels may be studied utilizing only one arterial puncture.

Pneumoencephalography involves injecting air into the subarachnoid space, ventricles, and basal cisterns through a puncture in the lumbar region or through a burr hole, with placement of a needle directly into the ventricle. This study is done primarily to study the anatomy of the ventricular spaces and cisterns.

Myelography with positive contrast medium is performed by injecting contrast material through a lumbar puncture into the subarachnoid space. The purpose of the study is to outline lesions causing compression on the spinal cord and thecal sac. The most common abnormality diagnosed by this method is a herniated intervertebral lumbar disc. A variant of myelography is posterior fossa cisternography, in which the patient is placed in a head-down position and contrast medium is allowed to flow through the foramen magnum into the basal cisterns of the brain. The purpose of this study is to outline suspected mass lesions, such as an acoustic neuroma, in the

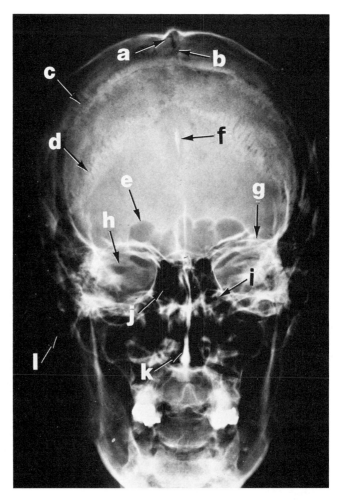

Fig. 11-1. Normal skull PA view. *a,* Groove for superior sagittal sinus; *b,* sagittal suture; *c,* coronal suture; *d,* lambdoidal suture; *e,* frontal sinus; *f,* calcified falx; *g,* roof of orbit; *h,* internal auditory canal; *i,* foramen rotundum; *j,* superimposed shadows of ethmoid and sphenoid sinuses; *k,* nasal septum; *l,* mastoid bone.

cerebropontine angle. Myelography may also be performed using air as the contrast medium.

Radioisotope studies of the head include the brain scan and cisternogram. The radioisotope brain scan is performed by intravenous injection of sodium pertechnitate (technetium-99m). A rapid-sequence examination is performed following the injection to detect vascular lesions and flow abnormalities. After a delay of 2 hours, a static scan is made of the head to search for other pathologic entities. This is considered a safe, inexpensive, and "noninvasive" method of studying the brain. The impact of cranial CT on the isotope brain scan is yet to be determined.

The isotope cisternogram is a study used to evaluate the dynamics of cerebrospinal fluid flow. In addition, the study is often done to diagnose and localize the site of a suspected dural tear that has resulted in cerebrospinal fluid rhinorrhea. In the first type of examination, the radioiodinated (^{131}I) serum albumin is injected into the thecal sac in the lumbar region and is followed by static scanning of the basal cistern area in the brain at intervals. In this way, flow dynamics may be assessed. Under normal circumstances, all the isotope is contained within the subarachnoid space over the brain after 48 hours, without concentration within the ventricular system. If the patient is being evaluated for cerebrospinal fluid (CSF) rhinorrhea, pledgets of cotton are placed within the nose. They are later measured for the presence of isotope. Radioactivity within these pledgets is indicative of a CSF leak into the nasal cavity.

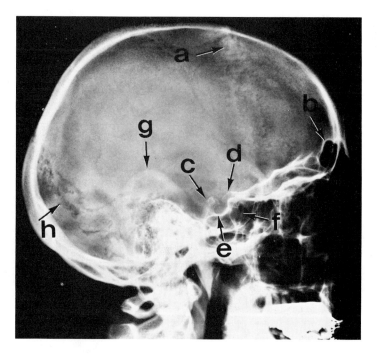

Fig. 11-2. Normal skull, lateral view. *a,* Coronal suture; *b,* frontal sinus; *c,* dorsum sellae; *d,* anterior clinoid process; *e,* floor of sella turcica; *f,* sphenoid sinus; *g,* shadow of earlobe; *h,* lambdoidal suture.

Skull examination

Several studies have shown that the skull examination is highly overused. The yield of positive findings is extremely low compared to the number of examinations made. You may validly request a skull examination, however, if you suspect a fracture, a destructive lesion, or anomalies of the skull. I concur with several authorities on cranial CT who believe that any patient with significant positive neurologic findings should be referred for a cranial CT examination as a *primary* study rather than having skull films. *Before ordering any skull film, consider whether or not the patient will need a CT examination, which will give you more definitive information.*

ANATOMIC CONSIDERATIONS

The basic views of the skull are the PA, lateral, AP half-axial (Towne), and base. Each view is designed to demonstrate particular areas of the skull: the PA view, either straight or with slight angulation of the x-ray tube, is designed to demonstrate the frontal bones, frontal and ethmoid sinuses, nasal cavity, superior orbital rims, and

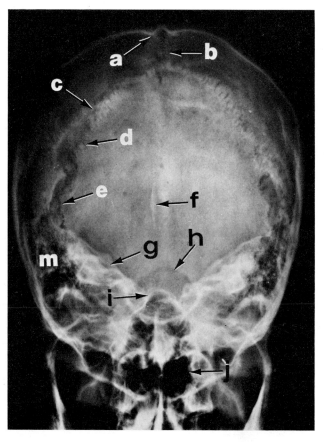

Fig. 11-3. Normal skull, Towne view. There is slight rotation on this film. *a,* Groove for superior sagittal sinus; *b,* sagittal suture; *c,* coronal suture; *d,* lambdoidal suture; *e,* occipitomastoid suture; *f,* calcified falx; *g,* internal auditory canal; *h,* foramen magnum; *i,* dorsum sellae; *j,* nasal cavity; *m,* mastoid air cells.

mandible (Fig. 11-1); the lateral view demonstrates the frontal, parietal, temporal, and occipital bones, the mastoid region, the sella turcica, the roofs of the orbits, and the lateral aspects of the facial bones (Fig. 11-2); the modified half-axial projection (Towne, occipital view) (Fig. 11-3) demonstrates the occipital bone, the mastoid and middle ear regions, the foramen magnum, and the zygomatic arches; the base view (Fig. 11-4) shows the basal structures of the skull, including the major foraminae.

Additional studies with which you should become familiar include stereoscopic examination of various views of the skull. This is particularly useful for localizing intracranial calcifications and for exact localization of bony defects. The occipito-mental (Waters) projection (Fig. 11-5) is used primarily to study the facial bones and sinuses. Other plain film studies of the skull include internal auditory canal views, views for the optic struts, mastoid series, and studies of the temporoman-dibular joint.

In reviewing a skull radiograph the near-perfect symmetry is quite helpful. It is

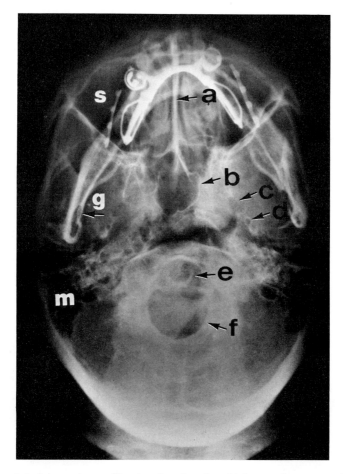

Fig. 11-4. Normal skull, base view. *a,* Nasal septum; *b,* sphenoid sinus; *c,* foramen ovale; *d,* foramen spinosum; *e,* dens of C2; *f,* foramen magnum; *g,* mandible; *m,* mastoid air cells; *s,* maxillary sinus. Note metallic dental prostheses.

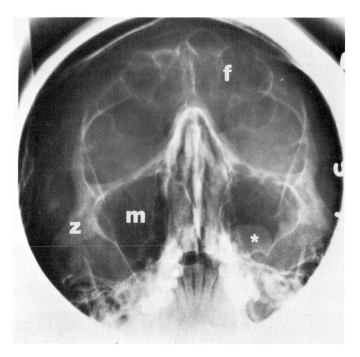

Fig. 11-5. Normal Waters view. Polyp (asterisk) is present within left maxillary sinus. *f,* Frontal sinus; *m,* maxillary sinus; *z,* zygomatic arch.

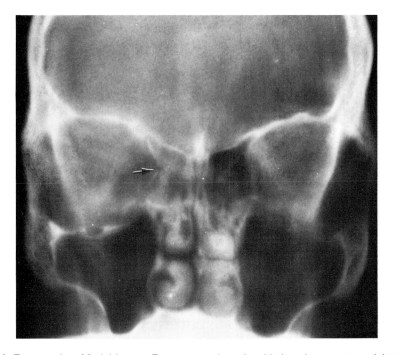

Fig. 11-6. Tomography of facial bones. Fracture entering ethmoid sinus is present on right (arrow).

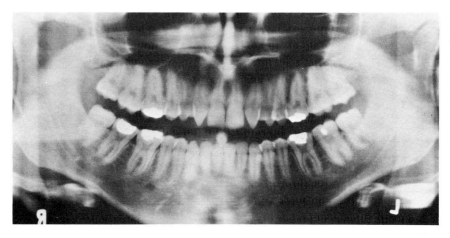

Fig. 11-7. Dental panoramic tomography (Panography).

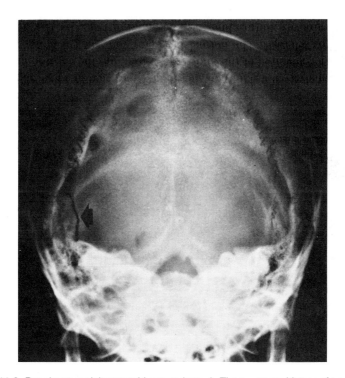

Fig. 11-8. Prominent occipitomastoid suture (arrow). There was no history of trauma.

therefore important for you to match findings on both sides of the skull before labeling a lucency or a dense shadow as an abnormality.

Special studies of the skull include tomography of the sella, facial bones (Fig. 11-6), and middle ear. Dentists and oral surgeons use a panoramic type of tomogram to study the mandible and facial bones (Fig. 11-7).

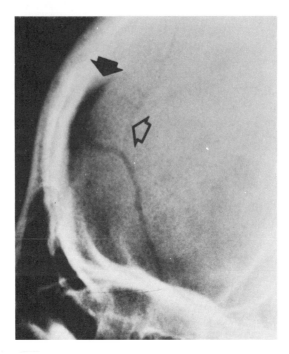

Fig. 11-9. Prominent vascular groove. Dark vascular groove ends in venous lake (solid arrow). Open arrow points to branch of vessel.

The analysis of a skull film should be conducted in a logical, orderly fashion, the same as for any area of the body. First, examine the calvaria for abnormal areas of lucency or sclerosis. The normal lucencies you will encounter are the sutures and vascular grooves. Suture lines, as illustrated in Fig. 11-1 to 11-3 have characteristic locations and fine interdigitations. They should not be difficult to recognize. Occasionally, however, the occipitomastoid suture (Fig. 11-8) may appear unusually prominent on one side of the skull and could be misinterpreted as a fracture. Vascular markings appear as gray shadows, often with sclerotic margins on either side. They gradually branch and taper toward their periphery. Occasionally a prominent vascular groove may be misinterpreted as a fracture (Fig. 11-9). However, these structures are often paired; fractures usually are not. Vascular markings usually occur in predictable locations such as those of the meningeal vessels. You must also be certain that a vascular marking is not enlarged, as may occur in meningioma (Fig. 11-10). Other lucencies normally present within the skull are the arachnoid granulations that occur in the parasagittal regions, small venous channels, and diploic lakes, which generally have vessels coursing to and from them. You must also search for any breaks in continuity of the bone, which would indicate a fracture (Fig. 11-11).

Next, examine the sella turcica. The size and configuration of the sella is subject to considerable variation. In general the upper limit of normal for a sella turcica is considered to be the size of a dime (18 mm); if you can fit a dime within the bony margins of the sella, it is enlarged (Fig. 11-12). The degree of mineralization of the sella will depend on the patient's age and physiologic state. The sella is frequently

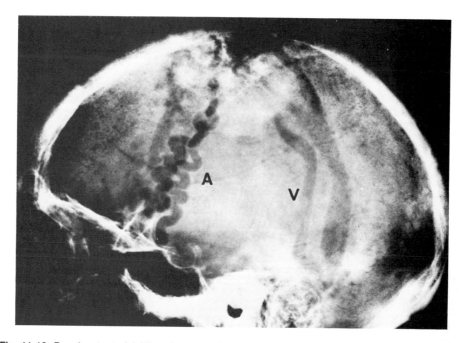

Fig. 11-10. Prominent arterial *(A)* and venous *(V)* markings in patient with parasagittal meningioma.

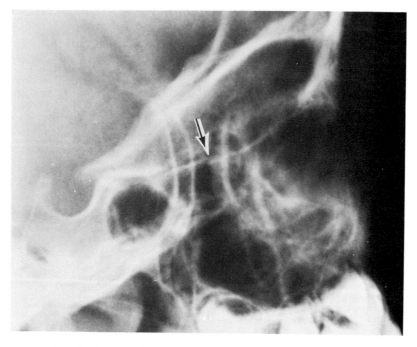

Fig. 11-11. Basal skull fracture. Note discontinuity of bone (arrow).

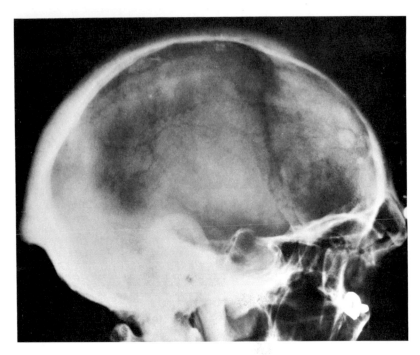

Fig. 11-12. Enlargement of sella turcica in patient with acromegaly. Compare sella in this patient with that of patient in Fig. 11-2.

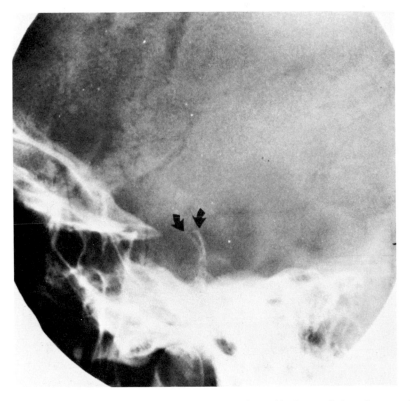

Fig. 11-13. Posterior displacement of dorsum sellae in patient with chromophobe adenoma. Arrows show double contour of dorsum.

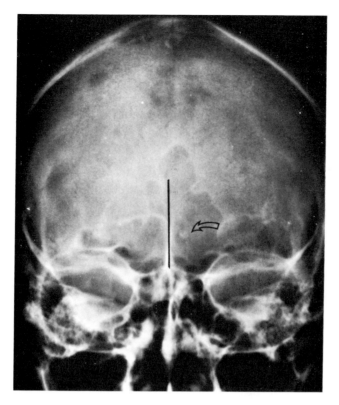

Fig. 11-14. Shifted pineal gland in patient with malignant glioma. Vertical line represents center. Arrow points to shifted pineal gland.

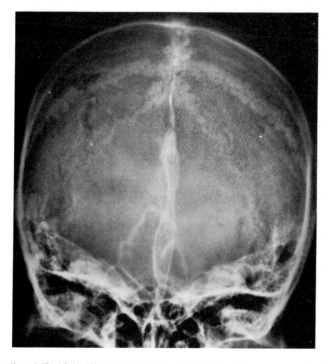

Fig. 11-15. Heavily calcified falx. Wavy contour and heavy calcification are normal variants. Compare with Figs. 11-1 and 11-3.

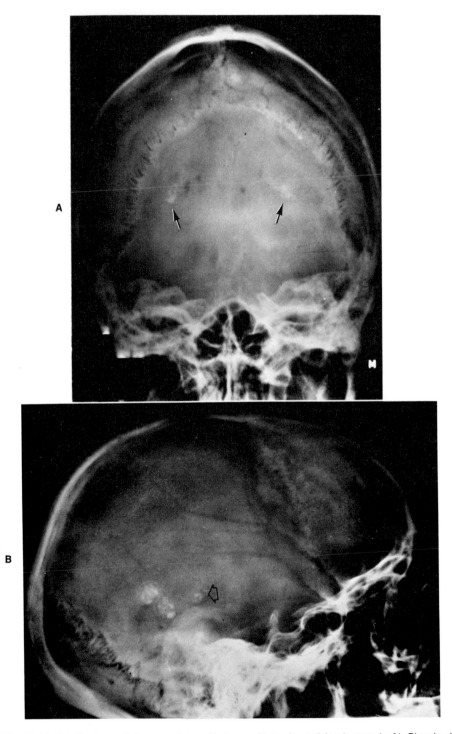

Fig. 11-16. Calcifications of glomera of choroid plexus of lateral ventricles (arrows in **A**). Pineal calcification is also seen on lateral view, **B** (open arrow).

osteoporotic in elderly individuals and alcoholics. In addition to enlargement of the sella, you must search for erosive lesions of either the floor or the dorsum (Fig. 11-13).

Next, look for intracranial calcifications. The most common intracranial calcification is the pineal gland. The incidence of calcification increases with age. In general, children and adolescents do not have calcified pineal glands. Approximately 20% of the population in the third decade and 70% in the eighth decade have a calcified pineal gland. The calcified pineal gland, which should be midline, may provide a valuable clue regarding intracranial mass lesions. In some instances a visible shift of the pineal gland may be found (Fig. 11-14). The calcified pineal gland is best located on the lateral view. If you cannot find it in this view, you certainly will not find it on the frontal view. The cerebral falx is often calcified and should be in the midline. You will not see this calcification on the lateral views. In the frontal view a calcified falx appears as a linear calcific streak in the midline extending nearly to the vault (Fig. 11-15). Calcifications of the glomera of the choroid plexuses of the lateral ventricles often appear somewhat punctate or flocculant and are generally bilateral and symmetric (Fig. 11-16). Occasionally there will be a slight variation in the size of the calcification. On the frontal film the calcifications are superimposed on the orbits. Carotid artery calcification is frequently seen adjacent to the sella in older individuals. This is a frequent site, however, for the location of carotid artery aneurysms, which also occur in this age group. Dural plaques appear as platelike calcifications over the surface of the brain. They are frequently located anteriorly. They should not be confused with hyperostosis interna (Fig. 11-17), which is a normal variant of bony thickening, particularly in the frontal region. Generally, all other intracranial cal-

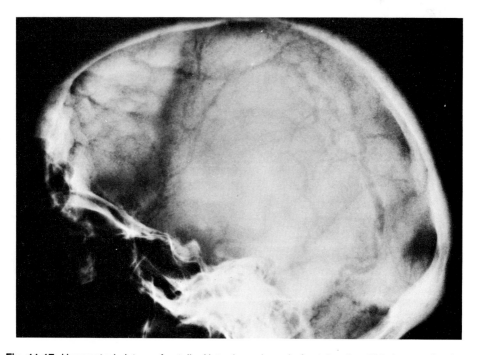

Fig. 11-17. Hyperostosis interna frontalis. Note dense bone in frontal region. This is normal variant.

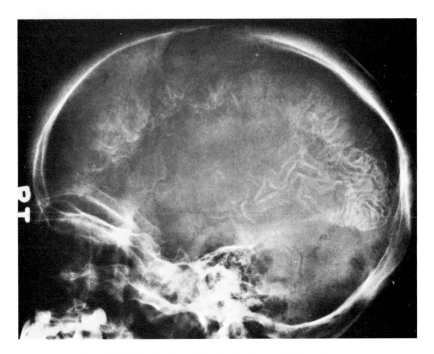

Fig. 11-18. Cerebral calcification in Sturge-Weber disease.

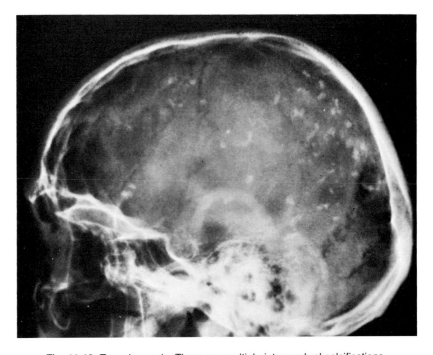

Fig. 11-19. Toxoplasmosis. There are multiple intracerebral calcifications.

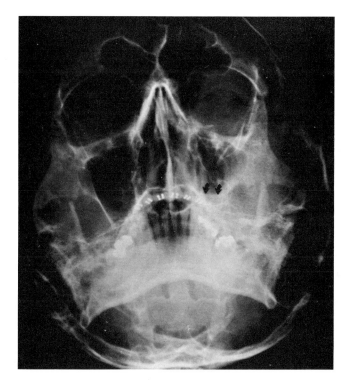

Fig. 11-20. Air-fluid level of left maxillary sinus (arrows) in patient with facial fractures.

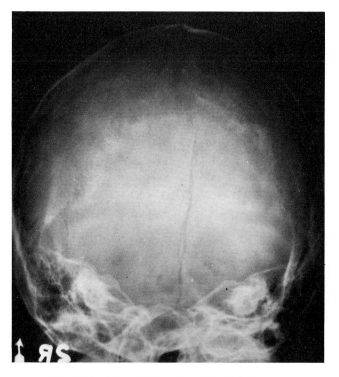

Fig. 11-21. Linear skull fracture of occipital bone.

cifications are considered abnormal. Some are nonspecific, such as those found in tumors. Others considered "diagnostic" include calcifications in Sturge-Weber disease (Fig. 11-18), tuberous sclerosis, toxoplasmosis (Fig. 11-19), and cytomegalic inclusion disease.

The base view should be examined for a widening of any of the foramina. Frequently, enlargement of the foramen spinosum may be seen with a meningioma. Tumors of the nasopharynx may extend posteriorly and erode the basilar foramina.

The sinuses should be studied for their degree of development, degree of aeration, and presence of air-fluid levels, which are suggestive of acute sinusitis (maxillary sinus) or a basilar skull fracture, when seen in the sphenoid sinus. An air-fluid level in the maxillary sinuses may also result from a fracture entering that sinus (Fig. 11-20).

PATHOLOGIC CONSIDERATIONS

The three most common pathologic states you will encounter in the nervous system radiologically are trauma, neoplasm, and vascular disease.

Trauma

Fractures of the skull and their sequelae are the best example of the statement I have made before: "A fracture is a *soft tissue* injury in which a bone is broken." No area has generated more controversy from a medical and legal standpoint than the evaluation of patients with head injuries. In recent years, attention has been directed by several authors to the utility and futility of skull films in every patient who has sustained a head injury. I side with the group saying "no" to routine skull films. The skull examination, as with any other diagnostic examination, should be performed only when indicated. Indications include signs and symptoms of neurologic abnormality: loss of consciousness and abnormal neurologic findings on examination. Since the treatment of skull fractures, with two notable exceptions, is directed toward treating the neurologic abnormality, the presence or absence of a fracture itself makes little difference in the management of the patient. You will encounter many patients in whom a skull fracture is present without neurologic findings or sequelae as well as cases of head injury without fracture where severe neurologic damage has occurred.

Two situations in which the skull fracture itself is significant are the depressed fracture and the fracture associated with penetration of a bullet or other foreign body. However, in both these instances there are usually associated neurologic abnormalities that will dictate corrective therapy. Figs. 11-21 through 11-25 illustrate a variety of skull fractures. Important findings to recognize are the lucency of skull fractures, their random appearance, the absence of sclerotic borders, and the lack of tendency to taper at their periphery.

A fracture is more likely to produce significant soft tissue (vascular, meningeal, or brain) damage in certain locations. A fracture that crosses a meningeal arterial groove such as that of the middle meningeal artery (Fig. 11-24) is likely to transect this vessel, resulting in an epidural hematoma. A fracture that crosses one of the dural venous sinuses may produce an acute rupture of that sinus and intracranial bleeding. A fracture through the frontal bone that traverses a sinus is likely to tear the dura, resulting in CSF leak into the sinuses and CSF rhinorrhea. A basilar skull fracture

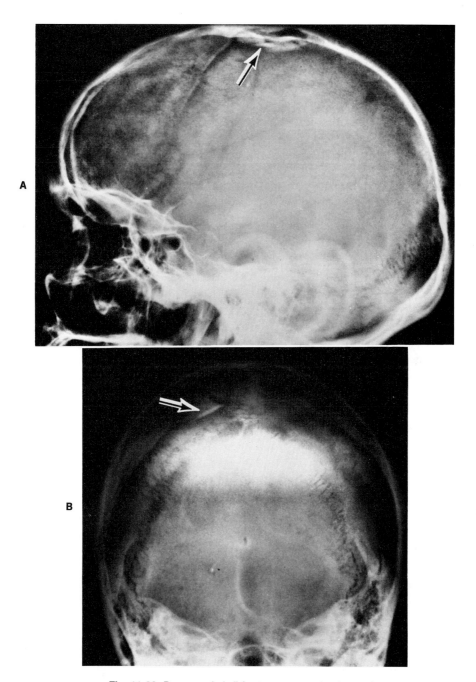

Fig. 11-22. Depressed skull fracture near vertex (arrows).

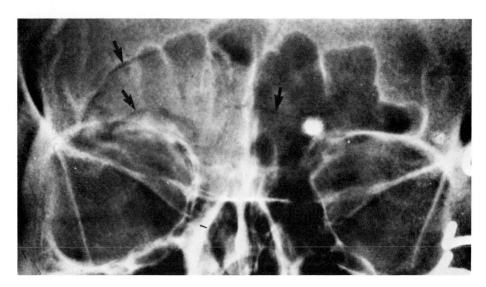

Fig. 11-23. Fractures through frontal sinus (arrows).

(often not recognized on the radiographs per se but seen as an air-fluid level in the sphenoid sinus) (Fig. 11-25) is generally associated with severe neurologic deficit and usually results in severe residual neurologic deficit or death.

Pseudofractures, usually the result of a group of normal markings, may mimic fractures in the patient who is evaluated for head trauma. Common pseudofractures include vascular channels, accessory sutures, persistent sutures, scalp lacerations, dressings, tape, and foreign material on the scalp. In addition, healing fractures or old fractures may occasionally be misinterpreted as acute fractures.

Vascular markings are the group most often mistaken for a true fracture. Venous channels in the diploic space, which are irregular and frequently terminate in the larger venous lakes, are common pseudofractures (Fig. 11-9). These have smooth margins that are often sclerotic and are less lucent than fractures. Arterial grooves may be particularly difficult to differentiate from fractures. Often these are paired and in a predictable location—coursing obliquely behind and superior to the sella turcica toward the midparietal region (Fig. 11-26). These are posterior branches of the middle meningeal artery and superior and posterior branches of the superficial temporal artery. They, too, taper near their ends and are less lucent than fractures. Learning their common location is important in establishing the proper diagnosis.

Accessory, or wormian, bones occur often in the occipital region and may be misinterpreted as a comminuted fracture. Once again, recognition of their common locations just below the lambda in the occipital bone or along the occipitomastoid suture helps you avoid a dangerous pitfall.

Other sutures may be misinterpreted as fractures. These are the mendosal and occipital sutures in the occipital bone and the metopic suture in the frontal bone. The mendosal suture, a fetal suture, separates the interparietal and suboccipital portions of the occipital bone. The occipital suture divides the occiput in the midsagittal

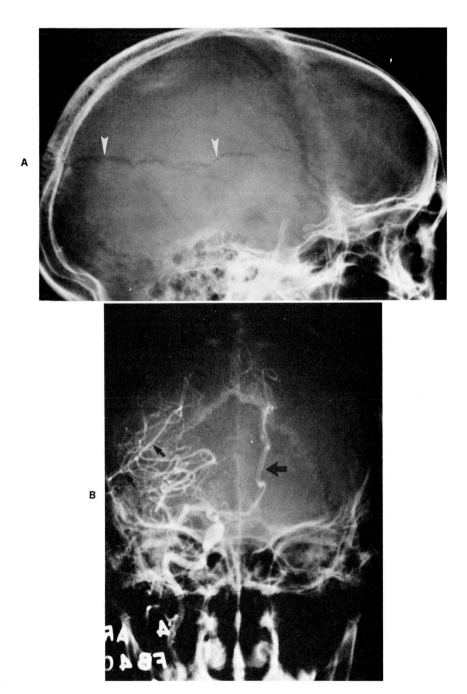

Fig. 11-24. A, Plain skull film shows fracture of parietal bone (arrowheads). **B,** Fracture resulted in epidural hematoma. Note shift of anterior cerebral artery (large arrow) and separation of surface vessels from inner table (small arrows) of skull.

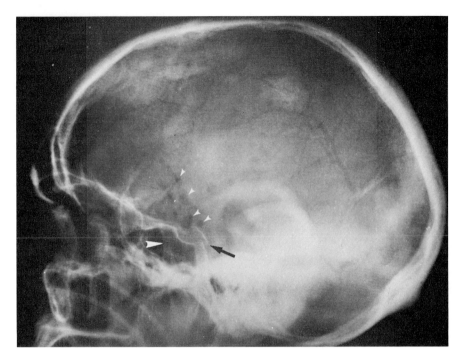

Fig. 11-25. Air-fluid level in sphenoid sinus (large arrowhead) in patient with basal skull fracture. There is fracture of dorsum sellae (arrow) and traumatic pneumocephalus (small arrowheads).

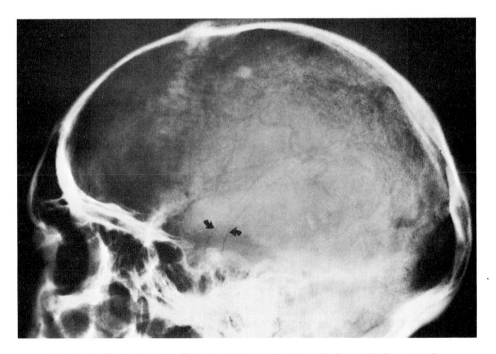

Fig. 11-26. Pseudofracture. Paired arterial grooves (arrows) rise vertically near sella.

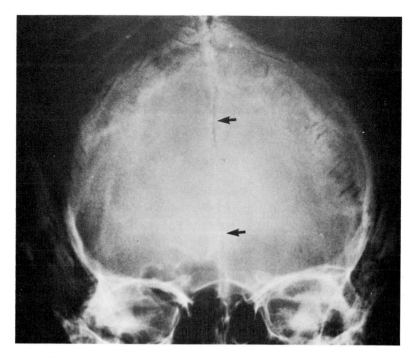

Fig. 11-27. Persistent metopic suture (arrows). Note sclerotic margin.

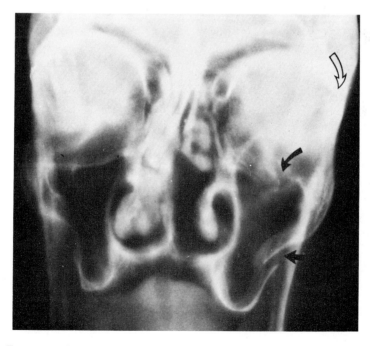

Fig. 11-28. Tomogram showing multiple facial fractures. There is fracture of lateral maxillary wall (straight arrow), floor of orbit (solid curved arrow), and frontozygomatic suture (open curved arrow).

plane. The metopic suture divides the frontal bone in a similar manner. Additionally, a rare persistent interparietal suture divides the parietal bone horizontally. All these sutures occur in the fetal skull, are seen occasionally in neonates, and rarely persist in the normal adult skull (Figs. 11-27).

Scalp lacerations, dressings, tape, and other foreign material have occasionally been misinterpreted as fracture. You are cautioned to examine your patient carefully and remove any of these foreign materials if possible before requesting a radiograph.

Skull fractures heal slowly in both children and adults. Fractures in children heal in 3 to 12 months. In adults, up to 3 or more years may ensue before the fracture heals. Confusion between an old fracture and a fresh one may occur, especially if the old films are not available for comparison. Fresh fractures have sharp, distinct margins and are quite lucent. A healing fracture is less distinct and less lucent. Quite often a fresh fracture will have soft tissue swelling over it.

Facial fractures occur in a variety of recognizable patterns. For example, a blow to the malar region (from a fist) is most likely to produce a so-called tripod fracture of the zygoma, wherein the zygoma fractures at the arch, at the frontozygomatic suture, and through the inferior orbital rim. Quite often this has accompanying fractures of the maxilla. Other more severe forms of facial trauma include various forms of maxillofacial separation (the Le Fort type fractures). Tomography is often required for complete evaluation of these patients (Figs. 11-6 and 11-28).

An associated abnormality that often occurs in patients with skull or facial trauma is cervical spine trauma. A direct blow to the skull or face is usually of sufficient force to produce enough stress on the cervical spine in flexion, extension, or lateral flexion to cause a fracture. At this medical center, all patients evaluated for skull or facial trauma also have a cervical spine examination.

Neoplasm

The diagnosis of brain tumors (primary or metastatic) has been greatly aided by the development of CT. Although some of your patients will undoubtedly have these lesions, the actual radiographic interpretation of studies of these patients will be vested in the hands of neuroradiologists, neurologists, and neurosurgeons. For this reason, the discussion of this area will be brief and will concentrate on the CT appearance.

Radiographically, neoplasms are recognized by four types of change they produce on plain skull films and specialized studies: bony changes, mass effect, vascular changes, and calcifications.

Although bone is seldom directly involved by brain tumors, there are certain abnormalities that are recognized as indirect signs of the presence of a tumor: erosions or hyperostosis, often produced by meningiomas (Fig. 11-29); signs of increased intracranial pressure such as erosion of the dorsum sellae or split sutures; and increased vascular markings, often seen with a meningioma (Fig. 11-10).

Changes caused by the mass itself include definition of the tumor mass on CT (Fig. 11-30) or on a pneumoencephalogram and hydrocephalus secondary to obstruction of the pathways of CSF flow. In addition, edema is produced by intracerebral tumors in various degrees. The mass itself or the edema may result in displacement

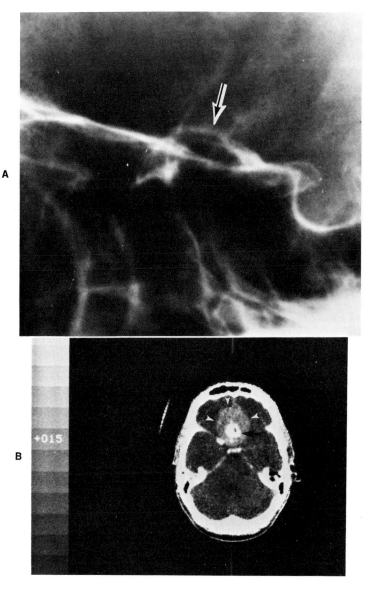

Fig. 11-29. Sphenoid ridge meningioma. **A,** Detail view of sellar region shows small area of hyperostotic blistering by tumor (arrow). **B,** CT scan shows hyperostotic area (small arrow) with overlying tumor (arrowheads).

of the pineal or ventricular structures as well as compression of adjacent normal brain tissues (Fig. 11-31). Multiple masses suggest metastases as the etiology. Similarly, metastasis is suggested if there is a large amount of edema surrounding the tumor.

Vascular changes of tumors include displacement of vessels (Fig. 11-32) and the presence of neovascularity (tumor vessels). One of the features of many brain tumors, because of their vascularity, is the ability to enhance on CT when the patient has had an intravenous injection of contrast material (Fig. 11-33).

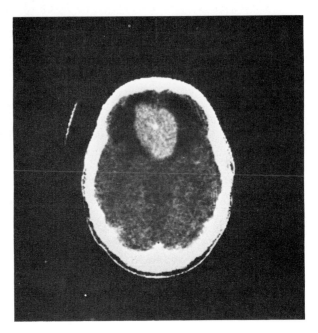

Fig. 11-30. Same patient as in Fig. 11-29. Tumor mass is well defined. Note low density zone of edema surrounding tumor.

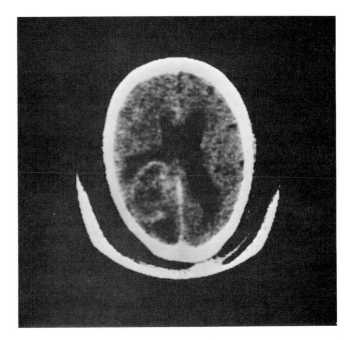

Fig. 11-31. Metastatic brain tumor on right. Note ventricular displacement.

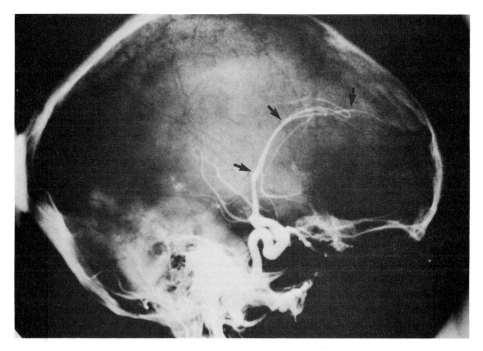

Fig. 11-32. Upward displacement of anterior cerebral vessels (arrows) in patient with sphenoid ridge meningioma.

Calcifications occur occasionally within cerebral neoplasms. These may be seen on the plain film as a small collection of calcium in an abnormal location (Fig. 11-34). Calcification is readily detectable within neoplasms on a CT scan.

Vascular disease

Vascular lesions probably constitute the most common abnormality of the brain and surrounding meninges. These include infarction secondary to atherosclerotic or embolic occlusions (Fig. 11-35), intracerebral hemorrhage (Fig. 11-36), arteriovenous malformations, and extracerebral hematomas (Fig. 11-37). All these are readily diagnosable by CT examination.

What should be the order of diagnostic studies in a patient with history, signs, and symptoms of neurologic disease? Three basic imaging examinations should be used: the lateral skull film, the isotope brain scan, and the CT brain scan. Invasive studies such as arteriography and pneumoencephalography should be reserved for those instances where the brain scans have not provided sufficient diagnostic information.

SUMMARY

The pertinent anatomy of the normal skull radiogram has been reviewed. Emphasis was placed on the impact cranial CT scanning has had on neuroradiology. Three pathologic entities—trauma, tumor, and vascular disease (the most commonly encountered that will produce an abnormal neuroradiologic study)—have been discussed briefly.

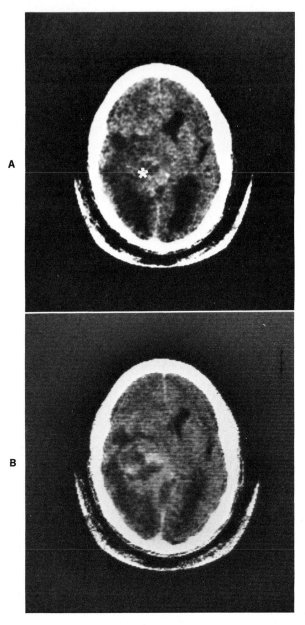

Fig. 11-33. Effect of vascular enhancement on CT scan. **A,** Unenhanced scan shows nondescript mass in midportion of brain (asterisk). **B,** After intravenous enhancement, there is better definition of tumor and surrounding edema.

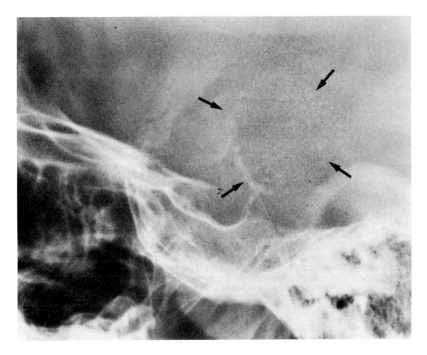

Fig. 11-34. Craniopharyngioma. There is flocculent calcification (arrows) in this child.

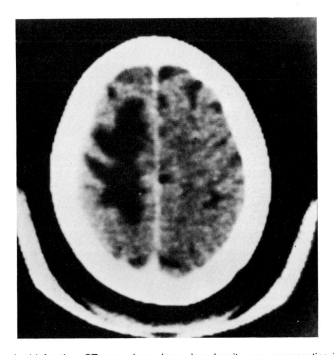

Fig. 11-35. Cerebral infarction. CT scan shows large, low density area representing infarcted brain.

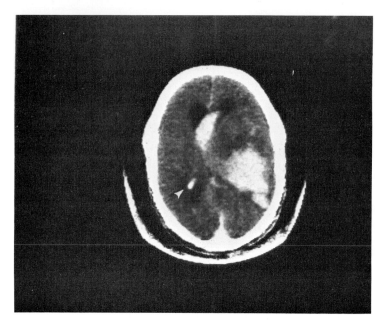

Fig. 11-36. Intracerebral hemorrhage. High density areas represent fresh blood within brain and ventricular system. There is shift of midline structures to right. Note calcification within choroid plexus on right (arrowhead).

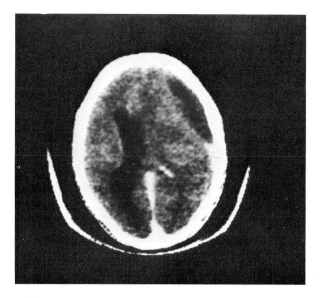

Fig. 11-37. Chronic subdural hematoma. There is shift of brain to right. Note lens-shaped, low density collection in left frontal region representing old hematoma. Recent hemorrhage would appear as area of increased density, as in Fig. 11-36.

Selected case studies

These cases illustrate the use of neuroradiologic studies in a group of patients who are being evaluated for their initial episode of major motor seizure.

Patient 1 is a 40-year-old alcoholic who was being treated for cirrhosis. He was observed by nursing personnel to have a major motor seizure on his third hospital day. Neurologic examination is normal. Representative views from his CT scan are shown in Case 11-1. *What are the findings? Would you order any additional studies?*

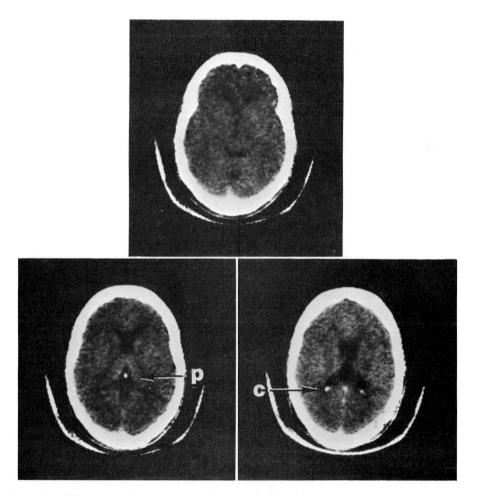

Case 11-1. CT scan of 40-year-old man with seizures. Note calcified pineal gland *(p)* and calcifications in choroid plexus *(c)*.

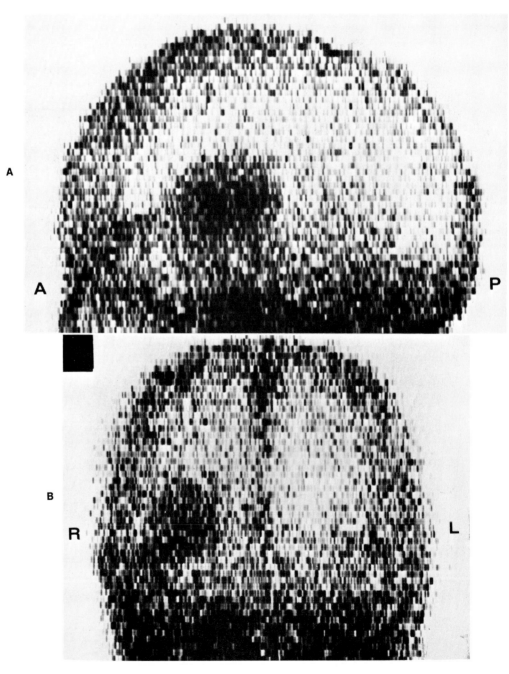

Case 11-2. **A,** AP and, **B,** lateral radionuclide brain scan of 35-year-old man with seizure. What is the main finding? **C,** CT scan on same patient. **D,** Same slice following injection of radiographic contrast material intravenously. What are the arrows pointing to?

Patient 2 is a 35-year-old man who was admitted after suffering a major motor seizure while at work. His past history is noncontributory. Neurologic examination reveals signs referrable to the left side of the brain. An isotope brain scan (Case 11-2, *A* and *B*) and a CT scan (Case 11-2, *C* and *D*) are shown. *What are the main findings? Are any additional studies indicated?*

C

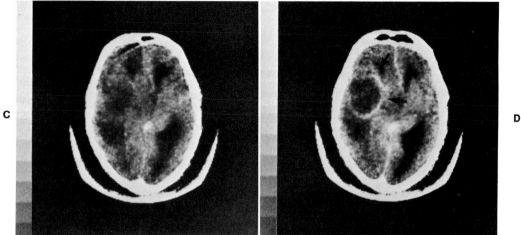

D

Case 11-2, cont'd. For legend see opposite page.

Patient 3 is a 50-year-old man who was admitted after suffering a major motor seizure while watching a football game. Past history includes heavy cigarette consumption (three packs a day for 25 years). An electroencephalographic study demonstrates diffuse abnormalities. His CT scan is shown in Case 11-3, *A* and *B*. *What are the findings? What additional studies should you order?*

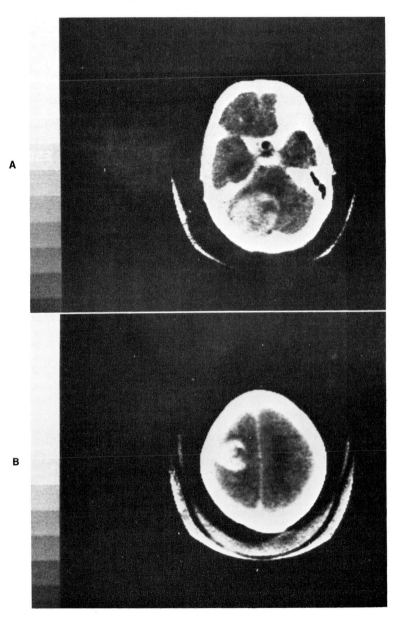

Case 11-3. CT scan of 50-year-old man with seizures. **A,** Level near base of skull. **B,** Level near convexity.

Patient 4 suffered a major motor seizure while driving to work and was involved in an automobile accident. Past history reveals a head injury 10 months previously when the outhouse he was repairing collapsed on him. On physical examination, he is comatose and has neurologic findings suggesting a right-sided lesion. A CT scan (Case 11-4, *A* and *B*) is shown. *What are the main findings? Would you order additional studies for this patient?*

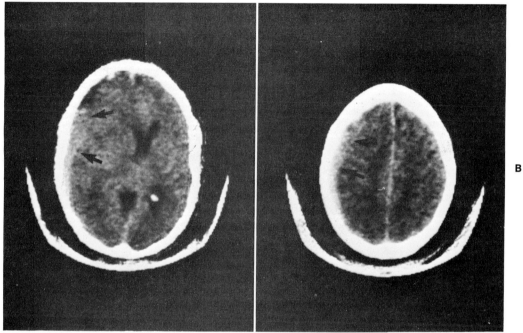

A   B

Case 11-4. A and **B,** CT scans of patient with seizure after head injury. What are the arrows pointing to? What other abnormalities are present?

Patient 5 is a 65-year-old diabetic man who suffered a major motor seizure while sitting in his physician's office. He is comatose on admission. Emergency CT scan (Case 11-5) is shown. *What are the main findings? What is your diagnosis?*

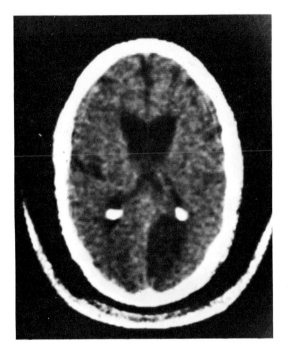

Case 11-5. CT scan of 65-year-old man who was comatose after seizure. What is the main abnormality?

ROENTGEN DIAGNOSIS

Patient 1. The CT scan on this patient was interpreted as being normal. In this instance the patient clinically proceeded into delirium tremens (DTs) shortly after his seizure. Neurologic workup was normal and no further diagnostic radiographic studies were performed. The final diagnosis was alcoholic withdrawal seizures. This scan is included for you as a normal to compare with the other scans.

Patient 2. The radioisotope brain scan shows an area of increased tracer uptake in the right frontotemporal area. The CT scan shows a cystic mass lesion surrounded by a large zone of edema that is displacing the midline structures to the left. A repeat study with intravenous injection of contrast material was performed (Case 11-2, *D*), revealing contrast enhancement of the lesion (indicating a vascular nature). Arteriography confirmed the diagnosis suggested by the CT findings. The patient was taken to surgery, where a malignant astrocytoma was found.

Patient 3. The CT scan in this patient reveals multiple mass densities surrounded by zones of edema. The admission chest radiograph (Case 11-3, *C*) revealed a large mass in the right hilum with right upper lobe collapse. The most likely diagnosis in this case is multiple metastases from bronchogenic carcinoma. A lung biopsy was performed and confirmed the diagnosis. No additional diagnostic imaging studies of the brain were performed. The CT scan was used in the ensuing months to follow the patient's progress.

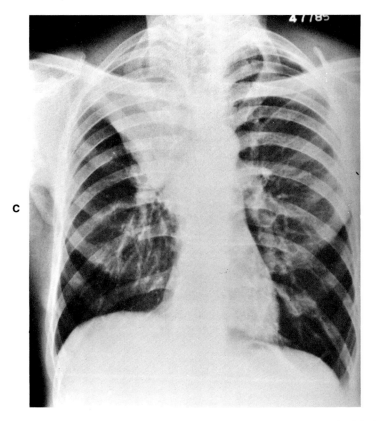

Case 11-3. Patient 3. **C,** Chest radiograph taken on admission shows large mass in right hilum with right upper lobe collapse. Diagnosis: bronchogenic carcinoma. Intracerebral lesions were metastases.

Patient 4. The CT scan reveals a convex area of *increased* density over the frontal and parietal regions on the right. The CT number of this density is that of fresh blood (CT No. 25). No other abnormalities are present. There is a slight shift of the midline structures to the left. The patient was taken to surgery, where an acute subdural hematoma was evacuated. A chronic subdural hematoma would appear biconcave (Case 11-4, *C*). The density of the abnormal collection would be lower than fresh blood (CT No. 10 to 15). The seizure in this patient was related to his brain damage from his *old* trauma. The hematoma resulted from the most recent episode of trauma.

Patient 5. The CT scan on this patient revealed a zone of decreased radiodensity in the left occipital lobe. There is no shift of midline structures. The findings are consistent with an infarct in this region. The patient was subsequently studied by arteriography and found to have an occlusion of the posterior cerebral artery on the left.

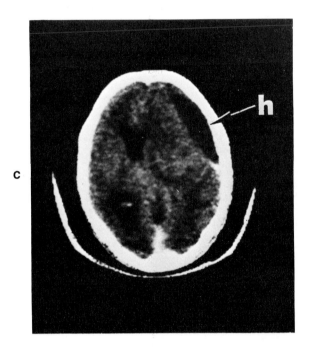

Case 11-4. C, CT scan of patient with chronic subdural hematoma in left frontal region. Note biconcave appearance of hematoma *(h)*. Note also displacement of left-sided brain structures to right.

References

Allen, W. E. III, Kier, E. L., and Rothman, S. L. G.: Pitfalls in the evaluation of skull trauma. A review, Radiol. Clin. North Am. 11:479, 1973.

Bell, R. S., and Loop, J. W.: The utility and futility of radiographic skull examination for trauma, N. Engl. J. Med. 284:236, 1971.

Daffner, R. H., Gehweiler, J. A., and Carden, T. S., Jr.: Case studies in radiology, New York, 1975, Appleton-Century-Crofts.

Dublin, A. B., French, B. N., and Rennick, J. M.: Computed tomography in head trauma, Radiology 122:365, 1977.

Harwood-Nash, D. C., Hendrick, E. B., and Hudson, A. R.: The significance of skull fractures in children. A study of 1187 patients, Radiology 101:151, 1971.

Holder, A. R.: Roentgenograms of head injuries, J.A.M.A. 222:613, 1972.

Koo, A. H., and LaRoque, R. L.: Evaluation of head trauma by computed tomography, Radiology 123:345, 1977.

Newton, T. H., and Potts, D. G.: Radiology of the skull and brain, vol. I. The skull, St. Louis, 1971, The C. V. Mosby Co.

Peterson, H. O., and Kieffer, S. A.: Introduction to neuroradiology, rev. ed., 1976, Harper & Row, Publishers.

Roberts, M. F., and Shopfner, C. E.: Plain film roentgenograms in children with head trauma, Am. J. Roentgenol. 114:230, 1972.

Robinson, A. E., Meares, B. M., and Goree, J. A.: Traumatic sphenoid sinus effusion. An analysis of 50 cases, Am. J. Roentgenol. 101:795, 1967.

Schoultz, T. W., Morrison, J. R., and Calhoun, J. D.: Atlas of the human brain for use in diagnosis by computer-assisted tomography, Surg. Neurol. 5:255, 1976.

Swischuk, L. E.: The normal pediatric skull. Variations and artefacts, Radiol. Clin. North Am. 10:277, 1972.

Taveras, J. M., and Wood, E. H.: Diagnostic neuroradiology, ed. 2, Baltimore, 1976, The Williams & Wilkins Co.

Weinstein, M. A., Alfidi, R. J., and Duchesneau, P. M.: Guest editorial: computed tomography versus skull radiography, Am. J. Roentgenol. 128:873, 1977.

Index*

*Boldface numbers indicate pages on which figures are found, and t indicates pages on which tables appear.